Author

Slávka Démuthová

SPECTRUM SLOVAKIA Series
Volume 41

Self-Harming Behaviour in Adolescent Age

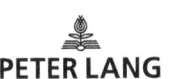

Bibliographic Information published by the Deutsche Nationalbibliothek
The Deutsche Nationalbibliothek lists this publication in the Deutsche Nationalbibliografie; detailed bibliographic data is available in the internet at http://dnb.d-nb.de.

Reviewers: doc. PhDr. Iva BUREŠOVÁ, Ph.D.
doc. Mgr. Elena LISÁ, Ph.D.

Author: Slávka DÉMUTHOVÁ

ISSN 2195-1845
ISBN 978-3-631-89835-2
ePDF 978-3-631-89945-8
ePub 978-3-631-89946-5
DOI 10.3726/b20680

ISBN 978-80-224-2009-9

© 2023 Peter Lang Group AG, Lausanne
Published by Peter Lang GmbH, Berlin, Deutschland

© VEDA, Publishing House of the Slovak Academy of Sciences
Bratislava 2023

All rights reserved.
Peter Lang – Lausanne • Berlin • Bruxelles • Chennai • New York • Oxford

All parts of this publication are protected by copyright. Any utilisation outside the strict limits of the copyright law, without the permission of the publisher, is forbidden and liable to prosecution. This applies in particular to reproductions, translations, microfilming, and storage and processing in electronic retrieval systems.

www.peterlang.com   www.veda.sav.sk

This work was supported by the Slovak Research and Development Agency under contract No. APVV-17-0123.

Contents

Foreword 7

1 The Definition of Self-Harm 11
   1.1 The History of Research into Self-Harm 13
   1.2 The Current Social Context 17
   1.3 The Terminology of Self-Harm 31
   1.4 The Definition of Self-Harm 41

2 Theoretical Bases 59
   2.1 Psychodynamic Concepts 61
   2.2 Interpersonal Concepts 65
   2.3 Biological Concepts 71
   2.4 Cognitivist Concepts 78
   2.5 Regulatory Concepts 91
   2.6 Integrative Concepts 95

3 The Occurrence of Self-Harm 99
   3.1 The Prevalence of Self-Harm in the World 101
   3.2 The Prevalence of Self-Harm in Slovakia 120
   3.3 Methods Used for the Study of the Prevalence of Self-Harm 125
   3.4 The Demographic Specificities of the Prevalence of Self-Harm 146

4 The Forms and Types of Self-Harm in Adolescence 159
   4.1 The Forms of Self-Harm 161
   4.2 The Prevalence of the Forms of Self-Harm 165
   4.3 The Types of Self-Harm 174
   4.4 The Prevalence of the Types of Self-Harm 180

5 The Characteristics of Self-Harming Adolescents 185
　　5.1　Mental Disorders 187
　　5.2　Personality 199
　　5.3　Temperament 208
　　5.4　Motivation 214
　　5.5　Cognition 221
　　5.6　Emotionality 229

Conclusion 239

References 243

About the Author 301

Foreword

Self-harm is a new phenomenon that threatens children and adolescents' physical and mental health. It is a form of high-risk behaviour that leads to individuals causing themselves intentional harm. Self-harm as such is not a completely unknown phenomenon – it is a part of the clinical symptoms of several mental disorders and also occurs in various specific subcultures. Recently, a significant spread of this phenomenon has been seen in the non-clinical population, and considering the data from physicians, teachers, psychologists and parents, there are signals that its prevalence is hugely widespread.

In order to plan effective interventions in the area of self-harm, several steps need to be taken – it is necessary to map out the prevalence of the phenomenon in the target population, the specificities of its occurrence, typical signs, risk and protective factors, intervening variables and the dynamics of its propagation and prognosis. There is a lack of basic research in all these areas – there is not enough data from any of them. There are also limited opportunities for the use of international data – there is no consensus as to the definition of the term "self-harm", there are vast differences in the methods of data collection and methodologies used, and what is more, the information gained on self-harm differs depending on the sample population participating in the research.

Given that there is no extensive scientific overview about self-harming behaviour in Slovakia, this monograph aims to present basic information related to the definition of the term "self-harm", its prevalence, forms and types which have been identified. Furthermore, it tries to present specific concepts that clarify its onset and retention in the repertoire of maladaptive reactions and uncover the typical characteristics of individuals who exhibit this behaviour. A specific characteristic of the monograph is the publication of the unique data from a multi-year research project into a group of Slovak adolescents, and in the context of the findings from the project, it highlights problematic areas that require further research.

1 The Definition of Self-Harm

1.1 The History of Research into Self-Harm

Research into self-harm and interest in this phenomenon is nothing novel. Records of acts of intentional harm that individuals have done to themselves, with the consequential pain or that lead to the deterioration of some important functional areas, as well as efforts to understand these actions, frequently occur in literature from areas such as culturology, history, sociology, religion and psychology. Cultural anthropologists have reported painful initiation rituals within indigenous tribes (such as the Sateré-Mawé in the Amazon – Bosmia et al. 2015), as well as procedures that lead to mutilation in the belief that they help an individual gain unique abilities. A fundamental concept of the cult of Shamanism is that through, often painful, interventions into the body, the individual ascends to a higher level of existence, which gives them the ability to heal themselves or others, as well as other abilities, such as extraordinary wisdom or ability to influence destiny (Favazza 2009). During the festival of Thaipusam, Hindus perform extreme forms of piercing (Lee et al. 2016), Shia Muslims believe that the harder the trials, pain and suffering they experience in life, the better they will be prepared for the journey to heaven (Favazza 2009). Self-harm of our own bodies is not uncommon in Western culture either – the history of Christianity reveals that in an effort to achieve spiritual cleanliness, it is better to "get rid of" the part of the body that prevents it (that tempts an individual to commit sins – Mt. 18 8–9). However, reasons for self-harm may also be symbolic – for example, tattoos may express an affiliation with a group or subculture (Ragmanauskaite et al. 2020).

What all these forms of self-harm share is that the individual gains something in return – enlightenment, spiritual strength, social importance, acceptance within a group, etc. But psychological research into self-harm[1] only focuses on the specific fraction

---

[1] Of course, psychology also studies the above-mentioned specific forms of behaviour. For instance, it addresses people's need for affiliation to a social group that increases their willingness to undergo even highly unpleasant and painful rituals; it addresses the mechanisms of the psychological effect of rewards and punishments, which, for example, explain the importance of these acts that allow them to gain recognition and status in a community, or the impact of social exclusion;

of these acts that lead to harm in certain important domains of the individual. An important defining criterion is the determination of the reason that the individual undergoes pain, suffering and harm. If they are the previously mentioned aesthetic, social, religious, and other similar reasons, it is not "true" self-harm (for the detailed criteria of the definition, see the following sections). The reason they perform self-harm is not for the pain/harm itself, but to gain power, to become part of a group, to experience a specific act or to improve their own aesthetic, etc. These motivations should not be included in a study of the phenomenon of self-harm, and actions that do not have, as their primary reason or motives, the desire to cause pain, harm or damage to themselves should also not be included among self-harming behaviours.

Despite this relatively large number of "limitations", self-harm occurs relatively often, even in its narrow sense. In the history of psychological research, self-harming behaviour was often described in terms of mental disorders. Various forms of self-harm are included in the symptomatology of mental retardation (van den Bogaard et al. 2018), autism (Maddox et al. 2017), alcoholism and substance addictions (Gupta et al. 2019), personality disorders (Hawton et al. 2013), schizophrenia (Haw et al. 2005), depression (Parker et al. 2005) and bipolar and anxiety disorders (Singhal et al. 2014). The analysis of patients hospitalised after injuries caused by self-harming behaviour revealed that up to 84% of the adults and 81% of the adolescents suffered from some of the mental illnesses of Axis I[2].

This data clearly shows that self-harming behaviour is a relatively frequent symptom of mental disorders or, at the very least, it

---

the impact of conformity as a form of pressure to adapt to the majority and its rules (and the preservation of traditions), as well as neural mechanisms activated during critical moments (a state of pain, mortal danger...) that have an impact on the experience of the individual.

2 Axis 1 is one of the five "categories" of mental disorders in the international DSM classification (Diagnostic and Statistical Manual of Mental Disorders). The present study reflects on the classification of the fourth revision of the manual (DSM-IV), and within Axis 1, it includes mental illnesses with the exception of personality disorders and mental retardation (American Psychiatric Association 1994). The prevalence of psychiatric diagnoses in the observed sample would, therefore, probably be greater if personality disorders or mental retardation were included in the study.

accompanies them[3]. In terms of defining self-harm as an intentional and conscious act that leads to harming yourself, it is necessary to address whether in all cases of self-harm with the presence of a mental disorder, the individual's primary and conscious intention is to cause pain or to harm themselves. The current level of awareness, the degree of detectability of danger and the ability to manage behaviour may be limited by many mental disorders (for instance, in the case of mental retardation, deliriums in addicts, hallucinations and delusions in schizophrenics, etc.). Hence, it can be disputed whether it is possible to clearly detect any intention or full awareness of consequences – which is necessary in our understanding of self-harm.

In spite of the extensive links between self-harming behaviour and mental disorders, this undesirable phenomenon has occurred far more often in the last few decades in the non-clinical population (Klonsky et al. 2003; Straiton et al. 2013) – that is in individuals who were not diagnosed with any mental disorder and do not currently suffer from any disorder. It is this population that has been in the spotlight of many recent studies – it is a modern phenomenon, especially in adolescents, and due to its extremely destructive nature, it may be considered to be a high-risk form of behaviour[4]. Interest in the topic of self-harm in this context was first sparked in the 1960s[5] – after the experience with patients hospitalised with cuts to their wrists, Harold Graff and Richard Malinn (1967) defined the syndrome of "wrist-cutter", which is described as an individual that suffers from, inter alia, deprivation of motherly love in their early childhood, and they suggested therapy that focused

---

[3] For more information on correlations between self-harm and mental disorders, see Chapter 5.
[4] The spectrum of self-harming behaviours not only include scratching, burning or cutting but also constantly reopening wounds with the subsequent infections, intentionally avoiding medication for chronic illnesses, poisoning and other life and health-threatening forms (for more details, see Chapter 4 "The Forms and Types of Self-Harm in Adolescence".
[5] Earlier records of self-harm appear in the 1940s in Karl Menninger's work, who was the first to start using a conceptually similar term, self-mutilation, to refer to self-harming behaviour without the intention of ending life. Interestingly, in his book Man Against Himself published in 1938, he considers this behaviour to be a coping strategy, the purpose of which is to prevent/avoid self-destruction in the form of suicide (Posner et al. 2014).

on support for giving and accepting love. During that period, studies were published that addressed the topic of self-harm in individuals who did not exhibit any psychiatric conditions – an often-mentioned group was that of single, attractive, intelligent young women (Adler & Adler 2011).

In the next phase of the development of studies into self-harm, awareness of self-harming behaviour spread from clinics and hospitals to the general public. In the 1990s, more and more individuals[6] began to speak, in public, about their problematic behaviour, and this period is considered a milestone from the perspective of the initiation of the debate around this phenomenon. It became clear that the problem not only concerns people who suffer from mental disorders, although most of the general public did not understand the true psychological reasons and mechanisms of self-harm. As a result of the "promotion" of this phenomenon, social imitation started to have a stronger impact – in particular, cutting oneself became a symbol of the punk or heavy-metal subcultures, and in contrast to individuals, for whom self-harm "solved" mental problems, there were groups for whom self-harm was a way of attracting attention by demonstrating affiliation to a subculture or lifestyle (Adler & Adler 2011). Partially due to these "untrue" motives[7] of self-harm, for some time the general public became convinced that self-harming individuals only wanted to attract attention. Nowadays, it is clear that manipulating others to gain attention is an unusual motivation for self-harm (Lewis & Heath 2013).

The turn of the millennia is considered by experts to have been the beginning of the "pandemic" of self-harm. Self-harming individuals were no longer only characteristic of specific subcultures, but they had spread to all (socio-economic, age, gender or ethnic…) groups of society (Adler & Adler 2011). Over the last two decades, the trend has not stagnated – the occurrence of self-harm is increasing worldwide. Experts have identified several circumstanc-

---

6 Including celebrities such as Drew Barrymore, Johnny Depp, Colin Farrell, Angelina Jolie, Courtney Love, Amy Winehouse or Princess Diana (Adler & Adler 2011).
7 "Untrue"; meaning that in these cases, the function of self-harm is to show affiliation to a subculture and as such its primary motive is not to cause pain or harm to oneself.

es that may have led to the large increase in the prevalence of this undesirable phenomenon – however, they are merely opinions and theories rather than the exact identification of decisive factors.

1.2 The Current Social Context

Over the last two decades, experts have reported an increase in self-harm (Cipriano et al. 2017; Morgan et al. 2017; Bae et al. 2020). New forms are emerging, and the prevalence is increasing, even in those groups where this phenomenon was less common. There are several reasons why so many individuals, particularly in adolescence, are currently resorting to this high-risk behaviour. They form a set of social, family or developmental specificities that create predispositions for adolescents to be more exposed to psychological burdens and subsequently to resort to maladaptive solutions.

The Internet and Social Media

To some extent, the upsurge in self-harm is thought to be linked to the widespread availability of the Internet – research shows that large numbers of young people in particular, who self-harm, are connecting to the internet to interact with other self-harming individuals. Although such behaviour may not, in itself, be the source of the problems (theoretically, it can provide a benefit in terms of support from peers), these activities often increase the risk of self-harm in young people (Lewis et al. 2012). Sharing stories, learning about new forms of self-harm and ways to effectively disguise it can lead to a higher frequency or severity of self-harm. In this regard, we cannot overlook the numerous online forums and groups that have been created to encourage such behaviour[8] or to directly entice individuals to join in.

---

[8] S. P. Lewis and T. G. Baker analysed the content of 71 different self-harm websites. Up to 91.55% of them promoted self-harm as an effective cognitive strategy (Lewis & Baker 2011).

Even in the absence of a direct intention on a social network/forum/website, it is still the case that the sharing of experiences and difficulties with peers, who seek the same maladaptive strategy to cope with the situation (self-harm), leads to the reinforcement of these behavioural patterns. The self-harming individuals themselves state (see Adler & Adler 2011) that many of these websites even have a strong aspect of competition and they glorify individuals who post examples of severe or high-risk forms of self-harm. Self-harming individuals also tell us that through visiting such websites, they have an increased desire and need to hurt themselves, to engage in the activities on these websites (e.g., by sharing a photograph or a story of an act of self-harm), and this subsequently leads them to constantly return to the websites and observe the reaction of others. If there is a reaction (admiration or compassion), they experience a sense of belonging and this reinforces their behaviour.

Contacting groups of individuals with the same experiences, who understand the adolescent and share the same problems, also leads to the individual forming social bonds with equally at-risk individuals at the expense of creating and strengthening social bonds with "healthy"[9] and real (non-virtual) peers. Adolescents, therefore, lose contact with the individuals who could provide them with examples of non-pathological coping strategies, as well as space to spend time away from risky topics. As a result of the principles of social imitation and contagion[10], exposure to self-harm, on its own, increases the likelihood and frequency of its occurrence. The registration of self-harm as a coping mechanism or as a prevalent behaviour among adolescents may engender contagion of such behaviour. Adolescence is a critical period characterized by significant reliance on social connections and peer interactions, therefore, observing and internalizing certain patterns or behaviour in the environment may lead to its imitation..

---

9 In the sense of non-self-harming peers.
10 For a more detailed analysis of the effects of these phenomena within self-harming behaviour, see the section "2.2 Interpersonal Concepts".

The Period of Adolescence

The phenomenon of imitation may provide some possible reasons why adolescents more often choose to solve their mental issues through self-harm. However, it fails to explain why adolescents suffer from mental disorders to such a great extent and are forced to cope with them. A partial answer is offered by the characteristics of this period of development and the developmental issues they have to deal with. Adolescence is a complex transitory developmental period between childhood and adulthood. Completing such important developmental tasks (e.g., biological and sexual maturity, the shaping of identity, the development of partnerships, building of autonomy and independence, choosing a career path... – Christie & Viner 2005) is not easy, and several complications occur in the process.

Cognition

The period of adolescence is characterised by a change in thinking and culminates in qualitative changes in cognition. Reaching the stage of formal operations (Piaget) allows the individual to think hypothetically, and with that change, the individual has the opportunity to think about the consequences of their decisions and attitudes. With this knowledge also comes responsibility for their actions, which is not easy to accept for inexperienced adolescents. In addition, the idealism of this period of development places a high demand on the consistency of thoughts and actions[11], which creates even more pressure. A critical view (due to idealism) of the attitudes and behaviours of the older generations, who act more pragmatically or are more open to compromise, leads to the rejection of parents, teachers and elders as figures of authority or role models, which leads the adolescent to lose their childlike faith in the wisdom and reliability of adults. Adolescents stop turning to their parents with requests for advice and help and much more often[12] turn to their peers. Making decisions based on their own consciousness and conscience may pose

---
11 Represented by, for example, a desire to not betray their own principles.
12 In comparison to previous developmental periods.

a serious dilemma for the adolescents – they are aware (unlike previously) that the many consequences of their decisions can seriously affect their future[13]. They want to make these decisions on their own, but at the same time, they are aware of their own lack of experience and also lack the certainty that these decisions are correct. Adolescents may not always be able to cope with these demands without some difficulties – depressive moods during this period are often accompanied by worries about the future or are related to the dysphoric nature of their relationships with their parents (Lundh et al. 2011). Adolescents can easily succumb to feelings of anxiety or worry about the future, which can paralyse them, but they can also (in an effort to put fear and uncertainty out of their minds) react in the completely opposite way with extremely reckless or even risky behaviour.

The Social Area

The independence and detachment from family ties, typical of the period of adolescence (Meeus et al. 2005), are not only the result of criticism of the older generations – they are an integral and natural part of this period. By the end, an individual should be mature and able to break away from the family and start to live their own life. However, an adolescent can only reach adulthood once they have successfully mastered various developmental tasks, which is not easy due to their number and severity. Apart from gaining a certain degree of freedom, independence also comes with responsibility – a reliance on parents is replaced by self-reliance. This transition is difficult and relatively long, and therefore, the adolescent temporarily shifts the focus of their interpersonal ties from the family to peer relationships in order to master some of the tasks[14]. Friends become important and the ties and relationships with them acquire a specific meaning[15] (Henneberger et al.

---

13 For example, choosing a profession, deciding to stay at home or going to stay/work outside of the family, how to manage intimacy and levels of commitment in their first more serious relationships (Gordon 1990)... etc.
14 In addition to independence, "intermediate steps" are also taken, for instance, in shaping identity.
15 In the case of a problematic family background, it is even more important than relationships with family members. In such cases, the adolescent is often willing

2021). For adolescents, friends represent significant social support, a frame of reference for behavioural responses, role models for decision-making (Andrews et al. 2020), and a community, in which they spend the majority of their time. This can become a risky situation if the peer relationships do not gain importance through natural developmental tendencies but as a consequence of bad relationships within the family. In such cases, the family no longer fulfils its support function, which is always necessary, despite developmental changes. Adolescents perceive the opportunity to become independent more as a necessity. The knowledge that when they experience difficulties, they do not or cannot turn to their family significantly increases distress in stressful situations. In this regard, peers are not able to help, give advice or manage the solution of the problems of their friends in the way that families or adults are able to. Another risk in this respect is that if an adolescent is critically dependent on a peer group, one will try to remain a part of the group even if it has behavioural models or value orientations, which are different from those preferred by the adolescent. Losing their position or no longer belonging to a group[16] would, for an adolescent, mean a loss (from one's point of view) of the only social ties, they currently have.

The Formation of Identity

Experts highlight the importance of the peer group even in the process of the formation of identity. It is one of the most important (Erikson 1972) and most complicated aspects of adolescence. It is during this period (as a result of qualitative changes in cognition) that the individual may incorporate ideas for the future, as opposed to simply the past and present, into their complex self-im-

---

to modify or violate their own internal standards in order to maintain friendly ties and relationships within the peer group.
16 The period of adolescence is also characterised by the fact that even individuals who live in optimal conditions with functional family backgrounds are hypersensitive to the negative effects of social exclusion in this period. For this reason, they intensely conform to the standards of the group; the effort to avoid the risk of social exclusion or the threat of leaving the group may also outweigh the potential negative consequences associated with risky or illegal behaviour (Blakemore 2018).

age (McAdams 2001). Changes in their physical appearance (Godina & Zadorozhnaya 2016), new social roles (Cadigan et al. 2019), new commitments stemming from their responsibility for key decisions (Greenberger 1984), new ideas and plans for the future, among others, create confusion and a constant need to answer the question: "Who am I?" (Tsang et al. 2012). In order to answer this question, it is necessary to consider changes in the biological, social, emotional, cognitive and other areas and over time to integrate them into their self-image. It is a difficult task, in which the adolescent must explore their inner self, they experiment with various alternatives of self-identity and the consequences of their behaviour. In this context, feedback from significant others is highly important – especially from their peers and in optimal circumstances also from their parents (Schacter & Margolin 2019). Based on this feedback, adolescents not only adapt their behaviour but also form their self-image. In this regard, the adolescent may discover inappropriate forms of behaviours from their peer group, which they copy in an effort to integrate with the group or to retain their status or affiliation to the group (the theory of social pressure and imitation explains the appearance and retention of self-harm in the repertoire of behavioural patterns). In addition, a negative self-image (saturated by feedback from adolescents) may create a basis for the formation and development of cognitive biases[17] that support self-harming behaviour. A negative self-image in various areas (physical attractiveness, evaluation of self-worth, the ability to solve problems, etc.) is closely linked to self-harming behaviour (Greydanus & Apple 2011; Batey et al. 2010; Townsend et al. 2001; Liu et al. 2016).

Other important aspects that have an impact on the formation of a new form of self-image are the hormonal changes in early adolescence. They not only cause a change in hormonal levels and the subsequent sexual maturation of the organism, but they also have a significant effect on the appearance of the individual. Accepting these changes can be quite difficult – not every adolescent feels they are prepared to accept changes in the composition and proportions of their own body, to accept the role of an individual

---

[17] Cognitive mechanisms of the formation and retention of self-harming behaviour are discussed in the section "2.4 Cognitivist Concepts".

who is capable of reproduction and face it responsibly. Some psychodynamic concepts explaining self-harming behaviour[18] see it as a way of gaining control over sexual urges (Nock 2009) and sexual maturity. They point out that the occurrence of self-harm (mainly in the form of cutting oneself) particularly increases at the beginning of sexual maturity (Stone 1987), and especially in girls who find it hard to accept that they have become a woman (Rosenthal et al. 1972). Psychodynamic models point to the parallels between menarche and bleeding when cutting oneself. In this context, menarche represents sexual maturity that is not accepted and that is often even rejected or unwanted. However, an adolescent woman has no control over it, so she attempts to gain symbolic control by cutting herself – only then can she decide when, to what extent, and how long the bleeding will last (as opposed to menarche) (Rosenthal et al. 1972). Although this is a relatively specific view on the topic of self-harm, it highlights a real problem and the difficulties that self-harming individuals may have with their own identity and self-acceptance.

Neurodevelopmental Changes

In addition to processes related to hormonal maturation, during adolescence, many changes also take place in several systems of the brain. It is assumed that the rise in the occurrence of risky behaviour during this period, including self-harm, may be related to neurodevelopmental changes. The results of studies that focused on specific forms of behaviour of adolescents suggest that high-risk behaviour is linked to an increase in the tendency to seek excitement and new impulses. This is characterised by individuals who exhibit a greater need to expose themselves to new and intense feelings and experiences in spite of the possible risks (Zuckerman & Kuhlman 2000; Steinberg 2008). This tendency rises during adolescence and peaks at the age 10–15 (Jaworska & MacQueen 2015). At the same time, adolescents are more sensitive to reward (Cservenka et al. 2013), which significantly increases the risk of the fixation of inappropriate behaviour (as well as self-harm as a maladaptive strategy to reduce emotional tension)

---

18 For more details, see the section "2.1 Psychodynamic Concepts".

during this period, if it is positively reinforced. Another important point is that impulsiveness also increases during adolescence. It is the tendency to act without thinking about the consequences (impulsive actions) or to choose smaller, more immediate rewards rather than greater, but delayed rewards (impulsive selection) (Romer et al. 2017). These impulsive actions may lead to the selection of non-optimal strategies for problem-solution and maladaptive forms of behaviour or responses to stress.

The above-mentioned deficits, which point to a certain "loss of control" over the regulation of impulses, stand in opposition to the increasingly more mature thought processes and improvements in executive functions. Neuroscientists claim that this apparent paradox (the increasing quality of cognitive and executive functions in contrast to impulsive, irresponsible and risky behaviour) stems from the asynchronous maturation of the subcortical and cortical brain areas. The limbic system and its connections that are responsible for emotional reactions develop more quickly than the connections in the prefrontal cortex, which acts as the control centre for long-term planning, the consideration of results and the regulation of behaviour (Steinbeis & Crone 2016; Mueller et al. 2017). The consequences of this imbalance include increased sensitivity to certain types of impulses[19]: impulsiveness, risky behaviour, succumbing to the influence of peers and emotional instability (National Academies of Sciences, Engineering, and Medicine 2019).

Emotions

Changes in hormonal levels and brain activity during the period of adolescence also result in dramatic changes in emotions. For instance, testosterone has a significant impact on emotional and social development (Vijayakumar et al. 2019); elevated levels of oestradiol are associated with more intense emotional experiences (Balzer et al. 2015). The amygdala (which modulates and integrates emotional reactions based on their relevance and the impact of the context of the situation) is subjected to extensive

---

19 See the following section on emotional development in adolescence.

change in early adolescence, forming new connections with other parts of the brain, such as the striatum and hippocampus (Scherf et al. 2013). Due to this sudden and intense development, adolescents react more intensely to threatening impulses than children or adults (Pattwell et al. 2012; Fuhrmann et al. 2015), which may lead to the individual having a more anxious and depressive mindset. Negative emotions are a typical trait of self-harming adolescents – research has reported a higher level of sadness and a lower level of happiness (compared to non-self-harming adolescents) (In-Albon et al. 2015), the presence of feelings of loneliness, hostility or self-hatred (Lloyd-Richardson et al. 2007). A significant indication of the level of emotionality of self-harming individuals is the instability of their emotions (Andover et al. 2014; Wolff et al. 2019) – self-harm often occurs comorbidly with disorders that are characterised by unstable emotions (such as borderline personality disorder – Reichl & Kaess 2021); however, even adolescents from the non-clinical population suggest that they perceive that their own emotions fluctuate, they are remarkably intense and they are not able to regulate them.

During this period, intense emotional reactions are also triggered by the increased vulnerability of an adolescent to criticism from others and due to the greater sensitivity of an adolescent to their self-image. It is also true that many situations occur for the first time during adolescence – for example, emotional experiences that involve intimacy, romantic love, jealousy, deliberate rejection or, on the contrary, acceptance by partners and peers… (Guyer et al. 2016). These experiences (due to their novelty) provoke stronger reactions than later in life when the individual experiences them again. Overly intense, variable or strongly negatively tainted emotions are a burden for the adolescent, which (due to a lack of experience, a lower number of coping mechanisms and their lower efficiency…) they are unable to process appropriately. Thus, they opt for the quickest, most accessible and, at the particular moment, the most effective coping strategies, which may, however, be significantly maladaptive and risky. Immediate relief from intense emotions through physical pain and deflecting attention from the current burden are temporary results of self-harm and the main reasons why adolescents perform self-harm in times of emotional burden.

In the context of changes during the period of adolescence, we may argue that the developmental characteristics of this period have always been present, so there is no reason to assume that the complications associated with maturing and reaching adulthood would result in an increase of problematic phenomena (such as self-harm). However, adolescence is the process of growing into certain criteria (adulthood), which are closely linked to the characteristics, requirements and conditions of the society in which the adolescent grows up. Societal changes are then reflected in the whole process of the maturation of the individual and may either facilitate this process or complicate it. Over the last two decades, in our modern-day society, it is possible to observe a highly intense shift in the onset and end of the period of adolescence. Early sexual maturation as a result of favourable conditions for the development of an organism[20] has shifted the onset of adolescence, which is currently stabilised at the age of 10 years (Sawyer et al. 2018). On the other hand, the need for longer preparation for a career and the socio-economic conditions that allow us to care for our offspring for longer, greater demands on the quality of romantic relationships, etc. are postponing the point of reaching adulthood[21] (Arnett 2018). The transition from childhood to adulthood is lengthy and, in many aspects, more complicated than in the past. Improving living conditions and our quality of life put ever greater demands on the satisfaction of people – it is no longer enough to have a job and a partner, to start a family; a young person wants to grow in their relationship (both romantic and professional), to grow as a person, to find satisfaction, to meet their various needs, which is why they are always more demanding in this aspect[22]. Hence, adolescence as a transition period between

---

20 High-quality food, the absence of serious diseases and other stressors that slow the biological maturation of the organism.
21 In this regard, Jeffrey Jensen Arnett suggested the implementation of a new period of development (emerging adulthood), which would reflect the need to provide young people with sufficient space to reach psychological adulthood after they have legally become adults (18–21 years). Based on several studies in economically developed countries, he suggested from 18 to 29 (Arnett 2014); through this, he highlights the need to deal with maturation for much longer than in the past.
22 Just two generations ago, it was not common to end an employment or romantic relationship due to personal dissatisfaction or because they failed to provide

childhood and adulthood along with its tasks and complications has changed from taking approximately 4 years (in the past, it was typically understood as the period from the age 15–18 (20) – Rican 1989) to an entire decade. The second aspect that complicates the transition from childhood to adulthood is the current characteristics of the social environment, in which the young person is formed – especially in terms of complications in the family background and the absence of stable relationship frameworks in the area of ideas/values.

The Liquid Modernity

Adolescence is apparently a difficult period full of complications. But adolescence as such does not explain the increased prevalence of mental problems over the last decades, including self-harm. Increased vulnerability to mental issues can be observed in several specificities of the function of society and social contacts in the 21st century. The whole setup of the society, where adolescent grows up and which is the space where they need to become integrated, where they search for their place and space, both in the present and future, is pivotal for the mental well-being and health of a young person.

In this context, society should provide the adolescent with space for them to successfully integrate and support, if the processes take place as we desire. Young persons should understand that they have the same opportunities as any other adolescent, that there is no discrimination and they are valued. On the other hand, society should be active in the formation of the individual, and if socio-pathological phenomena, undesirable reactions or risky forms of behaviour occur, it should provide the adolescent with unambiguous feedback about the unacceptability of these actions and should have role models who provide information on accept-

---

enough mutual understanding or fulfilment of our own ambitions and personal development. It was important to have a job and a partner, and satisfaction was mostly a bonus rather than a necessity. Currently, satisfaction is one of the most decisive factors of stability and continuing a romantic or employment relationship.

able alternatives or the possibility of support if they are unable to effectively control their experiences and behaviour in a desirable form. However, the present generation of adolescents is growing up in a society that is referred to as a "liquid" period/society/culture[23] by experts (Franklin 2012; Sen 2016; Alonse-Stuyck 2019). "Liquid" because it keeps changing in most key areas. Society prefers short-term values over permanent ones, immediate over the long-term and practical over anything else (Palese, 2013). Adolescents are forced to search for their own identity, to generate their own overview of the world, to adopt stances and to find their own values, at a time when society only provides them with a few clues or support points as a basis for building their own position both now and for the future. Young people lack certainty and clear-cut positions which could define them, so they have to navigate their way through this critical period in life alone and, given the plurality of opinions and ambiguity of attitudes, in a considerably more difficult manner. According to Bauman, liquid modernity gives adolescents intense feelings of insecurity, instability and vulnerability (Bauman 2000, 160).

A Performance-Oriented Society

The complex nature of adolescence is further enhanced by another characteristic of most societies of the 21st century – an extreme focus on performance. It puts pressure on the achievement of results, with the evaluation of performance being significantly formalised (Stark 2020). It supports materialism and competitiveness, and the value of a person is more determined by what they do than who they are. Harmonious relationships disappear into the background under the influence of rivalry and competitiveness, and individualism is valued. Society is full of competition; there is little willingness to make a sacrifice for the benefit of others, which leads to tension and insecurity in interpersonal relationships. Facing these pressures, individuals prefer more practical values and the immediate fulfilment of needs over long-term values and work

---

23 The term "liquid modernity" was coined by the Polish sociologist Zygmund Bauman at the turn of the millennia (Bauman 2000).

whose results are seen in the long term or are uncertain. Moreover, adolescents grow up in an "interconnected" world with the extremely fast transfer of knowledge and information, which increases the demand for never-ending adaptation and thus the risk of failure (Committee on Improving Health 2015).

Self-fulfilment and the self-respect of members of these societies is closely linked to the progress and improvement achieved by the individual (Ye et al. 2015). As a result of these high demands, which go hand in hand with higher levels of failure, the adolescent is aware that it is their performance which is evaluated and valued, thus their self-evaluation is primarily tied to their success. Each failure, each percentage point less than a hundred in their performance, is a reason for the individual to be convinced of their own lack of ability. This substantially enhances the formation and reinforcement of cognitive distortions related to self-image, which are typical of self-harming adolescents.[24] They are convinced of their lack of ability, convinced that they are a burden to others, that they do not meet expectations and thus are unworthy of love and affection.

The Loss of Family Certainties

Another pitfall of our present-day society is the absence of a stable family environment, which is the source of primary socialisation and certainty, especially in childhood and adolescence (Craigie et al. 2012; Goldberg & Carlson 2014). Up to 41% of children in OECD countries are born outside of marriage. Furthermore, statistics report that the divorce rate[25] in EU member states is at 44% (PORDATA 2020). Today, most adolescents grow up in family systems which are not composed of both biological parents – either in single-parent families or in families with a step-father or mother with step-sisters and brothers. The high divorce rate, information on the frequency of domestic violence (Lepistö 2010), the occurrence of addiction and other pathological phenomena that intervene in the function of the family suggest that many of

---

24 This is more closely discussed in the section "2.4 Cognitivist Concepts ".
25 The data was collected in 2016.

the adolescents who live in families with both biological parents and siblings grow up in malfunctioning families. The link between risky behaviour and malfunctioning families has been demonstrated by numerous studies (Muyibi et al. 2010; Fomby & Osborne 2017; Sitnik-Warchulska et al. 2018; Alm et al. 2019). Self-harm is no exception – direct (sexual abuse, child abuse, etc.) and indirect (neglect, exposing the child to a violent environment), violence in the family (Armiento et al. 2016), tense relationships between family members, conflicts between the mother and child, a lack of affection from parents (Brunner et al. 2014) and more discrete problems such as insufficiently sensitive or consistent parenting (Nock 2008) are well-known risk factors for self-harm. It should be noted here that the increase in the occurrence of self-harm does not have to be directly caused by traumatic experiences in the family; even the fact that the adolescent does not feel they have sufficient support from their parents, or is worried about how they might react, or their parents are not available because they are always busy and have a high level of mental stress as a result of their own problems, or they communicate with the adolescent in an incorrect manner... all these may be reasons why the adolescent does not consider themselves to have a safe family environment, one that is supportive, that provides certainty, or why they might not ask parents for help when problems occur and thus opt for maladaptive solutions to problems or do not disclose their problems (with self-harm) to parents, and as a result, they receive no help in this regard.

The complicated period of adolescence, along with negative societal pressures and the absence of basic certainties, creates a high-risk environment, where successfully resolving the demands that result from the developmental needs of adolescents as well as the problems encountered by adolescents is very challenging. As a consequence of unfavourable life experiences, there is a greater probability of the use of maladaptive strategies to cope with mental burdens which, combined with other factors (e.g., negative patterns, distorted self-image or depressive mood), may become self-harm.

1.3 The Terminology of Self-Harm

Self-harm is one of many terms that describe an intentional self-oriented activity that leads to a deterioration of an area within the health or well-being of an individual. The meaning of the term may significantly vary, depending on which of the many diverse areas this term covers and which activities it relates to; this may be reflected in the terminology, that is in the specific form of the term that refers to a specific phenomenon (Burešová 2016). In psychology, self-harming behaviour has many different names.

Parasuicide

One of the older terms that has appeared in scientific literature is parasuicide. It was initially used to refer to an attempt to commit suicide, since psychiatrists mainly dealt with the consequences of self-harming activities within patients at clinics who had been hospitalised after an attempted suicide. However, a closer analysis of some of these patients revealed a proportion of cases that did not primarily include an unsuccessful attempt at suicide. Consequently, as early as the 1970s, experts used parasuicide as an umbrella term for the wide range of self-harming behaviours (Henderson et al. 1977). Hirsch et al. (1983) defined parasuicide as a non-fatal act of deliberate self-injury that resembled suicide but that did not lead to death. Other authors, in their works, employed the term "parasuicide" as well, to mean, inter alia, intentional self-harm – for instance, Brooksbank (1985), who analysed this phenomenon in children and adolescents, or Henderson and Lance (1979), who classified "wrist-cutters" (who had previous experience with self-harm) in the typology of their patients. Ferreira de Castro et al. (1998), when observing the co-morbidities of parasuicide, suggested it was necessary to differentiate between patients who had intended to die and those that had not. But the truth is that most published scientific works utilise the term "parasuicide" as a synonym for attempted suicide (see, for instance, Black et al. 1982; McGaughey et al. 1995; Liu et al. 1996; Bai et al. 1997).

Self-Wounding

This term is seldomly used – it is mentioned in the studies of, for example, Huband and Tantam, who define it as "a subset of self-harm" (Huband & Tantam 2004, 413). When describing and characterising this behaviour, they use information obtained from scientific literature, but the literature itself uses different terms – self-mutilation (e.g., Favazza 1998), deliberate self-harm (Allen 1995) or self-destructive behaviour (Figueroa 1988). D. Tantam repeatedly uses this term in his work with J. Whittaker, in which they observed the prevalence of personality disorders in self-harming individuals (Tantam & Whittaker 1992). They understand self-wounding as a subset of self-harming behaviour, and it is in this work that they published the main differences they had identified between self-wounding and self-mutilation as another subset of self-harm (Table 1).

Table 1. Characteristics of different types of self-injury

	Self-Mutilation			Self-Wounding		
	Patho-logical	Reli-gious	Motiva-ted	Reactive /habitual	Depre-ssive	Motiva-ted
Associated with:						
Unequivocal depression	-	-	-	-	+	-
Borderline phenomena	-	-	-	+	-	+/-
Psychosis	+	-	-	-	-	-
Other habit disorders	-	-	-	+	-	-
Tendency to repeat many times	-	-	-	+	-	-
Much commoner in youth	-	-	-	+	-	+
Surgical correction often needed	+	+	+	-	+	-
Major anatomical change	+	-	+	-	-	-
May affect vital structures	+	-	-			
Commonly life-threatening				-	+	-
Medical care rejected	-	-	-	+	-	-
Cause of injury concealed	-	-	+	-	-	+

Source: Tantam & Whittaker (1992, 452)

An almost identical term is self-inflicted wounding used by, for example, C. Moffatt (2000). As a result of its aetiology, which evokes wounds, the term "self-inflicted wounding" refers more to direct and visible physical forms of self-harm – hence, it is only related to a proportion of the relatively wide range of self-harming behaviours. Its meaning is closer to the term which is preferred today, non-suicidal self-injury, as per the definition suggested by DSM-5[26], except for the inclusion of attempted suicide, which DSM-5 excludes from its definition of the forms of self-harm.

Wrist-Cutting Syndrome

A relatively specific term that was particularly used in the early days of research into self-harm[27] is a wrist-cutting syndrome. At the same time, other parallel expressions were also used, including wrist slashing (Grunebaum & Klerman 1967), self-wrist cutting (Gu & Jeong 2012) and self-inflicted wrist slashing (Harris & Rai 1976). Scientific literature (see e.g., Graff & Malinn 1967) had already described the wrist-cutting syndrome in the 1960s (Offer & Barglow 1960). It was identified in hospitalised individuals, especially young women, who tried to convey signals to others through this behaviour – according to the psychiatrists of that time, these gestures carried little risk of suicide (Rosentahl et al. 1972). Apart from cutting wrists, the first studies had already reported cutting other body parts (e.g., forearm, legs, stomach), and in approximately half of the observed subjects, they reported the simultaneous occurrence of other forms of self-harm (such as burning by cigarettes, scratching) (Rosenthal et al. 1972). Thus, it appears that the term "wrist-cutting syndrome" was named for a dominant but certainly not a singular expression of self-harm. In the 1990s, wrist-cutting syndrome appeared under a new set

---

26 The fifth revision of the Diagnostic and Statistical Manual of Mental Disorders (DSM) of the American Psychiatric Association, which describes the non-suicidal self-injury (NSSI) in the last part of section III (Emerging Measures and Models) entitled Conditions for Further Study (APA 2013). More details are available in the following section.
27 For more details, see the previous section "1.1 The History of Research into Self-Harm".

of circumstances – S. M. Lena and S. Bijoor (1990) described the phenomenon of group cutting in an adolescent population without sufficient adult supervision, which mostly originated in problematic (low-income) environments. Occasionally, the term "wrist-cutting" also appears in the new millennium (Matsumoto et al. 2004; Gu & Jeong 2012; Ersen et al. 2017; Cho & Choi 2020; Kim et al. 2021) – it has mostly occurred in the literature coming from Eastern countries (Turkey, Korea, Japan, etc.). As in the case of self-injury, wrist-cutting syndrome mostly involves a form of self-harm that results in a visible disturbance to an individual's tissues.

Dermatitis Artefacta

In the context of self-harm that causes a disturbance to the skin (cutting, burning, scratching, etching, causing frostbite, etc.), a fairly large number of specifically medical terms that are used to designate those wounds that result from the intentional activity of the individual are employed in scientific literature. These include dermatitis artefacta, which is defined as a dermatological state caused by the individual themselves that is understood to be an act of self-harm (Saha et al. 2015). This is not only reported in adults in the scientific literature (Reis et al. 1997) but also in children (Finore et al. 2007) and adolescents (Boyd & Dewan 2015). A similar (albeit more generally formulated) term is an artefactual skin disease[28] (Mohandas et al. 2018). It is defined as a fictitious skin disorder, or artificial dermatitis, which is self-inflicted by the individual. There are also expressions that reflect the specific orientation of the individual medical fields which encounter the consequences of self-harm, and these are used in their professional literature (for instance, plastic surgeons use the term "self-induced skin lesions" – Gattu et al. 2009). Generally speaking, these terms refer to a relatively narrow and specific range of forms of self-harm, which focus on the skin and cause superficial injuries.

---

28 The U.S. Centers for Disease Control and Prevention in their coding system SNOMED-CT reported artefactual skin disease (disorder) under number 402737007, and various phenomena are classified under this diagnosis, including factitious blistering (disorder), or self-inflicted caustic burns (disorder) (CDC 2021).

Deliberate Self-Poisoning

Another specific term used to denote a form of self-harm is deliberate self-poisoning (or simply self-poisoning). Since it is only a single form of self-harm, it rarely draws any attention as a separate phenomenon. It is most often mentioned in combination with other forms of self-harm, such as self-injury (Kessel & McCulloch 1996) or the more general term "self-mutilation" (Teixeira & Luis 1997). However, deliberate self-poisoning, just like other forms of self-harm, may or may not be motivated by a desire to end one's own life[29]. Studies of self-harming behaviour mostly focus on non-fatal cases, and their analysis has revealed that this type of self-harm occurs most often in women with depressive symptoms at secondary schools or universities/colleges who have a family background that exhibits signs of dysfunction (Lifshitz & Gavrilov (2002). Preliminary analyses of the prevalence of the individual forms of self-harm in the Slovak adolescent population[30] revealed that 5.3% of self-harmers have abused prescribed medication, 4% have overdosed deliberately, and up to 43.4% abused alcohol with the intent to hurt themselves[31] (Démuthová & Démuth 2019a). In the case of deliberate self-poisoning, they use various substances – the substance selected both depends not only on availability but also on "popularity", which often depends on the state of development of the country or the degree of urbanisation of the environment in which the individual lives (Eddleston 2000). Pesticides are the most frequently used poison in tropical areas and are associated with high levels of lethality. Self-poisoning using medications such as benzodiazepines or antidepressants is common in urban areas but is linked to a small number of deaths. Poisoning using the antimalarial drug chloroquine is frequent in Africa and the Pacific

---

29 In this respect, Y. Finkelstein et al. (2015) state that almost a quarter (23.4%) of the patients after terminating their hospitalisation resulting from deliberate self-poisoning will later (in 585 days on average) commit suicide. Risk factors include a higher age, male sex, multiple self-poisoning episodes, higher socio-economic status, depression and recent psychiatric care.
30 A detailed analysis of the occurrence of self-harm forms is provided in the section "4.2 The Prevalence of the Forms of Self-Harm".
31 They did not use it to induce intoxication, to copy a behaviour of a group, to impress peers, etc. but specifically with the aim to harm oneself and cause damage to oneself.

and is also often fatal. Self-poisoning by ingesting parts of plants is fairly common on a global scale, but it is locally highly popular in certain regions of the world (such as Sub-Saharan Africa and certain Asian islands) (Eddleston 2000). In the context of the selection of the toxic substance, it is important to mention the studies of M. Eddelston et al. (2006) who reported that most individuals in Sri Lanka who deliberately poisoned themselves did so half an hour after their initial decision, with the toxicity of the substance playing an insignificant role in their choice. Thus, the current availability of a substance appears to be the decisive factor in their choice. Self-poisoning, in the context of the hitherto presented terms, is specific because it is a form of self-harm which does not cause any visible wounds or tissue damage – it is a concealed or indirect form of self-harm, which means that even these forms may significantly contribute to self-harming behaviour.

Self-Inflicted Injury

A somewhat wider range of forms of self-harm is covered by the term "self-inflicted injury". Apart from the term "self-inflicted injury" (Sluga & Grünberger 1969; Sneddon & Sneddon 1975), international scientific literature also uses the term "self-injurious behaviour" (LeBlanc 1993; Kern et al. 1997), which, as opposed to self-wounding, does not necessarily result in visible wounds. Such an injury may include a fractured bone, which does not appear to be a wound, thus this term may be used more broadly than the above-mentioned self-wounding. The term "injury" is broader than wound. The broader understanding of this term is also documented by several studies in this field – for example, Peterson et al. (2019) utilised this term in their analysis of the occurrence of intentional cuts, burns, drowning, burning, suffocation, poisoning, etc. Similarly, Skinner et al. (2016) mention drowning, burning oneself, intentional injuries in traffic, falls or poisonings as forms of deliberate self-harm, using the term "self-inflicted injury" to jointly refer to them. Moreover, self-injurious behaviour is also defined as a broad class of behaviours that directly and deliberately harm one's own body (Son et al. 2021). Nevertheless, it is apparent that these terms refer to physical forms (either visible or concealed) of self-harm and do not take mental forms of self-harm into consideration.

Self-Destructiveness

When it comes to forms of self-harm, the term "self-destructiveness" (see e.g., Green 1978; van der Kolk et al. 1991; Noshpitz 1994; D'Alessandro & Lester 2000) is relatively broad. Its specificity rather lies in its reference to the intent of the behaviour, which is the destruction of oneself[32]. Hence, it describes a more serious involvement in self-harm in terms of its intended consequences. Considering the fact that this term covers a large variety of self-harming activities, there have been efforts to categorise it in the scientific literature. It differentiates between direct and indirect self-destructiveness – direct self-destructiveness refers to actions that lead to auto-mutilation, such as self-harm, attempted suicide or committing suicide. Indirect self-destructiveness is understood as taking or abandoning specific actions, for the individual to place themselves into hazardous or high-risk situations (the active form) or to threaten their safety or health by neglecting certain activities (the passive form) (Tsirigotis 2016). Moreover, with indirect self-destructiveness, the harm does not occur immediately, but after a period of time – mostly depending on how quickly the consequences of these actions have an impact on the individual (Suchańska, 1998, 2001). Generally, there are several categories of indirect self-destructive behaviour: it may include various activities that bring various degrees of risk; poor preservation of health, neglecting or harming health; social and interpersonal self-neglect; personal and social neglect; and intentional passivity in the solution of problems/difficult situations. Indirect self-destructiveness also includes high-risk behaviours such as dangerous driving, gambling or the search for life-threatening situations (Zanarini et al. 2008; Tsirigotis 2016).

---

[32] A conceptually similar term is self-destruction or its synonym auto-destruction, both of which are used in the work of A. Suchańska (1998, 2001).

Automutilation

Automutilation is a term that primarily occurs in psychiatric terminology. It was extensively used, especially in the second half of the last century, as a scientific term that referred to the wide range of self-harming behaviours, and not only abroad (as automutilation – Tiggelaar 1958; De Smet et al. 1997 or self-mutilation[33] – Zerbe 1988; Katz & Levendusky 1990; Favazza 1998) but was also adopted in Slovakia (Izáková et al. 2006; Bošiaková 2013). Automutilation is defined as "deliberate harm inflicted upon one's own health, which has pathological and often psychotically altered motivation" (Bošiaková 2013, 66) and has a habitual nature (Izáková et al. 2006). It is commonly used as a synonym for the term "self-harm", which is more widespread and comprehensible for a wider audience, but, considering the etymology of the term "automutilation", there are certain differences between these expressions. In Latin the word "mutilo" means to shorten, to chip away (Špaňár & Hrabovský 1998), to cripple, and as such, it still implies physical damage to the body. On the other hand, "harm" is understood more broadly – it is possible to cause harm even in "nonmaterial" areas (mental health, prestige, status, the reputation of an individual...). This may also be reflected in other definitions of the term "automutilation" – for example, M. Oumaya et al. (2008, 452) characterise it as "the deliberate direct destruction or alteration of one's body tissue without conscious suicidal intent".

Self-Harm

Probably the most frequent term that denotes behaviours through which an individual causes harm to oneself is self-harm. Apart from the term "self-harm" (Skegg 2005; Ougrin et al. 2012; Bailey et al. 2017), international scientific literature also uses the term "self-harming behavio(u)r" (Low et a. 2000; Schützmann et al. 2009), and there are also terms that highlight any of its aspects – such as its deliberateness (deliberate self-harm & Arendt et al.

---

[33] In rare cases, an even more specific term "superficial/moderate self-mutilation" is used (Favazza 1996).

2019; Lai et al. 2021). Considering the relatively wider meaning of the term "self-harm", we may encounter a great deal of variability in the forms that individual authors cover with it. For instance, Skegg (2005, 1471) defines self-harm as a "wide range of behaviours and intentions including attempted hanging, impulsive self-poisoning, and superficial cutting in response to intolerable tension"; Bailey et al. (2017) as simply harming oneself; Lauw et al. (2015, 306) as "the intentional act of causing physical injury to oneself without wanting to die". Therefore, it is clear that certain authors limit the term "self-harm" to activities that do not include signs of attempted suicide, while others cover a wider range of self-harm forms, including the possibility of mental self-harm, in addition to harm inflicted upon physical health. For example, Sansone et al. (2006) or Jarahi (2021) include deliberately torturing oneself by self-defeating thoughts or deliberate alienation from significant others.

Non-suicidal Self-Injury

A specific term related to self-harm is non-suicidal self-injury (NSSI). It is probably the most widely used term in the psychological literature to denote self-harming behaviour, and one of its specific features is that it was selected by experts, who wished to introduce it into psychological terminology, as a consequence of the alarming and ever-increasing number of cases, especially among adolescents. This undesirable trend has led to the proposition formulated in the fifth revision of the Diagnostic and Statistical Manual of Mental Disorders (DSM-5) and included in the Appendix Conditions for Further Study, which proposes the following definition:

"A. In the last year, the individual has, on 5 or more days, engaged in intentional self-inflicted damage to the surface of his or her body of a sort likely to induce bleeding, bruising or pain (e.g., cutting, burning, stabbing, hitting, excessive rubbing), with the expectation that the injury will lead to only minor or moderate physical harm (i.e., there is no suicidal intent).

Note: The absence of suicidal intent has either been stated by the individual or can be inferred by the individual's repeated

engagement in a behavior that the individual knows, or has learned, is not likely to result in death.
B. The individual engages in the self-injurious behavior with one or more of the following expectations:
   1. To obtain relief from a negative feeling or cognitive state.
   2. To resolve an interpersonal difficulty.
   3. To induce a positive feeling state.
   Note: The desired relief or response is experienced during or shortly after the self-injury, and the individual may display patterns of behavior suggesting a dependence on repeatedly engaging in it.
C. The intentional self-injury is associated with at least one of the following:
   1. Interpersonal difficulties or negative feelings or thoughts, such as depression, anxiety, tension, anger, generalized distress or self-criticism, occurring in the period immediately prior to the self-injurious act.
   2. Prior to engaging in the act, a period of preoccupation with the intended behaviour that is difficult to control.
   3. Thinking about self-injury that occurs frequently, even when it is not acted upon.
D. The behavior is not socially sanctioned (e.g., body piercing, tattooing, part of a religious or cultural ritual) and is not restricted to picking a scab or nail biting.
E. The behavior or its consequences cause clinically significant distress or interference in interpersonal, academic, or other important areas of functioning.
F. The behavior does not occur exclusively during psychotic episodes, delirium, substance intoxication, or substance withdrawal. In individuals with a neurodevelopmental disorder, the behavior is not part of a pattern of repetitive stereotypies. The behaviour is not better explained by another mental disorder or medical condition (e.g., psychotic disorder, autism spectrum disorder, intellectual disability, Lesch-Nyhan syndrome, stereotypic movement disorder with self-injury, trichotillomania [hair-pulling disorder], excoriation [skin-picking] disorder)" (APA 2013, 803).

This text is clearly an attempt to set out standardised criteria for the clinical diagnosis of this phenomenon, which takes the key features of self-harm into consideration from various perspectives – its recurring character; its differentiation from other diagnoses, in which self-harm occurs as a concomitant symptom; or its differentiation from specifically motivated actions. On the other hand, the problem of this approach lies in the range of self-harm forms considered, it fails to take anything other than physical forms into consideration or to even mention indirect forms of self-harm (poisoning, suffocation, starvation...) and it strictly excludes individuals who attempt suicide. However, several studies (see e.g., Müller et al. 2016; Démuthová & Démuth 2019b) suggest that indirect and mental forms of self-harm are a common component of self-harming behaviour, and attempted suicide is a more extreme expression rather than a completely separate phenomenon (Tørmoen et al. 2013).[34] It is also apparent that the motivation and aim of self-harming behaviour are not only limited to relief from negative feelings, ideas and relationship problems or to achieve a positive emotional state, but it also includes other areas (such as self-punishment). Despite these objections, which may serve as an important impulse for further studies and the subsequent improvement of the proposed definition, the effort to introduce this undesirable and high-risk behaviour into clinical-psychological manuals is commendable, since it poses a serious problem with increasing prevalence.

1.4 The Definition of Self-Harm

The multitude of terms and variants of the definitions of similar behaviours suggest that it is necessary to clarify the terminology used in this field[35]. The previous definitions highlighted a few

---

34 For further analyses of the prevalence of attempted suicide in self-harming behaviour, see the subsequent part "The Aim".
35 The reason that there is a need for the clarification of the terminology is not the multitude of similar terms (and thus an attempt to make their use more consistent), but if different experts use different definitions for similar, yet not identical, determinations, it will be impossible to observe the development of this phenomenon over time or to compare its prevalence in the real world – whether it be in different countries or different populations.

of the important aspects that must be considered in the proposed definition; these include the agent (who does it), the object (what is affected), the intent (what was the intention) and the aim (what was supposed to happen). With regard to the object, it appears equally important[36] to define the extent (what the self-harm may involve) and to separate it from the most extreme form of self-harm, attempted suicide or suicide.

The Agent

The first impression suggests that in the use of terms associated with self-harm, the agent is always the individual involved in the self-harm. And in many cases, that is the case. Chapter 4 provides an overview of the forms and types of self-harm, and in most cases, it is an activity directly taken by an individual (cutting, burning, hitting oneself, etc.), or deliberate neglect (again, by the individual) leading to the deterioration of health – both physical (such as deliberately skipping medication when treating an illness) and mental (deliberately inducing unpleasant mental states). However, there are also some forms in which the harm to the individual is performed by another person – for instance, some people are mentally or physically abused. Although it may seem that this kind of action cannot be considered self-harm (since it is not the individual who harms themselves, but they are harmed by someone else), even these types of cases could be included in the wide range of forms of self-harm. The reason for this is that the individuals concerned admit that they provoke the situation that lead to their rejection, humiliation or harm in contact with others. They also confess to deliberately provoking aggressive people around them in order to become the target of an attack. They do not run from toxic, violent and pathological relationships; they do not defend themselves, quite the opposite; they remain in them for the exact same reasons that they also

---

36 Even considering the relatively narrow view of the proposal of DSM-5, which strictly defines self-harm as deliberate physical self-harm in the absence of suicidal intent (APA 2013).

perform other forms of self-harm[37]. Self-harming individuals also state that they intentionally enter relationships when they know, or assume, that they will be victims of various types of violence or mistreatment. Research conducted in Slovakia on a sample of adolescents also reports that in spontaneous occurrences of other forms of self-harm[38], the adolescents in question suggested many other forms that were characterised by the deliberate provocation of situations that might lead to them suffering harm from others, for example, they deliberately fail to defend their rights if they are wronged; they let other people believe they did something that they were not responsible for; they deliberately present unflattering information about themselves in order for others to spread this around and harm their social status; they deliberately provoke arguments with those close to them, to make them angry at them or to punish them, etc. Considering that the individuals are actively involved in the process, or they deliberately provoke it by their lack of activity, they should be considered the agents of self-harm in these cases.

The Object

The object of self-harm is the individual themselves – this is evident in most of the terms related to self-harming behaviour and equally obvious is the degree of agreement in this respect between the various definitions of the terms of self-injury, automutilation, self-harm, etc. However, the damage that may be suffered by the

---

[37] Common reasons include the conviction that they are unworthy of love, that they deserve to be mistreated, that others should treat them badly because they deserve it... If others do this, they do not defend themselves, and so the other people involved believe that this form of interaction is adequate, and they may do it in the future and keep doing so. The recurrent aggressive/humiliating approach from others is confirmation of the distorted conviction that they deserve this behaviour, and if others treat them badly, it is because they consider the individual less valuable or bad.

[38] The identification of the presence of various forms of self-harm was conducted in two ways – on one hand, the adolescents were given a modified SHI questionnaire (Self-harm Inventory – Sansone & Sansone, 2010), but they were also given the opportunity to freely add other forms of self-harm that they had performed that were not listed in the questionnaire.

object is quite actively debated. One approach follows the latest (fifth) revision of the Diagnostic and Statistical Manual of Mental Disorders of the American Psychiatric Association (APA 2013), the final part of Section III (Emerging Measures and Models) entitled Conditions for Further Study describes the so-called non-suicidal self-injury. It is characterised as "intentional self-inflicted damage to the surface of his or her body of a sort likely to induce bleeding, bruising, or pain (e.g., cutting, burning, stabbing, hitting, excessive rubbing), with the expectation that the injury will lead to only minor or moderate physical harm (i.e., there is no suicidal intent)" (APA 2013, 803). According to this definition, self-harm should only affect the surface of the body of the individual and only cause minor (or moderate) injuries. By accepting this perspective, we not only eliminate attempted suicide and other, more serious forms of harm from the various forms of self-harm but also many bodily injuries and damage to health caused by the consumption of indigestible objects; deliberate self-poisoning using medicine, alcohol, food or chemical substances, etc., or the abuse of these substances with the intention of harming oneself; rejecting food or deliberately overeating with the intention of inducing nausea, refusing to sleep or overexercising so as to become exhausted; not taking prescribed medication. Nor would it cover strangling, suffocation, jumps from height with the subsequent internal injuries and many other forms of self-harm, which, although they affect the body, are not visible on the surface.

In addition to this very narrow perspective, DSM-5 fails to consider other forms of self-harm which primarily affect the mental health of the individual. The reason is that the individual may not only harm themselves physically but also mentally, and the mental pain and suffering may be even more intense than the physical pain. It is also common for these individuals to harm themselves in other important areas of their lives as well – for instance, they intentionally provoke negative reactions towards themselves; they behave in a way that leads them to be rejected by others or that causes others to feel aversion, hostility or aggression towards them; they deliberately reduce their own social status or destroy social bonds. It is, therefore, beneficial to include those forms in which the object of self-harm is not exclusively their physical bodies – the individual may harm themselves in many other ways and feel pain in many diverse forms. Then the question is what could represent the target of self-harm (of course, while maintaining the main claim that the object is the individual that produces the self-harm).

The Aim

Based on the numerous studies that have observed various forms of self-harm, it is very clear that the prevalence of this behaviour includes not only deliberate superficial bodily harm but also many other forms that harm the somatic health of an individual (Sansone et al. 2006; Lloyd-Richardson et al. 2007; Hooley et al. 2020) including attempted suicide (Grandclerc et al. 2016; Harris et al. 2019; Knipe et al. 2019) as well as other forms that cause deterioration of the mental and social aspects of the quality of life of the individual (Sansone et al. 2006; Mülleret al. 2018; Jarahi et al. 2021). This is why we believe that the definition of self-harm should not be strictly limited to the consideration of forms which have the surface of the body as their only target, but that it should be understood in broader terms – ideally so that it covers the whole range of forms of self-harming behaviour. The reason for this "broad" definition of self-harm is that it is also (and will also be) a diagnostic tool for experts, and as such it will determine who will be considered to be a self-harming individual and who will not. Consequently, it leads to the decision of whether or not the individual will be provided (based on the diagnosis) psychological/psychiatric support, whether their treatment will be provided by professionals or whether they fail to meet the diagnostic criteria. At the same time, it is appropriate to limit the number of symptoms examined to the absolutely necessary minimum in order to ensure the effectiveness of diagnostic tools. The principle of Occam's razor in science postulates that the optimal strategy requires one to work with the smallest number of elements possible in any given situation. This means that the best definition (determination) should be as brief as possible, yet provide cover to the necessary extent.

This is why we should ask ourselves what would be the impact of narrowing down the diagnostic criteria (or accepting a narrower definition resulting from the proposition formulated in Appendix

III DSM-5) on the detection of real cases of self-harm. If narrower criteria were practical but would lead to the drop-out of an overly large number of cases, it would be inappropriate. On the other hand, observing too many symptoms and signs would be impractical and lead to even less clarity of diagnosis. It is apparent that there is a large number of forms of self-harm, and it is those, in particular, that are not listed in DSM-5 that represent a relatively large fraction of the possible self-harming activities. Previous surveys into this issue have revealed that visible physical damage to the surface of the body and other forms, as defined in DSM-5, was found in 38.7% of adolescents, while indirect forms of physical self-harm[39] were found in 46.3% of cases (Démuth & Démuthová 2019). Forms of mental self-harm[40] are also relatively frequent among adolescents – for instance, deliberate torture with self-defeating thoughts is indicated as a form of self-harm by 33.6% of adolescents (Démuthová & Démuth 2019a). It is, therefore, obvious that forms which are not defined in DSM-5 represent a significant fraction of the spectrum of self-harming behaviours. The question is whether these forms appear as an addition to direct physical forms or they also exist independently. The real risk that individuals that behave in this way may not be diagnosed with self-harm would occur in cases where those individuals do not exhibit any of the forms of self-harm listed in DSM-5.[41] In order to provide the correct incentive to expand the definition of self-harming behaviour, an analysis needs to be performed which will demonstrate how individual adolescents would (or would not) be identified as self-harmers depending on the use of various diagnostic approaches.

---

39 Indirect forms of physical self-harm include activities that may lead to somatic harm, but are not directly visible on the surface of the body (e.g. the above-mentioned consumption of indigestible objects; deliberate self-poisoning through medicine, alcohol, food, chemical substances, etc., or their abuse with the intention to harm oneself; rejecting food or deliberately overeating with the intention of inducing nausea, refusing to sleep or overexercising with the intention of becoming exhausted; skipping prescribed medications and many others). For more information on the individual forms and types of self-harm, see Chapter 3.
40 This, for example, includes deliberate alienation from close ones, inducing unpleasant, emotionally burdening mental states, convincing themselves of their lack of abilities and inferiority, etc.
41 If they exhibited at least one form listed by DSM-5 in addition to a large number of indirect physical forms or mental forms, they would be diagnosed.

For this purpose, an analysis[42] was conducted on a sample of 1,823 adolescents, and the prevalence of self-harm was observed using three approaches – the first was the narrowest and it used the definition proposed by the fifth revision of the Diagnostic and Statistical Manual of Mental Disorders of the American Psychiatric Association. The second used the criteria which can be implicitly identified in the ICD-10 diagnostic system (International Classification of Diseases and Related Health Problems, Tenth Revision) (ICD-10, 2021). In chapter XX (External Causes of Morbidity and Mortality – codes V01 – Y98), it defines the category of intentional self-harm (under codes X71 – X83), with the extent of the individual types of self-harming behaviour being much wider – it includes (as opposed to DSM-5) hidden/indirect physical self-harm, such as intentional self-poisoning and exposure to toxic substances, self-harm by hot vapours and hot objects, by jumping from a high place, etc. In the X83 category (Intentional Self-Harm by Other Specified Means), it leaves space to include other forms of self-harm; moreover, it also includes suicide and attempted suicide as forms of intentional self-harm (ICD-10 2016). Unlike DSM-5, the International Classification of Diseases has an expanded definition of forms of self-harm, but finally, it only considers somatic forms.

The third perspective is represented by approaches that view self-harm as any intentional act that results in damage to health – whether physical or mental. An example of such an approach is the creation of a methodology to measure self-harm – the SHI questionnaire (Self-Harm Inventory – Sansone and Sansone 2010), which has the broadest scope – it has the potential to identify various types and forms of this behaviour.

Following these three approaches, the conducted analysis focused on the number of adolescents who would be identified as self-harmers based on the criteria listed in DSM-5 (direct, visible self-harm), ICD-10 (any physical self-harm) and the SHI questionnaire (physical and mental self-harm). The SHI questionnaire[43]

---

[42] Detailed results are presented in the study: Démuthová, S., & Spasovski, O. (2020). The Analysis of Drop-Out in the Potential Diagnostic Systems for Self-Harm in the Adolescent Population. AD ALTA: Journal of Interdisciplinary Research, 10(2), 51-55.

[43] The modified version of the Self-Harm Inventory (SHI – Sansone & Sansone, 2010) includes twenty questions observing the presence and frequency (never –

(with the broadest scope) identified 830 self-harmers in the sample of 1,823 adolescents (with a prevalence of 45.5%). As opposed to this result, the other two diagnostic systems (DSM-5 and ICD-10) identified fewer self-harmers (see Table 2).

Table 2. The number of cases of self-harm detected by the three diagnostic systems

System	Detected Cases		Undetected Cases	
	n	%	n	%
SHI	830	100	0	0
ICD-10	803	96.7	27	3.3
DSM-5	701	84.5	129	15.5

Source: author

The total drop-out rate when using the IDC-10 diagnostic criteria (as opposed to the broadest SHI system) is moderate – it is only 3.3% of cases. The difference is caused by the omission of mental forms of self-harm in IDC-10; however, it should be noted that out of the twenty different forms of self-harm listed in the questionnaire, there were only four mental forms (which is a fifth of the forms of self-harm observed). With regard to these forms, adolescents most often indicated that they deliberately entered a relationship in which they were abused and that they deliberately tortured themselves with self-defeating thoughts. It is possible that an adequate representation of mental forms of self-harm with regard to the other forms (direct and indirect physical forms) would increase this rate; but even if it did not, a drop-out rate of 3.3% within a self-harming population with a prevalence

---

rarely – sometimes – often) of the most common forms of self-harming behaviour. The original SHI questionnaire was slightly modified in order to correspond to the age group of the study sample (adolescence) and to monitor the occurrence of the most common forms of self-harm in the observed population; the good internal consistency of the modified methodology was confirmed (Cronbach's α = 0.809 – Démuthová & Doktorová 2019). Participants were included in the group of self-harming individuals if they included the frequency "sometimes" or "often" of at least one form of self-harm (meaning an individual performed the behaviour several times), or if they indicated a frequency "rarely" in several forms of self-harm.

1 The Definition of Self-Harm

of 45.5% among adolescents aged 11–19 years adds up to[44] 7,317 undiagnosed adolescents.

If the criteria in line with DSM-5 were used to identify self-harming adolescents, 15.5% of cases would be undiagnosed. This would result in 34,369 adolescents who would not be identified as self-harmers, who consequently would not receive treatment or be provided with adequate support/intervention. Statistical analyses (Table 3) demonstrated that the decrease in the identified cases using the DSM-5 criteria was statistically significant (sig. = 0.000).

Table 3. The differences in the number of cases detected using the ICD-10 and DSM-5 criteria

	Cases Undetected by ICD-10 (n/%)	Cases Detected by ICD-10 (n/%)	Total (n/%)	Chi-Square test	
Cases Undetected by DSM-5	27/3.3	102/12.3	129/15.5	Pearson coef. 151.65	Sig. .000
Cases Detected by DSM-5	0/0.0	701/84.5	701/84.5		
Total	27/3.3	803/96.8	830/100.0		

Therefore, it is obvious that mental forms of self-harm, which are not included in ICD-10, together with indirect forms of self-harm, which are missing in DSM-5, represent a significant proportion of self-harming behaviours and may have a very high prevalence, even on their own. Thus, these forms should be taken into account in assessments of self-harm and based on the results of other studies in this field[45]; the definition of the term should be reconsidered and a new one proposed for the diagnosis of this high-risk behaviour.

---

44 According to the public database STATdat, in 2020, there were 487,310 adolescents between the ages of 11 and 19 in the Slovak Republic (http://statdat.statistics.sk/).
45 An overview of the prevalence of individual forms of self-harm in the population of Slovak adolescents is provided in the section "4.2 The Prevalence of the Forms of Self-Harm".

The Intent

Another significant feature of self-harming behaviour is its intent. In order to correctly define the term, it is necessary to analyse this feature from several perspectives.

First, damage may be (and often is) inflicted upon one's own body unintentionally, by coincidence, as a result of an accident. Obviously, in such a case, there is no intent to harm oneself; thus, this kind of behaviour cannot be included in self-harming activities. It is a relatively clear distinction, which may not always be so clear. Problems occur when adolescents indulge in various risky forms of behaviour[46], being aware of the risk of harm and willing to take the risk. This may include various activities – ranging from risky driving with the possibility of an accident, through the consumption of large amounts of alcohol with the knowledge there is a possibility of alcohol poisoning, up to experimentation with psychotropic substances (medications, drugs...) with the risk of uncontrollable consequences. The extent of the intent to harming oneself remains questionable. If the primary motive for these high-risk activities is curiosity, an effort to be accepted by peers or the desire to have fun or find excitement, even if they are aware of the possibly dangerous consequences, it is not true self-harm. However, if the high-risk behaviour is a part of a complex of self-harm, in the sense that the individual performs these activities, especially due to their potential to cause harm, associated pain or even lethality, meaning that they perform them with the intention to hurt themselves (physically or mentally), they should be identified as self-harm. That being said, the intent of the adolescent may not be easy to identify, since the adolescent may conceal it or in some cases, even they do not clearly understand their motivations – but it must be noted that in order to label the behaviour as self-harm, its primary intent must be to cause harm. It is this intent (purpose) that differentiates it from similar (or even the same) forms of behaviour.

---

[46] In fact, high-risk behaviour is very typical of the period of adolescence (Steinberg 2008; Lerner & Ohannessian 2014; Duell et al. 2018); it stems from the intense tendency to seek new and exciting impulses (Maslowsky et al. 2019), the incomplete development of the regulation of impulses (Kahn & Graham 2019) or the tendency to explore one's own possibilities and boundaries.

Second, it should be emphasised that there is a group of activities, which indisputably result in harm – even in a way that would be considered to be deliberate self-harm, even using the DSM-5 diagnostic criteria, but which should not be labelled as self-harm. This includes tattooing or piercings which cause painful tissue damage or even much larger injuries, which are parts of an initiation ritual within various (sub)cultures[47]. In cases like these, there is an apparent shift in terms of the intent of the behaviour – although the harm is accompanied by pain, the intent is not to feel pain but rather to enhance the attractiveness of the physical appearance (tattoos, piercings and other forms of intrusions into their body[48]), to enhance social prestige (gaining membership or a position in a social group) or to demonstrate other characteristics that are praised by others (enduring pain, courage, bravery). As such, the primary motives are not the pain itself; thus, these activities should not be considered to be self-harm.

Studying the intent or primary motive of self-harm is also crucial in other cases – individuals may willingly undergo various painful procedures or even inflict damage upon their bodies in order to ultimately (or potentially) achieve an improvement in their health. A classic example is the use of chemotherapeutic treatment, which, in itself, is toxic for the organism; it triggers pain and nausea, but the individual is willing to suffer these "harms" because they assume that from a long-term perspective, the benefits (the possibility that they may overcome, slow down/stop the disease) are worth the suffering. The development of medications and the administration of analgesics or medications that reduce nausea is proof enough that if it were possible to reduce/eliminate the pain, the patient would choose this form. Causing oneself harm (albeit deliberately) is only a "necessary" evil in this case. In the case of self-harm, the individual performs these activities because they cause pain/harm.

However, in this context, we should highlight the very subtle differences in terms of the categorisation of the primary intent in self-harm. According to many authors, one of the fundamental functions of self-harm is affect regulation (Klonsky 2007; Houben

---

47 A more detailed description of these rituals is provided in section 1.1.
48 Including very painful liposuction or undergoing invasive plastic surgery.

et al. 2017; Wolff et al. 2019; Brausch et al. 2019). It means that the individual uses self-harm to reduce an acute negative affect or an aversive affective excitement that they cannot (either as a result of their own deficiencies or the height of the intensity of the emotions) cope with in another way. The act of self-harm that aims to provide affect regulation is effective[49] for several reasons. The need to prepare for the act, its painful nature, and the need to take care of the wound after the act shift the attention of the individual from the emotional burden they are experiencing. It also allows them to hide their emotional pain behind the physical pain, which alleviates the mental burden (albeit only temporary). Finally – as opposed to the emotional burden, which the individual is unable to influence, since they are affected by it – they are able to control the intensity and duration of the physical pain; thus, the individual has it under control (as opposed to their emotions)[50]. Hence, it is possible that just as a patient undergoes painful medical procedures (chemotherapy, surgeries) in an effort to cure a health issue (an illness), the individual undergoes physical pain in order to cure the problem (emotional pain), which they consider to be considerably more serious (more traumatic, painful, less bearable). Looking at the problem from this perspective, it might seem that as to the intent of the individual, there would be no difference in the way illnesses and emotional problems are "cured". Thus, when defining and characterising self-harm, it is necessary to assess the intent from a long-term perspective. In medical procedures, the potential benefit of painful treatments (slowing, halting the progress of or eliminating the illness) must outweigh the negatives associated with the continued presence of the illness, and painful treatments

---

49 However, it is undesirable and maladaptive despite its effectiveness.
50 Yet, they only assume they have this control. This happens when the consequences of self-harm are more serious or even more lethal than the individual initially intended, but it also stems from the fact that this approach to solving problem is highly addictive. Releasing tension through self-harm, transferring emotional pain to physical pain and manipulating it act as a strong element in the negative reinforcement of this behaviour (Victor et al. 2012), leading it to become fixated and a tendency to repeat it. The strong addictiveness of self-harm is one of its features that is emphasised by many of the experts that study this maladaptive strategy (Blasco-Fontecillaet al. 2016; Guérin-Marion et al. 2018; Matera et al. 2021). Since self-harm becomes an addiction, it is difficult to discuss any "control" over this behaviour.

1 The Definition of Self-Harm   53

are only indicated if there is a conviction that their administration will have a positive effect[51]. On the contrary, we cannot claim that self-harm will lead to the elimination of emotional problems. An intervention in the form of self-harm is not focused on the sources of emotional burden and pain; it does not result in the "treatment" or solution of these problems. Quite the opposite – from a long-term perspective, it leads to even greater problems, whether in the form of physical injuries, or further mental problems that are associated with the consequences of self-harm[52].

The Extent

The question of the extent of self-harming activities is directly linked to the aim of self-harm. From the section "1.3 The Terminology of Self-Harm", it is obvious that the extent of self-harm can greatly vary. It has not been determined whether self-harm should only include visible injuries to the surface of the skin of moderate to high severity, or if the extent ought to be sufficiently broad to even include highly frequent indirect forms of self-harm or even mental forms. The analyses conducted under the section "The Aim" in this chapter suggest the consequences of various approaches, and a detailed analysis of the prevalence of the different forms and types of self-harm can be found in Chapter 4. The studies carried out until now have proven that indirect and mental forms of self-harm represent a significant proportion of the spectrum of this high-risk behaviour. The nature of the forms with a relatively high reported prevalence (see Table 4) suggests that self-harm occurs in various areas – physical, mental, social and religious.

The wide range of targets of self-harm could give the impression that it is virtually impossible to verbalise all the potential areas that could be intentionally damaged by such actions. However, it is evident that the specific areas are important to the individual,

---

[51] It is a medical principle ("primum nihil nocere"), which focuses on the avoidance of harm to the patient (see, e.g., Smith 2005; Valentin 2006). It also applies to very serious, deadly illnesses – if the negatives of the treatment outweigh the potential positives, these procedures (treatments) cannot continue. Usually, this is the moment of transition from causal to symptomatic treatment.

[52] This includes worsening social isolation or addiction to self-harm.

Table 4. The prevalence of selected forms of self-harm in the population of Slovak adolescents
Have you ever intentionally, or on purpose, done any of the following:

[Form of self-harm]:	%
Abused alcohol to hurt yourself	43.4
Not slept enough to hurt yourself	42.2
Tortured yourself with self-defeating thoughts	33.6
Over-exercised to hurt yourself	21.5
Starved yourself to hurt yourself	14.4
Made medical situations worse on purpose (e.g., skipped medication)	12.6
Engaged in emotionally abusive relationships	9.6
Distanced yourself from God as a punishment	6.5
Abused prescription medication	5.3
Overdosed	4.0
Set yourself up in a relationship to be rejected	3.2
Abused laxatives to hurt yourself	2.3

Source: Démuthová & Démuth (2019a, 43)

and based on their context, we may assume that they are part of what we would term "health", as it is defined by the World Health Organisation: a state of complete physical, mental and social well-being (WHO, 2021). Therefore, self-harm can be (in terms of its range) simply defined as damage to health, and if we accept the definition of self-harmed proposed by the WHO, it includes physical, mental and social domains.

Another robust problem concerning the extent of self-harm is the question of whether attempted suicide can be included in the spectrum of self-harming behaviours or if they should be strictly excluded. The term "non-suicidal self-injury" as well as the proposed diagnostic criteria ("the injury will lead to only minor or moderate physical harm (i.e., there is no suicidal intent)" – APA 2013, 803) from DSM-5 refuse to include behaviour, with the presence of attempted suicide, as self-harm. The support of this stance stems from the fact that although self-harm may, at its core, be maladaptive, it is a self-preserving behaviour; on the contrary, attempted suicide is aimed at the termination of life. That being said, clinical practice and scientific studies report frequent co-occurrence of self-harming and suicidal behaviour (Hamza et al. 2012; Kapur et al. 2013; Grandclerc et al. 2016). Thus, the question is what differentiates individuals who have attempted suicide from those who have not, and why it is important to separate them from the population of self-harmers.

Several studies have attempted to observe the differences between self-harming individuals who have not attempted suicide and those who have. They suggest that individuals who have attempted suicide, in comparison to those who have not, exhibit lower levels of self-confidence and rationality, along with higher levels of hopelessness (Kienhorst et al. 1990); a higher occurrence of depressive symptoms and suicidal thoughts (Muehlenkamp & Gutierrez 2007); and they more commonly meet the diagnostic criteria for a depressive disorder or post-traumatic stress disorder (Jacobson et al. 2008) along with feeling that they have less support from their parents (Brausch & Gutierrez 2010). The studies that have been conducted on the Slovak population of adolescents (see: Démuthová & Václaviková 2019; Démuthová & Démuth 2019b; Démuthová & Rojková 2019) focused on several variables – personality characteristics, age, motivation for self-harm, forms of self-harm and their frequency (Table 5).

The results suggest that self-harming adolescents who have attempted suicide start to self-harm earlier than those who have not attempted suicide. They have lower levels of extraversion and exhibit higher levels of neuroticism and psychoticism. There is no difference in the forms of self-harm[53] between the two groups, and also they do not have different motivations[54]; however, the number and the intensity of the occurrence of individual forms and motives are significantly greater in the group of self-harming adoles-

---

53 Except for attempted suicide, the two groups were differentiated based on these criteria.
54 To find the motivation for self-harm, the second part of the self-reporting ISAS (Inventory of Statements about Self-Injury – Klonsky & Glenn 2009) was used. The inventory maps thirteen potential motives (functions) of self-harm (affect regulation, preventing dissociation, preventing suicide, autonomy, interpersonal boundaries, interpersonal impact, demonstrating distress, securing relationships with peers, revenge, self-care, self-punishment, seeking excitement and roughness), with all of these thirteen areas covered through the evaluation of three statements (items), with the option to rate them on a three-degree scale.

Table 5. The statistically significant differences in selected variables between self-harming adolescents who have attempted suicide and those who have not

	Attempted Suicide	n	Mean Rank	Mann-Whitney U	Asymp. Sig.
Age at the Onset of Self-Harm[a]	No	201	153.83	7,472.00	0.016*
	Yes	90	128.52		
	Total	291			
Extroversion[b]	No	217	140.41	3,600	0,001***
	Yes	48	99.51		
	Total	265			
Neuroticism[b]	No	217	125.27	3,530	0,000***
	Yes	48	167.96		
	Total	265			
Psychotism[b]	No	217	119.80	2,344	0,000***
	Yes	48	192.67		
	Total	265			

Note: * $p \leq 0.05$; *** $p \leq 0.001$
Source: [a] Démuthová & Démuth (2019b); [b] Démuthová & Rojková (2019)

cents who have attempted suicide (Démuthová & Démuth 2019b; Démuthová & Václaviková 2019). It appears that self-harming individuals who have attempted suicide differ from individuals who have not attempted suicide through some quantitative (rather than qualitative) parameters – their self-harm is more intense; they tend to have several mental problems and difficulties in their relationship with themselves, as well as with others; they start to self-harm earlier; the problematic characteristics in their personalities are more pronounced. The interpretation of the differences between the observed groups seems to suggest that the occurrence of attempted suicide rises as the intensity of self-harm and the number of complications increases. The absence of qualitative differences implies that self-harming individuals who have attempted suicide cannot be strictly separated from those who have not; suicidal expressions (thoughts and attempts) are more of an accompanying sign of a greater intensity of self-harm. Similar conclusions have also been reached by international studies – for example, Hawton et al. (2012) stated that self-harming behaviour has a tendency to become chronic; it continuously evolves towards other forms of self-harming behaviour, including attempts to commit suicide. Tørmoen et al. (2013) probably put it in the clearest possible way, arguing that non-suicidal self-injury (NSSI) and suicidal self-injury are parts of the same construct. The possible differences mostly concern the degree, not the type.

In light of the above, individuals who have attempted suicide (but of course, only if their attempts co-occur with other forms of self-harm and not without any other forms of self-harm) should not be excluded from the diagnosis of self-harm. In this regard, Kapur et al. (2013) quite clearly claim that the term "non-suicidal self-injury" (NSSI) is inaccurate[55], since self-harm has high comorbidity with suicidal behaviour, and they argue that even self-harming individuals cannot always clearly determine whether their actions have a self-preserving (i.e., non-suicidal) or self-destructive (suicidal) character. This significantly questions the extent to which NSSI is truly non-suicidal.

The Term and Its Definition

Considering the above, the following sections of this work will employ the term "self-harm", since it most accurately captures the behaviour we are trying to describe. The content of the term is intended to express that the individual causes their own change of state (the prefix "self-"), and this change is negative ("harm"). Since our contemporary knowledge does not suggest it appropriate to exclude attempted suicide from the range of self-harming behaviours, we will not use the adjective "non-suicidal" when describing this behaviour.

When defining self-harm, we took several of the above-mentioned factors into consideration, especially the intent and aim of such actions. It is not our ambition to replace the DSM-5 diagnos-

---

55 Some authors even claim that to separate non-suicidal self-harm as a separate nosological unit is a "false dichotomy", since they consider the distinction between non-suicidal and suicidal self-harm to be artificial (Kapur et al. 2013).

tic criteria with this definition; rather, we are attempting to remove ambiguities and create a clear image of its contents.

Our understanding is that the term "self-harm" is the repeated infliction of harm on our health (in its physical/psychological/social domain) with the intention to harm oneself directly or indirectly or to provoke pain.

2 Theoretical Bases

If we look at self-harm as a type of behaviour which is highly risky, yet does not primarily result from a mental illness, we may identify several non-pathological mental mechanisms and models, which could potentially clarify its initiation and retention in the repertoire of reactions of an individual. Through the aspects that all these concepts highlight in their explanation, they allow us to have an insight into the interpretative frameworks of specific fields and mechanisms having an impact on self-harming; however, none of them provides a universal explanation for all cases of this high-risk behaviour. Yet, all of them can be applied in the interpretation of findings obtained through the available empirical data on self-harm.

2.1 Psychodynamic Concepts

Psychodynamic models are one of the first, in the ontogenesis of the study of self-harming behaviour, that have attempted to clarify the reasons for this self-destructive behaviour. They primarily stem from psychoanalytic concepts, which means that they rely on the perennially mentioned conflict between the life drive and the death drive postulated by Sigmund Freud. According to this concept, the objective of human existence is to establish absolute equilibrium, which stems from the initial inorganic state and which the individual finds again in a state of non-existence. The death drive (Thanatos) is linked to this goal and tries to find the shortest possible way to death and decomposition (Freud 2005). In opposition to the death drive is the life drive (Eros) and libidinous preferences, which creates a continuous conflict that accompanies an individual from the moment of conception. In accordance with the principles of lust, libidinous energy forces an individual to preserve their existence, to provide enough energy for the life drive and acts in opposition to the death drive (Thanatos).

The Substitution of Self-Destruction

Psychodynamic models of one of the possible explanations of self-harming behaviour work with the dynamism of these two forces. An individual is under pressure from the death drive, but the life drive prevents them from succumbing to it and terminating their existence. Psychodynamically oriented theoreticians point out that self-harming behaviour is often performed as a replacement for absolute destruction – and this is not only theoretical; self-harming individuals themselves state that they perform self-harm while experiencing an urge to end their lives, in order to avoid suicidal thoughts and tendencies or to divert (channel) the forces that lead to death. In this concept, self-harm is a result of the fight between Eros and Thanatos, when the life-preserving force keeps the individual from succumbing to the force that leads to the termination of their existence, and to avoid this, the individual seeks a substitute solution (compromise). In practice, this interpretation is common among the authors of the first scientific studies[56] on non-suicidal self-harm (Menninger 1938) as well as in later works – for instance, Asch (1971) develops Menninger's concept of focal suicide, in which the extent of self-destruction is concentrated on a single place, and he compares cutting with the bleeding to a minor suicide. In this context, cutting was perceived as a symbol of suicide – sufficiently visible to be seen and not lethal enough to represent a real attempt to end one's life.

Control over Sexual Urges

Psychodynamic theoreticians also suggest that self-harm might be one of the ways that we gain control over sexual urges (Nock 2009). This topic is very extensive especially in psychoanalysis[57], with the two most significant objects in these interpretations being skin and blood. When an individual cuts themselves, the blood symbolises a purge or is a parallel to menarche. In the first case,

---

56 See the initial section "1.1 The History of Research into Self-Harm" and references to Karl Menninger's work.
57 Sigmund Freud was generally well-known for his pansexualism.

the purging ritual should rid the body of the defilement caused by sexual desires that occur with greater intensity in the post-puberty period. The superego, formed by social pressures (unacceptable sex in adolescence, taboos associated with sexuality, etc.), reacts to these desires with specific mechanisms (moral and neurotic anxiety) that try to prevent these sexual thoughts, fantasies, desires and activities. However, all of these occur naturally during puberty, so the adolescent experiences anxiety. The adolescent often reacts through self-punishment, which may take the form of self-harm by cutting. In this case, it is a maladaptive strategy to cope with states of anxiety that result from the newly acquired sexual maturity and the newly activated associated drives (Jacobson & Batejan 2014).

In the period that the psychodynamic theories were dominant, several studies highlighted the occurrence of self-harm (especially cutting) in the early period of sexual maturity (Stone 1987), especially in girls, who had negative reactions after their menarche (e.g., disgust, worries) (Rosenthal et al. 1972). Accepting sexual maturity and dealing with the new life role of a woman, integrating it into their personal identity... are the tasks faced by adolescents which pose real difficulties in this developmental period (Greig & Ulman 1982). Self-harm is one of the inappropriate strategies (in addition to commonly seen eating disorders, as a reaction to changes in bodily proportions) which are used to cope with the mental burden caused by problems in accepting developmental changes. Psychodynamic models point to the parallels between menarche and bleeding when cutting oneself. In this context, menarche represents sexual maturity that is not accepted and is often even rejected or unwanted. However, an adolescent woman has no control over it[58], she can only gain symbolic control by cutting

---

[58] A certain way of controlling and rejecting the new role is intentional weight loss, which has two "desirable" (from the perspective of an adolescent rejecting the developmental milestones) effects: the loss of menarche and typical female body shape. By doing so, she triggers an artificial regression – her figure returns back to an "asexual" shape, and in the sense of sexual development, she re-enters the previous period, characterised by sexual immaturity (the inability to reproduce). The consequence of this behaviour is just as undesirable as self-harm – besides the obvious health consequences, these adolescents often also suffer from mental anorexia.

herself – when she is able to decide the timing of the bleeding and its extent and duration for herself (as opposed to her menarche). In this regard, self-harm is a way to change the passive (menstrual bleeding) into the active (transfer it to a different place), where it can be seen and controlled (Rosenthal et al. 1972).

In a psychodynamic context, the skin is an important organ, as tactile stimulation or irritation can be a source of pleasure. Cutting and damaging the skin are thus a mixture of arousal and pleasure, and at the same time, a punishment for the act, which evokes satisfaction (Daldin 1988). While previous concepts only considered self-harm amongst girls (young women) and reflected a period when self-harm was strongly oriented towards being a problem of the female gender (Milard 2013), drawing attention to the skin enables the interpretative framework to be extended to both sexes. However, unlike previous concepts, these do not find a great deal of support in the empirical data. Although some authors see an increased incidence of self-harm during the period of sexual maturation, when adolescents explore their sexuality, inter alia, through the discovery of erogenous zones on the surface of their bodies, as indirect evidence, these interpretations are not sufficiently convincing. Psychodynamic approaches also see the skin as an object that forms the boundary between the outer and the inner, between the body and the mind, and between the individual and others. By cutting it, the barrier is breached and the inner contents of the psyche, feelings, the individual themselves... have the opportunity to break free; the wound opens a symbolic path for communication with the outside world (Yakeley & Burbridge-James 2018). The motif of the skin as a place where the outer meets the inner, the organ that forms the boundary between the individual and the environment, is also elaborated in interpersonal models of self-harm[59].

The Concept of Auto-Aggression

Another explanatory framework is the concept of auto-aggression. In classical psychoanalysis (see e.g., Freud 1917), which

---

[59] See the following section 2.2.

focuses on childhood experiences, self-harm is the solution to the inner conflict caused by anger or hatred towards a loved one (or important person). Such negative emotions can occur in a child after they have experienced abandonment, betrayal, harm or illtreatment by a loved one, and are inherently natural. However, the dependence on these people and the fact that they were/are a source of love and the satisfaction of needs (ergo of pleasure) evokes ambivalent feelings – the child feels anger, disappointment and, at the same time, guilt for being angry at a loved one/significant person. The predominantly unconscious mechanisms of the psyche will resolve this confusion by internalising the negative feelings as a part of our "evil self", allowing the child to maintain an image of the loved one/significant person as a good person (Yakeley & Burnbridge-James 2018). The subsequent self-harm then becomes self-punishment for the negative feelings and thoughts (for the "evil self") towards the loved one. These interpretations have long been supported by research highlighting the high incidence of self-harm among abused children (van der Kolk et al. 1991, Romans et al. 1995); at present, however, self-harm as a symptom of the reaction to sexual abuse has been re-evaluated and is no longer considered to be important (Klonsky & Moyer 2008). The motive of self-punishment, however, has not disappeared from the issue of self-harm – it is one of the reasons frequently reported by adolescents[60]. Currently, however, it is predominantly associated with low self-worth, self-esteem and a negative relationship with themselves, which are characteristic of self-harming adolescents.

2.2 Interpersonal Concepts

Although self-harm may appear to be a behaviour that solely pertains to a specific individual (the self-harming individual is both the aggressor and the victim at the same time), in its causes

---

[60] Research focused on the motives for self-harm among adults shows that self-punishment is almost non-existent in this population (Briere & Gill 1998; Osuch et al. 1999).

and effects, it is also linked to a wide range of interpersonal relationships. Interpersonal models analyse the social interactions which are behind the emergence, occurrence and persistence of this high-risk behaviour in the repertoire of an adolescent, as well as the consequences of the self-harming behaviour of an individual on their relationships with others. Therefore, they deal with a wide variety of phenomena in interpersonal interactions.

The Model of Boundaries

Following on from psychodynamic models and utilising their interpretative framework, another concept that is quite frequently used to explain self-harm is the so-called model of boundaries (the boundaries model[61]). In this case, self-harm is understood as a violation of the body's boundaries, either by cutting the skin, which forms a barrier between the outer and the inner worlds, or by ingesting medication (indigestible objects, harmful substances...) through the mouth, which is a "gateway" that connects the outside environment to the inside of an organism. Disruption of the physical barrier is an objectification of problems which self-harming individuals experience in relation to their surroundings (inside vs. outside world). Self-harm is then a symbolic expression of a wide range of difficulties which stem from the relationship between the individual (his/her "self") and others. From the point of view of depth psychology, these boundaries represent a place of transition – whether at a real or symbolic level. A breach of the skin with penetration results in bleeding, which is some form of cleansing, a way to eliminate the unwanted and bad from the body (Yakeley & Burbridge-James 2018). Self-harming individuals often report that they release their internal tension and get rid of unbearable feelings by cutting (Laye-Gindhu & Schonert-Reichl 2005). At a symbolic level, these boundaries represent all kinds of transi-

---

61 The name "boundaries model" has no connection to borderline personality disorder, which includes self-harm in its symptomatology (APA 2015). It refers to the boundaries between the individual and the environment, and the resulting characteristics of the relationships which self-harming individuals form with other people.

tions – the transition between periods of development, life roles and events, which – if they have been burdened by trauma or were not properly processed – can be objectified through self-harm. However, most frequently, the boundary is perceived, in an interpersonal context, as something which excludes the individual from the outside world. Interactions with this boundary, in the form of self-harm, are thus, from the point of view of the interpersonal approach, an attempt to define oneself in relation to the surrounding environment, by emphasising the boundary between "self" and the environment. The need to exclude oneself in such a way stems from the fact that self-harming individuals suffer from difficulties with self-perception – they often underestimate themselves, they do not have a positive relationship with themselves and have difficulty perceiving themselves as unique beings (Suyemoto 1998). For them, self-harm represents a way to clearly exclude themselves, to make their boundaries real or to feel their existence through pain.

The Search for Identity

When self-harming adolescents verbalise their motivation, they often talk about feeling pain and that through it they feel they are real. Self-harm can pull them out of their feelings of emptiness and numbness, and at the same time, through pain, remind them that they exist and makes them feel "real" (Peterson et al. 2008); they establish contact with themselves, and at the same time, as unique people, they exclude themselves from the outside world. It can be said that in times of uncertainty, exploration and self-discovery[62], self-harm can be a very effective (albeit undesirable and high-risk) way to find our identity – to integrate our problematic experiences, through this behaviour, into a comprehensive and (for the individual) meaningful whole. The problem of seeking and finding ourselves, our identity and uniqueness through self-harm is not only that the behaviour is harmful and high risk but also that an individual finds their identity through events of self-harm, and primarily through such behaviour – thus they become a self-harming individual and they identify as such (Jacobson & Batejan

---

[62] Which has a key role in the development of adolescence.

2014). Abandoning this type of harmful behaviour could mean they abandon their identity and lose themselves again.

A Means of Communication

Within interpersonal interactions, self-harm can also have a communicative function. Especially in the past, this behaviour was perceived as an attempt by an adolescent to seek attention, by making their mental pain visible, especially through bodily injury[63]. Such tendencies fall under the, so-called, Social-Positive Reinforcement (SPR) theory (Jacobson & Batejan 2014), which assumes that self-harm is an attempt to seek attention from those around them or is an effort to gain access to other resources (not only attention but also compassion, interest or any[64] other reaction) (Nock & Prinstein 2005). By gaining a reward (in the form of a reaction, attention), such behaviour is positively reinforced, which leads to repetition and then fixation as a form of maladaptive response to critical situations. Some studies (see e.g., Nixon et al. 2002) highlight an increase in the incidence of SPR in self-harm among girls. The difference is understandable, considering that the female sex has a higher tendency to seek some form of social support in the solution of problems than men (Melendez

---

63 It is true that sometimes self-harm performs this function; however, most research studies, by various researchers who employed different methods in diverse populations, have shown that self-harm is rarely about seeking attention (Klonsky et al. 2014). The results show that self-harm is most frequently done in private, as a way of quickly reducing negative emotions (Nock & Prinstein 2004; Chapman et al. 2006). Nevertheless, the effects of the view of self-harm as attention-seeking behaviour can still be seen, for example, in the form of a tendency, that is still strong, to perceive self-harm as a behaviour and action which results in "damage to the surface of his or her body of a sort likely to induce bleeding, bruising, or pain (e.g., cutting, burning, stabbing, hitting, excessive rubbing), with the expectation that the injury will lead to only minor or moderate physical harm" (DSM-5 2015, 845), thus behaviour that almost exclusively leads to external, visible injuries. Hidden forms of self-harm (the consumption of indigestible objects, not allowing oneself to sleep, not taking medications...) and potential psychological forms (tormenting oneself with self-destructive thoughts, intentional entering into relationships in which an individual expects to be victim of violence...) are either missing in the definitions of this behaviour or are considered as "associated" forms.
64 Even negative ones (Llyod-Richardson et al. 2007).

et al. 2012). SPR is also frequently found in those with borderline personality disorder, where Brown et al. (2002) report that the motivation to self-harm to acquire an interpersonal influence, for example, to begin to communicate with others or to get help from others, had a prevalence of up to 61%. In addition to SPR, experts have also identified a second variant where self-harm is used as a tool to solve the needs that arise from interpersonal interactions – Social-Negative Reinforcement (SNR). In particular, this is found when the self-harm is a reaction to unmanageable interpersonal demands or as an escape from interpersonal interactions. For example, a characteristic emotion might be anger – Briere and Gil (1998) state that up to 56% of individuals felt anger towards others before the act of self-harm, while only 2% of respondents felt this way after an act of self-harm.

The communicative function of self-harm is not only manifested towards potential providers of help, attention, interest…, thus towards adults, but it is also important in peer relationships. Through self-harm (which is less hidden in the community of peers than, e.g., in contact with adults), adolescents show their peers that they are suffering and signal their alignment with other self-harmers. However, the purpose of such signals is not only an external expression of their problems but to also try to find contacts with those around them, to find "congenial" peers. Subsequently, they can share their problems and talk about them with someone who understands, who is in the same situation. The establishment of contact between self-harming individuals has, however, its risks – they can become competitive and compare the number and severity of injuries (Simpson 1980). Therefore, the initial search for understanding can turn into a high-risk contact, which leads to the reinforcement of self-harming behaviour[65].

---

65 Self-harm support groups who are mainly created with the intention to provide help to self-harming individuals do not always achieve such a result – and unfortunately – also bear such risks. A problem particularly occurs when the group lacks an expert, who would steer the discussions and guide the group dynamic (self-help groups). ("I looked for help in the voluntary sector and attended a support group for women who self-harmed. Here I began to solely focus upon myself as a self-harmer. I was exposed to the harming of others, and this made my harming much worse during this time. In my experience, support groups are unhelpful unless they are well moderated; for me it was an arena in which competitive urges towards self-destruction could arise. Due to this I ended up in A&E

Social Learning and Contagion

Another explanatory framework is the theory of social learning and contagion. The theory of social learning highlights the possibility that self-harm will be shaped through the reinforcement of specific modes of behaviour from an early age. An injury or pain suffered by children traditionally produces a wide range of responses from those around them, including a greater level of attention, care, soothing of pain, distracting the child from the pain of the injury by providing entertainment, etc., all the way up to the gifting of benefits – for example, getting presents, to be relieved of their responsibilities, a greater degree of tolerance of undesirable behaviours (irritability, anger, moodiness...). However, the most common response will draw attention, care and a display of affection to the child, which provides important information to the child about how those around them respond to injuries. During a problematic period within adolescence, when they are already ashamed to directly ask for displays of affection or care, or during a crisis situation, when the adolescent does not know how to ask, or cannot ask for help, they can (often unknowingly) start to behave in a particular way that is a consequence of social strengthening and learning mechanisms that are associated, in their personal history, with the desired responses from those around them. According to this concept, the individual, through self-harm, seeks (mostly unknowingly) to generate care or interest from those around them.

Social learning is not only effective in early childhood, but its mechanisms are also present throughout the whole of our lives – for example, during adolescence, when, to them, the most important people are their peers, self-harm can be the result of observations of friends or classmates, who provide a "guide to the solution" of problems in this way. There is a lot of discussion regarding the so-called effect of contagion[66], which, via peer contact, explains

---

countless times for treatment for the cuts and for overdosing" National Collaborating Centre for Mental Health 2012.)
66 Contagion effect is based on the assumption that every exposure of a healthy (in our case non-self-harming) individual to an infected (exhibiting self-harming behaviour) friend leads to the chance that this behaviour will transfer to the initially healthy individual. The probability of a healthy individual getting "infected"

another possible mechanism of interpersonal interactions that leads to an increased incidence of self-harm among adolescents. The contagion effect presupposes that, due to the importance of peer relationships and contacts in adolescence, it is possible that self-harm is "contagious" in this community, meaning that the patterns the adolescent sees in their environment are strong enough to lead them to imitation, even in such areas as the solution of problems and strategies to manage difficult situations. Several scientific studies, in connection with self-harm, have highlighted the very strong influence of peer groups[67] (Nixon et al. 2002, Prinstein et al. 2009) – either through direct (personal) contact or through the media (especially social networks[68]).

2.3 Biological Concepts

Biological contexts for the interpretation of the occurrence of self-harming behaviour essentially attempt to identify the mechanisms of the biological principles of the function of the psyche that may contribute to the formation, retention and escalation of this type of high-risk behaviour. Several scientific studies that have highlighted a biological basis of self-harm have often been conducted on patients at a psychiatric clinic or at the outpatient clinics of clinical psychologists or psychiatrists (Jacobson & Batejan, 2014). The reason for this is first the need for medical intervention

---

increases with the number of times they are exposed to the undesirable phenomenon, which may ultimately cause a massive spread of the particular behaviour to a substantial proportion of the population (Hodas & Lerman 2014).

67 Not only at the level of "contagion" – the power of the peer group may be so intense that in the effort to join this group, the individual will also start to self-harm even if they had no such tendencies prior to joining the group. This submission to group pressure is more typical of boys than girls (Nixon et al. 2002).

68 In the context of self-harm, on-line spaces pose several risks (see e.g., Lewis et al. 2012, Marchant et al. 2021). Although it may convey information that leads to finding help, many websites support this behaviour and create communities that focus on advice and ways of performing or concealing self-harm, etc. Moreover, even the contact of a self-harmer with the topic of self-harm may trigger this high-risk behaviour.

in this type of high-risk behaviour, and second that it is frequently associated with other conditions – such as dissociative identity disorder (Webermann et al. 2016), borderline personality disorder (Jacobson & Batejan 2014), post-traumatic stress disorder (Alharbi, et al. 2020), eating disorders (Islam et al. 2015), depression (Nitkowski & Petermann 2011), obsessive-compulsive disorder (Bolognini et al. 2003), autism (Maddox 2017) and mental retardation (van den Bogaard et al. 2018), with a history of sexual abuse (Klonsky et al. 2014) or anxiety disorders (Kiekens et al. 2018), which tend to have a strong biological basis. The potential for biological circumstances that contribute to self-harm is supported by the fact that it often occurs in individuals with accentuated degrees of impulsiveness, which is also significantly biologically saturated (Mitchell & Potenza 2014). In addition to a large number of studies on a clinical population, there are also enough studies that demonstrated the validity of certain biological concepts on a non-clinical population. When generalising these findings, it is important to bear in mind that many studies may have been affected, to a certain extent, by intervening factors that stem from mental health disorders (Jacobson & Batejan 2014).

Genetic Influences

Studies conducted until now suggest that from the wide range of possible biological factors, those with the most important role have genetic influences (e.g., T-allele of GN3 gene) or are changes in levels of important chemical substances as a result of negative experiences (e.g., chronic stress, abuse), which trigger an increased degree of vulnerability to maladaptive reactions to stress (e.g., in the form of self-harm). The integrated model of self-harming behaviour (Figure 1) includes several biological concepts (Sher & Stanley 2009).

The first significant factor in this model is genetic predispositions. These are supported by a small number of studies that suggest, for example, the potential impact of the T-allele of G-protein β3 (GN β3) on the occurrence of self-harm (Joyce et al. 2006), or on the presence of self-harming behaviour as a characteristic of genetically dependent Lesch-Nyhan syndrome (Stanley et al. 2010).

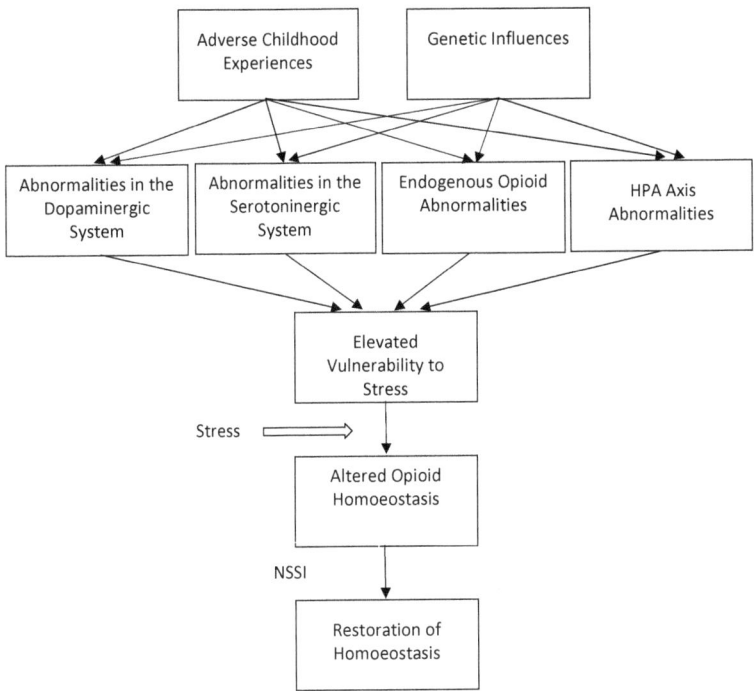

Figure 1. A biological model of self-harm
Source: Sher & Stanley (2009, 107)

The Dopaminergic System

Another factor often discussed in the context of the presence of self-harm, but still not sufficiently supported, is the impact of abnormalities in the dopaminergic system. Multiple studies suggest a plausible impact of the monoamine oxidase A gene (MAOA) situated on chromosome X (Xp11.23–11.4), which is one of the dopaminergic genes. It encodes the enzyme responsible for the activity of neurotransmitters in the brain, including noradrenaline, dopamine (DA) and serotonin (5-HT) (Gao et al. 2021). In the case of self-harm, it is believed that dysregulation of monoamine neurotransmissions plays a key role; this affects both emotional regulation and reactions to mental stress (Sher & Stanley 2009), which is something that is often problematic for self-harming individuals. It appears that the combination of stress, adverse family history and specific dysregulation of the dopaminergic system significantly contribute to the occurrence of self-harm. This assumption is confirmed by a study by Y. Gao et al. (2021), which concludes that the MAOA gene plays the role of a moderating factor between bad treatment in childhood and the consequent occurrence of self-harming behaviour in adolescence[69]. A similar effect has also been shown for another gene – COMT (catechol-o-methyltransferase), which is also a key gene within the dopaminergic system of the brain (Gao et al. 2021). We may, therefore, assume that adolescents exhibit varying degrees of sensitivity to adverse experiences due to the variability in the MAOA (Caspi et al. 2002) and the COMT gene pool, which may consequently (especially in stressful situations) lead to self-harm.

The Serotoninergic System

Besides the dopaminergic system, self-harm may also be based on abnormalities of the serotoninergic system. Research in this field most commonly builds on the assumption that 5-HTTLPR (serotonin-transporter-linked promoter region) – the gene that encodes the serotonin transporter – interacts with chronic stress (especially in the interpersonal domain) and significantly raises the probability of the occurrence of self-harming behaviour (Hankin et al. 2015). In this regard, T. I. Fikke et al. (2013) discovered that a reduction in the function of serotonin may lead to self-harm in emotionally stressful situations[70]. As with the effects of abnormalities in the dopaminergic system, it appears that even in the case of serotonin the biologically determined nature of self-harm does not lie in the presence of a special "self-harm gene" but that various deviations in brain activity lead to predispositions for maladaptive responses to mental burdens. Deviations in the activity of various brain systems may be caused by a specific development of CNS during intrauterine development or (which is typically the case in individuals who do not suffer from a mental disorder) from increased exposure to maladaptive, traumatic or burdensome situations in childhood.

---

[69] The authors particularly observed this link in male participants.
[70] In this case, the link was manifested in female participants.

Endogenous Opioids

The next biologically determined concept for the occurrence of self-harm – the opioid model – can be perceived in a similar way. The assumption is that people who self-harm through this mechanism have atypical levels of opioids in their CNS. The model is based on two fundamental and correlating assumptions – the first being that individuals who exhibit self-harming behaviour have low opioid levels, and the second that by self-harming the levels of opioids increase, which restores the correct balance (Heilbron et al. 2014). Stanley et al. (2010) discovered that patients with a history of self-harm exhibited lower levels of beta-endorphin and met-enkephalin in comparison to those who did not. Low opioid levels (especially beta-endorphin and metenkephalin) may be caused by chronic stress in childhood and adolescence, by traumatic experiences, abuse or neglect (Sher & Stanley 2009). This corresponds with the frequency that these events are found within the family history of self-harming individuals. Exposing oneself to pain through self-harm leads the organism to react and increase the production of endogenous opioids. This model has still not been sufficiently verified – there are several theories that question its consistency[71].

The Hypothalamic-Pituitary-Adrenal Axis

HPA (hypothalamic-pituitary-adrenal) axis abnormalities may result from stressful reactions to adverse or traumatising experiences in early childhood. These abnormalities may increase the probability of self-harm in stressful situations. Research shows that the cortisol levels in self-harming individuals have specific

---

71 For example, if a low level of opioids is a reaction to frequent pain and chronic stress... and therefore, a kind of adaptation of the organism to adverse conditions, why would the organism increase opioid levels back into "balance" and counteract the adaptation mechanisms already used? How is the organism capable of detecting lower opioid levels as opposed to "optimal" levels? Why does it activate behaviour which may increase these levels, but with far more destructive consequences than the low values present in the first place? (For more arguments, see Heilbron et al. 2014).

deviations in comparison with control samples from healthy (non-self-harming) individuals. For instance, C. Reichl et al. (2016) reported a greater response to waking, which took the form of higher cortisol levels, in self-harming individuals in comparison to the control group. They suggest that these elevated levels occur as self-harming individuals have higher expectations of mental stress when they wake up in the morning, which suggests a possible link with adverse life experiences. A more straightforward correlation between elevated cortisol levels and self-harming behaviour is documented by an older case study by Sachsse et al. (2002), in which female patient suffering from borderline personality disorder experienced episodes of self-harm after increases in her cortisol level. After her episode of self-harm passed, her cortisol level decreased to a below-average level for a long period of time. These fluctuations[72] are explained in the findings of studies which, on the contrary, recorded lower cortisol levels in self-harming individuals compared to the control group (see e.g., Klimes-Dougan et al. 2019). In self-harming individuals, the level of cortisol and its excretion during a stressful situation may be affected by environmental influences – for instance, it appears that adverse life circumstances and childhood experiences not only trigger the dysregulation of the HPA axis but also the dysregulation of cortisol production (Gartland et al. 2022). Disparities in cortisol levels measured in self-harming individuals from various studies could be explained by more recent studies, which have highlighted the possible concurrent effect of depressive states which often have co-morbidity with self-harm. In this context, B. Peng et al. suggest that self-harming adolescents, who are diagnosed with depression, have more adverse childhood experiences in their history and lower levels of cortisol. More detailed analyses revealed that there was a significant link between lower levels of cortisol and adverse childhood experiences, but not with depressive symptoms. Furthermore, lower cortisol levels, depressive symptoms and emotional neglect were all risk factors for NSSI in adolescents suffering from depression (Peng et al. 2022).

---

[72] The observed patient experienced a range of 2 to 30 μg, with a level of 20 μg triggering self-harm (Sachsse_2002).

Positive Valence Systems

In addition to systems that are dependent on specific chemicals, it is also necessary to mention brain mechanisms that are responsible for rewarding and forming habits. Clinical psychologists often point out that self-harm is a maladaptive strategy of coping with mental stress (Andover 2012), with one of the most commonly identified motives being a reduction of negative emotions and intolerable stress (In-Albon et al. 2013). Although self-harm causes harm to the organism, self-harmers explain that the physical pain is more bearable and effectively reduces, relieves or replaces the emotional or mental pain (Molaie et al. 2019). Hence, self-harm is a relief mechanism (associated with negative reinforcement), and as such, it has two significant consequences. First, behaviours that lead to relief activate the reward systems of the brain[73], which reinforces their impact. The second consequence is based on the mechanism of negative reinforcement, meaning that behaviours that lead to the activation of the reward systems of the brain are very quickly and intensely fixed, leading to addiction. The formation, retention and reinforcement of self-harm are thus, to a significant extent, supported by positive valence systems, and these generally include phases of seeking, achieving, fulfilling and retaining rewards (Westlund Schreiner et al. 2015).

In the light of the above, many experts consider self-harm to be an addictive behaviour (Victor et al. 2012; Blasco-Fontecilla et al. 2016; Guérin-Marion et al. 2018). In studies of the course of self-harm, experts have identified many symptoms that are typical of addiction in the experience and behaviour of self-harmers (Nixon et al. 2002) – for example: states that precede "attacks" of self-harm resemble withdrawal symptoms in drug addicts (Faye 1995); and the desire to cause harm is the equivalent of cravings (Washburn et al. 2010). It must be noted that as a result of specific cognitive biases, self-harming individuals have a limited repertoire of solutions for problems[74]; thus, they repeat their existing schemes

---

73 The reward systems of the brain include areas, such as the ventral tegmental area, nucleus accumbens, dorsal striatum and their associated connections to the ventral prefrontal cortex (Kalivas & Nakamura 1999).
74 See the following section "2.4 Cognitivist Concepts".

and fixed behaviours. Repeating the same behaviour then leads to self-harm, even in situations where other coping strategies would be far more effective and even when self-harm is completely maladaptive. This behaviour is then further reinforced even in those situations where it is not "appropriate"[75].

2.4 Cognitivist Concepts

Cognitivist concepts highlight those characteristics in the aetiology of self-harming behaviour, which are linked to either the mechanisms of the specific way that an individual processes information, or to the personality traits of the individual, which modify the way they process and interpret information. These tend to include the personality traits of the individual (e.g. perfectionism); specific cognitive mechanisms (e.g. deficits in problem-solving); incorrect processing of information (e.g. dichotomous thinking); cognitive biases (e.g. implicit associations), or other factors that may seemingly stem from the characteristics of the surrounding environment (loneliness, unbearable problems), but their problematic nature lies more in their subjectively perceived burden than in objective complications. The cognitive burden is mainly reported in severe cases of self-harm – it is more common in individuals who suffer with suicidal thoughts or with past attempts at suicide in their history of self-harm (Brausch & Gutierrez 2010; Wolff et al. 2013).

Perfectionism

Perfectionism as a personality trait means the constant tendency of an individual to attempt to achieve the best possible results, even in situations that do not require it. These characteristics are not inherently considered risky by society, quite the opposite –

---

[75] Appropriate in the sense of its ability to relieve mental pain. Despite the positive impact of self-harm on reducing mental pain, this form is still considered maladaptive and, therefore, inappropriate.

they may be highly praised, which increases the probability of fixation in a personality (especially in adolescents who are still evolving). Even scientific literature (see e.g., Bieling et al. 2004) speaks of both negative and positive perfectionism, although several studies warn that positive and negative perfectionism do not exist separately, but they co-occur and are mutually dependent (Gaudreau & Thompson 2010; Afshar et al. 2011; Limburg et al. 2017). The effort to excel in all areas is problematic, as it is associated with unrealistic goals, which leads to chronic stress in perfectionists (Xie et al. 2019). What is more, perfectionists usually derive their value from their productivity and the quality of their performance; they are extremely self-critical, with standards that are high and even unattainable, which consequently leads to a fear of making mistakes, self-doubt, feelings of failure, inadequacy or shame. A result of this set of cognitive automatisms is a vicious circle of dissatisfaction with themselves and their performance, which leads to a further increase in unrealistic expectations, which inherently lead to failure or further discontent. One possible maladaptive reaction[76] is self-harm which, in addition to the aspect of self-punishment, objectifies negative attitudes and emotions. The link between perfectionism and self-harm has been proven by several studies (for an overview, see Gyori & Balazs 2021). The situation is even more complicated, as perfectionists also need to reflect the achievement of excellence in their self-image; thus, they conceal their emotions, vulnerability, worries and pain, and they only seek a minimal amount of help. This mindset significantly complicates any possible intervention in the case of self-harm.

Hopelessness

In psychology, the concept of hopelessness was explored in detail by Aaron T. Beck[77], especially in the context of depression

---

[76] In addition to self-harm, there is a wide range of other mental problems associated with perfectionism – depression and anxiety disorder (Afshar et al. 2011), eating disorders (Peterson et al. 2018) or obsessive-compulsive disorders (Limburg et al. 2017).
[77] Beck's self-rating depression inventory is well known (Gottfried 2019), and it is based on the original Beck Hopelessness Scale (Beck 1988).

(Beck 1988; Beck et al. 1989, 1990). Hopelessness is the cognitive mindset of an individual who stereotypically sees their future in a negative light, which leads to a major loss of motivation and the absence of positive expectations for the future (Beck 1988). According to A. T. Beck, this mindset can be the result of burdensome situations in childhood combined with long-lasting stressors, which due to the specificities of the function of the brain[78] lead to a negative cognitive mindset. The individual then perceives both neutral and positive stimuli in a negative light and has mostly negative expectations of the future[79]. It is a highly robust factor (when it comes to its impact on the experiences, behaviour and emotional life of an individual) introducing not only self-harming behaviour but also depression as well as suicidal behaviour[80]. A negative perception of the future does not only influence the aspirations of an individual – it is also a significant stress factor when it comes to dealing with present hardships. If the individual sees their future negatively, they assume that the results of the solution of any problem will not be favourable. It is therefore a personal mindset of an

---

[78] A. T. Beck assumes that an increased prevalence of cognitive biases and dysfunctional convictions results from a hypersensitive amygdala, which if combined with hypoactive prefrontal areas that reduce the ability for adequate assessment creates conditions for the negative (depressive) mindset of an individual. Furthermore, the situation can become more complicated due to genetic anomalies contributing to an excessive reaction to stress (Beck 2008).

[79] In the observations and research into the concept of hopelessness, scientists primarily looked at the perception of the future among self-harming individuals. It was assumed that a negativist cognitive mindset would lead to a higher tendency to perceive one's future pessimistically and a higher degree of anticipation of problems. This assumption was confirmed in terms of the concept of hopelessness, but research revealed other interesting circumstances. It was also discovered that individuals with self-destructive tendencies differ from the unaffected population to an even greater extent in their ability to anticipate positive (as opposed to negative) events (Wenzel & Spokas 2014). This means that compared to non-self-harming individuals, they are incapable of identifying and anticipating positive expectations of the future.

[80] Many studies (see e.g., Klonsky et al. 2012; Wolfe et al. 2019; Berardelli et al. 2019) suggest the impact of hopelessness on suicidal behaviour in the long term – they describe hopelessness as a cognitive mindset that modulates the perception and interpretation of cognitive stimuli towards chronically negativistic attitudes. However, some studies warn that in addition to the long-term negativistic view of the future (which contributes to the overall depressive mindset of the individual), an acute state of hopelessness may directly trigger an acute suicidal crisis (see e.g., Young et al. 1996; Wenzel et al. 2009).

individual, which, on one hand, demotivates them to a great extent (they do not see any point in solving problems, to spend their time and energy as they are convinced the situation will only end badly), but it also substantially influences the way in which situations are resolved – the individual is exposed to negative emotions; as a result of a low level of motivation, they have to invest far more energy in the solution; the anticipation of negative results then increases anxiety, etc. Thus, there is a whole range of consequences due to which a hopeless individual may find that difficult situations are just too complicated to cope with, moreover, they are permanently frustrated by their conviction that things will never get any better. This mental pressure has a significant contribution to the maladaptive solution of problems. Hopelessness is considered a major factor within the formation, retention and escalation of high-risk behaviour (Fox et al. 2015; Pérez Rodríguez et a. 2017; Brausch et al. 2020).

Unbearability

The concept of unbearability is closely linked to hopelessness and future hopes. In cognitive psychology, it is classified as a type of cognitive distortions, which are called catastrophic scenarios because they are the situations that the individual evaluates as unbearable, overwhelming or unmanageable, or that exceed their capabilities... Even though, in reality, they are merely unpleasant (Chand et al. 2021). As a result of this cognitive mindset, self-harming individuals tend to be in situations where they are convinced that they cannot and are not able to cope with problematic situations. In addition to a low degree of motivation to resolve the situation[81], a feeling of unbearability paralyses the potential methods to cope with the situation; it triggers anxiety and shifts attention towards the worst possible scenarios, which, subsequently, reduces any real capacity the individual might have to cope with the burden. Unbearability and unmanageability do not only refer to problematic situations in life, but these words are also used by

---

[81] as a result of the conviction that it is unbearable and exceeds the possibilities of the individual.

self-harmers to describe their emotional experiences and mental pain. In this case, self-harm is an act that allows them to escape the stressful and unbearable situation (Dennis et al. 2007), especially through the transformation of mental pain into physical pain (Matera et al. 2021). Through this transformation, self-harming individuals get their pain (in its physical form) "under control" – they can determine its extent and duration, and they can decide to end it, something that is certainly not true for mental and emotional pain. The function of these mechanisms has been confirmed by several studies[82], for instance, I. Beatens et al. (2013) discovered that almost half of self-harming adolescents use self-harm as a way of gaining control over their emotions and transforming their emotional pain into physical pain.

Self-harm accompanied by suicidal thoughts and attempts is associated with a cluster of characteristics that describe the specific cognitive mindset of self-harming individuals – these include feelings of hopelessness, unbearability, entrapment[83], the feeling of burdensomeness, being unloved and not belonging (Siddaway et al. 2019). Unbearability and a feeling of not belonging are the strongest predictors of suicidal behaviour (Hallensleben et al. 2016).

A Lack of Belongingness

A lack (or a thwarted feeling) of belongingness is a concept similar to loneliness. While most lonely people do not have a sufficient number or quality of social contacts, in the case of a lack of belongingness, individuals may have many interpersonal interactions, but they do not feel that they are a sufficiently valid or important member of the social groups (e.g., among friends or in the family) to which they belong. While loneliness is relatively objective (it can be quantified in terms of the number of social interactions), the experience of a lack of belongingness is subjective, and the person feels estranged from others that they are not integrated

---

[82] Adolescents in our study which focused on the motivations that lead to self-harm also stated that their most frequent motivation is to regulate their emotions (Démuthová & Démuth 2019c).

[83] The feeling that a person is "caught in a trap" from which there is no escape.

2 Theoretical Bases

into the circle of family, friends or other social groups important to them (Joiner et al. 2009), even if these group members provide sufficient levels of contact. B. L. Assavedo and M. D. Anestis (2015) studied the correlation between the frequency of NSSI and a lack of belongingness and found statistically significant positive correlations. Since self-harming individuals, apart from a high presence of thwarted belongingness, are often clinically diagnosed with other mental problems[84], the next steps of their analyses examined the symptoms of depression and borderline personality disorder. A further significant correlation was found between the frequency of self-harming behaviour and lack of belongingness (Assavedo & Anestis, 2015). More specific findings were discovered by C. Chu et al. (2016), who identified a lack of belongingness[85] as a mediator between self-harming behaviour and the occurrence of suicidal thoughts (see Figure 2).

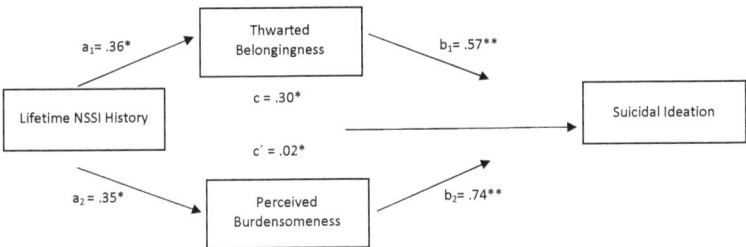

Figure 2. Standardised regression coefficients for the relationship between a history of self-harm and suicidal thoughts mediated by non-belongingness and the perceived burden[86]
Note: * $p \leq 0.05$, ** $p \leq 0.001$
Source: Chu et al. (2016, 576)

Self-Image

Many cognitive distortions in self-harming individuals concern their self-perception. Convictions bound to the self-image of an individual often belong to the "core convictions", the key worldviews,

---

84 Such as depression or borderline personality disorder.
85 As well as the perceived burden, see the following paragraph.
86 The concept of perceived burden refers to the conviction of an individual that they are a burden on others.

which consequently have an impact on their beliefs in other areas. These problematic beliefs, in self-harming individuals, include the ideas that the individual is unloved or unlovable, unworthy of affection, incapable and a burden to others. These core convictions consequently affect their view of their own value, their importance to others and their own abilities and skills.

For a young person to perceive themselves as a burden can have especially severe consequences because the social support and feelings of connection, during this period of life, still stem from the family unit[87] and peer groups (Muehlenkamp et al. 2015). If the adolescent is convinced that they are a burden to these key people, the likelihood of a feeling of not belonging or being unloved increases and the likelihood of using social support in stressful situations or when searching for help with self-harm decreases.

The feeling that an adolescent is unloved[88] is found in case studies of self-harming individuals (see e.g., Gulbas et al. 2015), as well as in quantitative studies (Sedgwick et al. 2019; Harman et al. 2021). This conviction is part of the cognitive biases that negatively influence the self-image of an individual and provide support to each other, reinforcing erroneous self-judgements.

Another typical characteristic found in the self-perception of self-harming adolescents is self-efficacy. The concept of self-efficacy was introduced into psychology by A. Bandura (1977, 1986 and 1997), and it represents an individual's image of their own ability to achieve goals or desirable behaviours. This concept allows us to understand why certain individuals[89] do not even attempt to reach their goals and give up without even trying. They are slowed down by the conviction that reaching the goal is beyond their abilities and that they will not be able to handle the required activity. This situation often involves another cognitive bias – entrapment, where the self-harming individual has the feeling that they are trapped in a situation without any possibility of escape or to free themselves. Since they see no possible escape, they are paralysed

---

87 J. C. Wolff et al. (2014) even discovered that in adolescence, social support from the family with regard to the occurrence of self-harming behaviour is perceived as more important than support from peers.
88 "It's like I don't fit in. I think [my mom] doesn't really love me" (Guilbas et al. 2015, 12).
89 In this case, these individuals will have low self-efficacy.

by hopelessness, and as a result of low self-efficacy, they do not even attempt to improve matters and stay trapped. These situations produce negative experiences accompanied by negative emotions, and as opposed to other individuals with good self-efficacy, self-harming individuals remain in these states considerably longer. As a result, the cognitive bias that the majority of situations in which the self-harmer finds themselves is extremely negative and unfavourable, without any possibility of escape, is further reinforced. The close link between self-harming behaviour and low self-efficacy has been demonstrated in several empirical studies (Hasking & Rose 2016; Dawkins et al. 2019).

Dichotomous Thinking

Dichotomous thinking is a specific way of processing and evaluating data, when an individual interprets the information as extremes – both in a positive and negative way. Facts, people, situations... are either good or bad, pleasant or unpleasant – the individual sees the world as "black-and-white" and ignores the whole scale of possibilities between these extremes. Another problem of self-harming individuals is that they pay different amounts of attention to negative and positive impulses and tend to ignore positive ones (Allen & Hooley, 2015). As a result, they especially notice negative stimuli, which not only leads to a negative emotional mindset (Hasking et al. 2017), but in combination with dichotomous thinking, it also changes the perception of reality in the self-harming individual towards extremely negative experiences. These then work as a validator of their negative convictions and close the vicious circle of biases. Dichotomous thinking is especially typical of individuals who have suicidal thoughts or have attempted suicide (Brausch & Gutierrez 2010; Wolff et al. 2013), and if self-harming individuals have actually experienced problems leading to attempted suicide, the higher the probability that their thinking will exhibit signs of dichotomy.

Problem-Solving

A result of many of the mindsets of self-harming individuals, that are outlined above, is that they find the solution of problems more complicated; these issues are also reinforced by, for example, a distorted self-image, low self-esteem, doubt in their abilities and qualities, hopelessness..., all of which create the image that the individual is incapable of solving problems, they do not have the necessary capacity to deal with them or the way they solve them is inappropriate. This initial mindset causes complications for the individual; it not only allows them to give up and abdicate from the solution of problems[90], but it also means they have to dedicate more energy to find the determination to resolve the issue and for the solution itself. Moreover, the solution of problems (if the self-harmer actually attempts to do it), for these individuals, is associated with higher levels of self-criticism, the methods used and the results are evaluated (due to the higher standards) more critically, which once again demotivates the individual and reinforces their conviction of their own deficits and weaknesses[91] in their ability to solve problems. Not only do difficulties in problem-solving stem from specific attitudes to oneself and one's own abilities, but they also influence these attitudes, which create a vicious circle of negative convictions and biases.

In addition to the above-mentioned difficulties, that are more caused by the attitude of the individual to solve problems rather than an inability to solve them, self-harming individuals also exhibit objective deficits and weaknesses in problem-solving (Pollock & Williams 2001; Townsend et al. 2001; Liu et al. 2016)[92]. These weak-

---

90 Individuals who perform severe self-harm often lack the ability to find any solution and may even become passive or avoid solving problems (Wenzel & Spokas 2014).

91 Which in fact do not have to be at a lower level than in non-self-harming individuals.

92 Deficits in the area of problem-solving are proven not only by studies but also by data from practical interventions provided to self-harming individuals by experts. An important component of psychological help is cognitive-behavioural therapy, which focuses on the elimination of obstacles and complications in thinking and improving the ability to solve problems. Manual-Assisted Cognitive-Behaviour Therapy (MACT) is a specific short-term psychotherapy specifically developed for self-harming individuals, and is used for both adults (Evans et al. 1999), as well as adolescents (Taylor et al. 2011).

nesses are demonstrated, for instance, when trying to find an efficient solution or reaching the desired outcome within the solution chosen for a particular problem (Wenzel & Spokas 2014) – in a lack of variation (versatility) in the solutions, in a higher tendency to avoid solutions, a higher prevalence of negative emotions and the choice of less relevant methods (Orbach et al. 1990). In the context of difficulties with problem-solving, it is also possible to apply the diathesis-stress model, which emphasises the vulnerability to the development of mental problems based on predispositions supported by environmental factors. In the case of problem-solving and self-harm, it is clear that deficits in problem-solving represent a risk factor that produces an elevated level of stress in difficult situations, as well as a higher risk of self-harm (Liu et al. 2016). The need to study the field of problem-solving has been documented by research that highlights the effectiveness of therapies that are focused on problem-solving – it was discovered that interventions focused on problem-solving led to a more significant improvement in mental problems (such as depressive symptoms, hopelessness) in self-harmers than other techniques (Townsend et al. 2001).

Deviations in the Memory Processes

Research into the difficulties that self-harming individuals have in problem-solving has also shown that some deficits that affect problem-solving may also be related to the specific way that information is stored. With regard to self-harming individuals, it was shown that their effective solution of problems was significantly limited by the function of their autobiographic memory (Pollock & Williams 2001). Several studies in this regard have pointed out the problem of an overgeneral memory[93]. Individuals that suffer from various mental problems[94] tend to rely on non-specific, overly general and neutral information when they recall

---

93 In foreign literature, it is referred to as overgeneral memory (OGM) in the sense of overgeneralisation, i.e., the low specificity of memory (see e.g., Jiang et al. 2020).

94 In addition to self-harm, this includes individuals with a history of attempted suicide, depressive individuals or individuals suffering from post-traumatic stress disorder (Barry et al. 2021).

memories, which is also typical for a number of other experiences. When they recall memories, these individuals appear to "stay on the surface" and do not go deeper into their memories, which at a deeper level show the specificities and how they differ from other memories. It is assumed that the origin of this process lies in the protective mechanisms of the psyche, which tries to suppress the recollection of negative and traumatic experiences or unpleasant memories (Wenzel & Spokas 2014). When recalling events, the individual stays in the safe space of the non-specific and general associations. By repeating this approach in their memories, the individual systematically avoids the involvement of areas which contain specific memories into the memory processes and limits them to a general level. This tendency then reinforces the memory traces and links between events, especially at this "generalised" level, and, on the contrary, specific memories are forgotten. What was originally a defence mechanism becomes a cognitive mindset, which not only influences the recollection of memories of events, places or people but also affects other processes that need to work with memories. Hence, even in those cases when an individual is dealing with a problem, they do not have access to the specific information from past experiences when they solved the same (or similar) specific problem; instead, they have access to generalised, non-specific solutions. Their overgeneral memory causes difficulties in the search for effective solutions, in reaching the desired outcome with the chosen solution (Wenzel & Spokas 2014) and is exhibited through a lack of diversity in the possible options or the choice of less relevant methods (Orbach et al. 1990).

Just as is the case of deficiencies in the solution of problems, it is also possible to perform effective interventions into cases of overgeneral memory, which, by using the mechanisms of cognitive-behavioural therapy, helps to rebuild inappropriate cognitive schemes and reduce their consequences in the process of processing key information. In this sense, MeST training (memory specificity training – Martens et al. 2019) has been shown to be effective and easily adapted, since through systematic training, it pushes the individual to focus on the specificities of their memories[95]

---

[95] Such as sensory-perceptual details (specific tastes, smells, sounds...) or contextual details (where, with whom, how...) (Barry et al. 2021).

(Barry et al. 2021) and to even activate those areas and contents of memory which were previously ignored.

Attention Focus

Within attention focus, the attention of the cognitive apparatus is drawn to a specific type of stimuli, while considerably less attention is paid to other stimuli. This is, in fact, a quite natural tendency often mentioned with regard to professional orientation[96], specific interests or the orientation[97] of the individual. But in more extreme cases, this may not only mean that the attention of the individual is attracted by a certain kind of stimuli but also that this process occurs to the detriment of other stimuli, which are ignored. In addition to natural situations, this cognitive bias is also described in several mental difficulties – for example, individuals who suffer from anxiety exhibit an attention bias towards threatening stimuli (Seymour 2016), while paying less attention to positive emotional stimuli (Jollant et al. 2011). A similar mindset has also been identified in individuals with self-harming and suicidal behaviour – they are overly sensitive in their reaction to impulses associated with their problems[98] (Wenzel & Spokas 2014).

---

[96] For example, a medical doctor automatically notices the symptoms of diseases, a fashion designer notices clothes, a car mechanic notices the sound of the engine, etc.
[97] For instance, parents who are expecting a child start to notice other pregnant women and have the impression that there are many more pregnant women around them than before.
[98] The experimental proof of this cognitive bias came from a variant of the Stroop test, in which conflicting information causes a perceptual load, which is only manageable by focusing attention. (In the Stroop test, the subject is instructed to notice the colour of the letters of a word, but the word describes a different colour than the one used to print it (e.g., the word "blue" is printed in red and the subject is expected to suppress the information contained in the meaning of the word ("blue") and instead to respond with the word "red").) In the variant that focuses on the observation of specific attention focus, the meaning of the test word was associated with the mental problems of the subject. In this case, their attention was significantly attracted by the meaning of the word (or its content, which was supposed to be suppressed) and the subject failed in terms of a longer reaction time and increased error rate. These expressions were absent in words that were neutral in meaning (MacLeod 2005).

An individual with a specific attention focus is mainly exposed to information associated with their mental problems, which further encourages other cognitive biases and convictions – and if they overly focus on their problems (due to a specific attention focus), they become even more convinced that the world is a complicated and hostile place full of hardship and problems. On the other hand, ignoring (neglecting) other signals through selective attention focus prevents the individual from having positive experiences, which could serve as a forming experience that would allow non-pathological ways to cope with problems. Furthermore, selective attention focus leads the individual to deal with their own problems more frequently; they are more often overwhelmed by them, which leads to a deterioration in their mental health. What is more, having to repeatedly cope with problems forces the individual to relive them, which may trigger self-harming behaviour.

Implicit Associations

A contribution to the formation and fixation of implicit associations comes from reliving problems and the consequent triggering of previous maladaptive patterns of behaviour. Implicit associations considerably contribute to the formation and retention of a negative self-image, which is associated with self-destruction and self-harm. Implicit associations are a set of various convictions, attitudes and opinions formed by an individual through their experiences, without the individual realising it (Sukhera et al. 2019). The study of implicit associations[99] may reveal the constructs that are linked to self-harm (its motives, consequences, triggers) and help us to understand the mutual links in the cognitive network of associations.

In the case of self-harming individuals, it was shown that test words, associated with self-harm, are closely tied to the experience of relief from emotional pain and distress (Gratz et al. 2016) or hopelessness (Gray et al. 2021), to their self-image as a self-harming individual (Glenn et al. 2016), to intense self-criticism (Nagy et al. 2021), or suicidal thoughts (Dickstein et al. 2015). It is also true

---

99 Mostly by the widely used Implicit Association Test (for examples of use in various fields, see: Nosek et al. 2014; Gratz et al. 2016; Sukhera et al. 2019).

that the more serious the self-harm, the more robust the system of implicit associations (Glenn et al. 2017). The system of implicit associations points to the deeply internalised problematic cognitive mindset of the individual, which leads to the formation of negative core convictions about oneself, even at the level of subconscious mechanisms.

2.5 Regulatory Concepts

Regulatory concepts are a set of theories and views that understand self-harming as a tool for regulating stressful emotions and cognitions[100]. Self-harm stems from the need to express or control anger, anxiety or pain, which cannot be expressed verbally or in other ways (Suyemoto 1998). When adolescents describe the circumstances of their self-harm, they often express feelings of unbearable tension, anxiety or the presence of intrusive thoughts that lead to intensive mental discomfort. The solution that the individual comes up with, either spontaneously or through social learning, imitation or information obtained from social networks[101] is to hurt themselves. Although self-harm is an inappropriate strategy, it is necessary to understand that at the same time, it is a very natural[102], efficient and available method for the reduction of emotional burdens. Its effects are immediate; thus, it is much more ef-

---

100 It has been reported that 63–78% of adolescents use self-harm to regulate their emotions (Taylor et al. 2018).
101 When feeling rage, the adolescent may vent their aggression by punches without an accurate estimate of their strength, and they may hit something with such force that they cause themselves intense pain, without intending to do so. This is followed by the discovery that the physical pain "drowns out" the emotional or mental pain and distracts them from feelings that the individual might not cope with at that moment. As a result of this experience, the adolescent may adopt this method of self-harm as a strategy to cope with any future intense mental burdens. However, it is more common for adolescents to opt for self-harm based on hearing about this strategy from their peers (or directly seeing it) or from social networks.
102 It is natural in the sense that self-harming activities are rather wide-spread ways of stimulating and calming one-self not only in humans but also in other animal species (Nock & Cha 2009).

fective than other methods. Moreover, no preparation is needed – the individual's own body is available at any time and owing to the wide range of forms and types of self-harm[103], there is always a form of self-harm immediately available[104].

The Regulation of Emotions

The experience of psychologists with self-harming adolescents frequently points to the presence of problems in the field of emotions. Self-harming individuals often exhibit deficits in emotional regulation, which means they have problems with recognising, understanding and/or managing their own emotions (Wolff et al. 2019). The regulation of emotions is a relatively complex and multilayered process that involves many areas, and the problems that lead to self-harm may appear at any phase within this process of regulation or from the mutual combination of multiple processes that function incorrectly. The model of the regulation of emotions (see e.g., Gross 1998) postulates that the main process in the initial phase is to become aware of one's own emotions. The correct identification of emotion (or emotions) is a common problem because (as several studies report – see, for instance, Greene et al. 2020, 2021; Iskric 2020) self-harm is frequently associated with alexithymia – the inability to identify and describe own emotions. Not only does this handicap prevent the individual from understanding their own experience (increasing anxiety, feelings of hopelessness and incapability), but it also prevents them from coping with their emotional state and selecting a suitable solution (Wester & Trepal 2017). Another step in the process of emotional regulation is

---

[103] The wide range of forms and types of self-harm are discussed in Chapter 4.
[104] It does not only have to be physical harm – adolescents also use other forms, such as self-harm and self-punishment by self-devaluation in a social or mental context. These forms of self-harm include, for example, behavioural expressions by adolescents that lead to rejection by others, friends, family, acquaintances…, when the adolescent is intentionally mean or unfriendly to others, their motive is not to vent their anger but to intentionally provoke rejection from others as a form of self-harm. Mental forms of self-harm include, for example, intentionally provoking thoughts about one's own inabilities, intentionally provoking a depressive mood, remaining in this state or causing its deterioration and other ways of punishing oneself so that the individual feels mentally unwell.

the management of emotions (e.g., by increasing[105] or decreasing the intensity of emotions). Self-harming individuals often fail in this phase, not only because they could not identify their emotions but also because the process of searching for possible strategies is ineffective and erroneous. As explained in the section 2.4, these individuals typically produce solutions with a lower degree of diversity or have a general tendency to avoid solutions completely (Orbach et al. 1990). Moreover, the specificities of the function of their memories do not provide access to sufficiently specific information about their previous experiences with the same (or similar) problems but instead provide generalised, non-specific coping strategies. A generalised memory then causes deficiencies in the search for effective solutions (Wenzel & Spokas 2014). The last phase of the process of regulation of emotions involves the effective implementation of adaptive strategies for reaching a goal (i.e., the regulation of emotions). As a result of several (previously mentioned) problems, self-harming individuals tend to avoid the solution of problems, and even if they actually do reach for a strategy, it is not effective or it is maladaptive. Problems with the search for strategies do not have to occur exclusively in the last phase of emotional regulation, but they are also typical of the period before the formation of an emotional reaction. A functional system for coping with burdens in a mentally healthy individual with adaptive and efficient mechanisms is able to prevent the occurrence of unmanageable emotional reactions based on experience and thus effectively intervene before they actually occur.

Due to these deficits, adolescents choose a maladaptive and highly risky strategy to cope with emotional burdens – self-harm. For adolescents, it has the desirable effect – numbing the mental or emotional pain[106], and since its effects immediately occur and

---

105 Self-harm is not only used to decrease overly intense emotions. Through self-harm, an adolescent may regulate their emotions by enhancing their affective experience. This especially happens when they feel emotionally "numb", "empty" or detached from others. The act of self-harm may help the teenager feel excited to stop their dissociative experience and bring back a feeling of being "real" (Peterson et al. 2008).

106 "I started burning myself with incense or candle wax as a way to deal with anger... I learned that pain can quickly dull emotions! I switched to cutting myself... as a way to deal with negative emotions quickly" (Wester & Trepal 2017, 23).

it is always available (Nock & Chia 2009), adolescents tend to return to it, further fixating it as a maladaptive strategy. It should be noted that self-harming individuals (as opposed to the rest of the population) have to regulate their intense emotions more frequently. They are more prone to distortions of self-image (Gulbas et al. 2015; Sedgwick et al. 2019, Harman et al. 2021), which provoke intense feelings of their own inabilities, their low self-worth or even self-hatred, and they also typically have depressive mindset (Andover et al. 2005; Burke et al. 2015; Maciejewski et al. 2019), which influences the experience and evaluation of most situations. As a result of these problems, they are more prone to intense negative emotions, which they have to deal with.

In fact, as a result of a failure in the regulation of emotions, self-harming individuals benefit from therapies that facilitate mindfulness focused on emotions (Heath et al. 2016). Thanks to this therapy, the sensitivity of the individual towards their own experience is enhanced and their ability to accept the present experience and not condemn it is strengthened (Schuman-Olivier et al. 2020). It is assumed that the practice of mindfulness has the potential to lead to behavioural changes as a result of the improvement of the ability of an individual to identify, understand and accept their own emotions.

Distracting Attention

Another common problem in terms of the experience of intense emotions is the simultaneous presence of a cognitive strategy – rumination (see e.g., Nicolai et al. 2016; Richmond et al. 2018) – which is the process of paying excessive attention to the current experience of the individual. As a result of the maladaptive degree of attention paid to the current problems they are experiencing, the individual becomes overwhelmed, and they relive their negative emotions over and over and immerse themselves in the problem, complicating the perception of the bigger picture that is necessary in the search for a solution. It has been suggested that it is rumination that is the key mediator that causes the adolescent to react to the occurrence of strong emotions with self-harm (Hasking et al. 2018). This suggestion has led to the formulation of the emotional cascade theory (Selby & Joiner 2009). According to this theory, rumination forces an individual to repeatedly pay attention to negative stimuli and the solution of problems. The individual relives the negative emotional burden, which once again draws the attention of the individual. By continuously dealing with the same problem, the individual is pulled into a vicious circle or into a so-called emotional cascade, which becomes more and more stressful, because, in this cycle, the negative emotions are reinforced. Considering the intensity of emotions, common techniques[107] used to distract attention are not effective, so the individual opts for more extreme techniques to disrupt the cycle (Hasking et al. 2018). Self-harm is highly effective in this regard – the intensity of the pain, the sight of their blood, the necessity to treat the wounds, shift attention away from the negativity to other stimuli. This attention shift disrupts the cycle of rumination and the consequent increase in emotional burden, reducing tension and the intensity of the emotions experienced (Selby et al. 2013). Reducing tension and intense emotions negatively reinforces the behaviour, which is why self-harm becomes a conditioned reaction to negative emotional stimuli or to intensely negative effects (Selby & Joiner 2009). The problem of such behaviour lies in its short-term effect, in its danger and even lethality that results from its destructive character and addictiveness.

2.6 Integrative Concepts

Integrative concepts are an effort to combine the various approaches and knowledge into a complex model, which would cover most of the areas necessary for the explanation of this phenomenon. Thus, integrative concepts of self-harm mostly work with several sources, motives, functions and mechanisms of this risky behaviour at the same time. They include, for example, genetic predispositions as well as environmental impacts; they work with

---

[107] For example, a walk or a discussion with a friend.

risk factors in the individual as well as with those that stem from interpersonal interactions and not only consider the typical symptomatology of self-harm but also, for example, the functions that this type of behaviour might fulfil.

Scientific literature that focuses on the issue of self-harm often works with the integrative model of the American psychologist Matthew K. Nock (Figure 3), who merges several components from the areas of risk factors, triggers and psychological mechanisms leading to the appearance, retention and enhancement of self-harming behaviour.

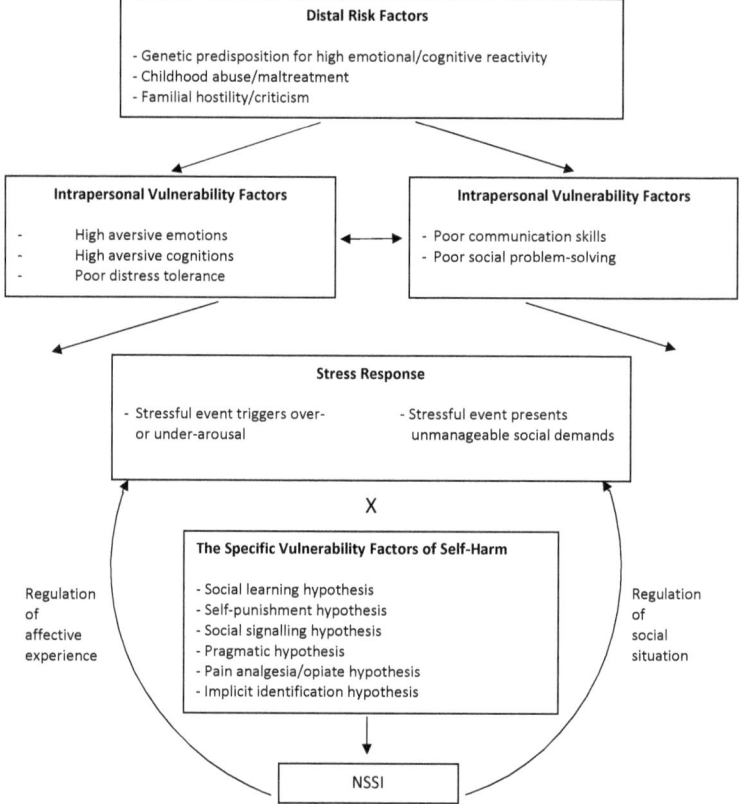

Figure 3. The integrated theoretical model of the development and maintenance of self-harm
Source: Nock (2009, 80)

Distal risk factors are circumstances from the past of the individual (they have a temporal distance from the present) and are highly likely to cause the initiation of self-harm in an individual. However, there are also other important variables between the distal risk factors and the appearance of self-harm, which are the various types of vulnerability to reactions in the form of self-harm. In his integrative model, M. K. Nock characterises self-harming behaviour as an effective way of immediately regulating aversive affective experiences and social situations. The model is based on the assumption that the risk of self-harm is increased by the presence of distal factors (such as bad treatment in childhood), which may lead to intrapersonal or interpersonal vulnerability (e.g., to weak communication skills) and the tendency to react to stressful life experiences through ineffective measures (such as ineffective methods of communicating the need for help). Although these risk factors may predispose a person to many forms of psychopathology, the likelihood of being involved in NSSI is increased by the additional set of factors of vulnerability to self-harm (such as the tendency to perform self-punishment) (Nock 2009). If self-harming behaviour appears as a reaction to a stressful situation, it has in return an effect on the selection of responses to stress, which fixes it in the repertoire of possible reactions.

Self-harm is studied from many perspectives, and various concepts offer a wide range of explanations for this negative and highly risky phenomenon. Although there are several different approaches, several important pieces of information are common to research findings and the practical experience of clinical psychologists. Self-harm is an effective yet maladaptive, coping strategy with a burden. It especially appears in individuals who had traumatic experiences in childhood or whose development was marked by circumstances that led to a specific way of processing information and a negative self-image. It is often accompanied by other complications, such as depressive mental states. Self-harming behaviour is maintained in the repertoire of reactions and preferred as a result of the impact of mechanisms of automatic and social reinforcement. As a result of the activation of the reward systems of the brain, self-harm may also become addictive.

3 The Occurrence of Self-Harm

In our observations of the occurrence of self-harm, we will focus on those types of behaviour which lack any religious, social or other cultural or aesthetic motives, which might encourage an individual to inflict injury and/or pain upon themselves – in an effort to gain social status, to undergo a ritual of acceptance into a group or social class, to become more attractive, etc. Thus, we will include activities which are performed by an individual in order to hurt themselves, to harm their health or to inflict pain upon themselves (both physical and mental). The prevalence of self-harm substantially differs in the various studies that have observed this undesirable phenomenon. This has happened for many reasons: the studies have worked with various different age groups; they have been conducted in various different social conditions, which may reinforce/reduce the prevalence of self-harm; they focus on various diverse groups (such as the clinical or general population). However, the main reason for the variation is that they do not use the same definition of the term, meaning that they have not observed the same types of behaviour. So, unless consensus is reached in the use and definition of the term "self-harm", the reported prevalence should be accompanied by as much data as possible with respect to the place where the data was collected, the method of collection, the study sample and the criteria employed.

3.1 The Prevalence of Self-Harm in the World

In many countries where research into self-harm has been conducted, they have pointed to a rise in the prevalence of this phenomenon. This trend has been striking over the last few decades (Carr et al. 2016; Morgan et al. 2017; Griffin et al. 2018; Borschmann & Kinner 2019), and the number of reported cases keeps increasing; this is also a result of the current situation[108] (Du et al. 2021; Henry et al. 2021). Data on the prevalence of self-harm differs in published studies (Muehlenkamp et al. 2012; Lim et al. 2019) – it

---

108 This work was created between 2019 and 2021, which was marked by the SARS-CoV-19 pandemic.

has been found to occur over a rather wide range from 3.3% (Jung et al. 2018) up to more than 50% (Calvete et al. 2015). In the following paragraphs, we will clarify the results of studies from some countries[109] (with an emphasis on Europe) as well as available data regarding the year when they were conducted, the study sample and the definition of self-harm.

Australia

In their extensive study of the prevalence of self-harm on a sample of Australian students (mean age 15.4 years), De Leo and Heller defined self-harm: "An act with a non-fatal outcome in which an individual deliberately did one or more of the following:

Initiated behaviour (e.g., self-cutting, jumping from a height), which they intended to cause self-harm;
- Ingested a substance in excess of the prescribed or generally recognised therapeutic dose;
- Ingested a recreational or illicit drug that was an act that the person regarded as self-harm;
- Ingested a non-ingestible substance or object" (De Leo & Heller 2004, 141).

The lifetime occurrence of self-harm reached 12.4%; over the previous 12 months, 6.2% had performed self-harm; the prevalence was higher among females and the most often reported methods included self-cutting (59.2%) and overdosing with medication (29.6%).

Asia and the Pacific

A complex study that mapped out the existing research into self-harm among high-school and university students in China was published by J. Lang and Y. Yao in 2018. They collected data that had been reported between 2000 and 2017; this ultimately

---

[109] To ensure clarity in this chapter, the countries are divided into geographic regions and are only grouped to orient a reader and do not always follow geopolitical classifications.

comprised of 26 studies with more than 150,000 students. The authors stated their observed prevalence of non-suicidal self-injury (NSSI), with a mean value of 22.4% (Lang & Yao 2018).

Jung et al. analysed five years (2011–2015) of reports of medical treatment of injuries to 250,000 young people in South Korea aged 11–29. In 3.3% of cases, the injury was classified as deliberate self-harm, which was defined as any non-lethal injury or poisoning which was reported by the patient or the physician as having been deliberately inflicted by the patient, regardless of the presence of any intent to cause death. The most common form of self-harm was self-poisoning/overdose (47.4%), followed by self-cutting (31.4%), self-hitting (8%) and jumping from heights (3.9%), with the highest prevalence of self-harm observed in the age range 16–19 (Jung et al. 2018).

N. Watanabe et al. observed the occurrence of self-harm over the previous twelve months on a rather extensive sample of adolescents in Japan (n = 18,104). The participants communicated their self-harming activity through an anonymous self-reporting questionnaire. The authors of the study analysed the results in two separate age groups – first, for younger adolescents (12–15 years of age) and then, for older adolescents (15–18 years of age). The reported prevalence of self-harming behaviour in the group of younger participants was 3.3%, whereas for the group of older adolescents it was 4.3%; in both cases, the prevalence was higher in the female subjects (the prevalence quadrupled) (Watanabe et al. 2012).

In 2015, a group of authors, led by J. A. Garisch, published the results of a cross-sectional and longitudinal study that focused on the prevalence of self-harm among adolescents in New Zealand. The study involved 1,162 adolescents with a mean age of 16.35. The lifelong prevalence of self-harm was studied through a short version of the DSHI questionnaire (Deliberate Self-Harm Inventory)[110], and they found a level of 48.7%. Interestingly, the most frequent form of self-harm was sticking sharp objects into the skin, and self-cutting was only in the fourth place (Garish et al. 2015).

---

110 A description along with the authors of this and other questionnaires mentioned in the following studies is provided in section 3.3.

Middle East

A team of scientists led by O. Somer conducted a study into the prevalence of self-harm on a representative sample of Turkish secondary schools. The analysis involved 1,565 adolescents with a mean age of 16.8. In order to map the prevalence of self-harming behaviour, the authors used the ISAS questionnaire created by Klonsky and Olino (2008)[111] (Inventory of Statements about Self-Injury), which captures twelve forms of deliberate self-injury and the lifetime prevalence. According to the results, in their lifetime history, 31.3% of students indicated the presence of at least a single form of self-harm in the ISAS (Somer et al. 2015). However, it is questionable to what extent a single (not repeated)[112] action intended to cause deliberate harm to their own health may be considered self-harm.

In this context, a specific and very current study is the research conducted on children living in the second largest city in Iran, Mashhad (approx. 1.5 mil. citizens), who are forced to work in order to survive and/or live on the streets. The authors (Jarahi et al. 2021) expected this population to be more vulnerable to pathological phenomena including self-harm. The study was performed on children up to 18 years of age, most of whom (due to the specific nature of the sample) were boys (71.4%), and the prevalence of self-harm was observed over the course of the previous four months using the SHI (Self-Harm Inventory – Sansone et al. 1998). The prevalence of self-harm was high – it was reported by 59% of children; but the forms of self-harm were also highly specific – the most frequent form was "God-distancing" (29.6%), followed by hitting (26.5%), deliberate self-starvation (23.5%) and self-cutting (21.4%) (Jarahi et al. 2021).

---

[111] The methods used in studies that are mentioned in this chapter are, in most cases, described in more detail in the following section 3.3.
[112] This is another reason why more attention should be paid to a clearer definition of self-harming behaviour.

North America

The prevalence of non-suicidal self-injury in the United States, as defined by the proposed criteria in DSM-5, was studied in a sample of children from 7 to 16 years of age by Barrocas et al. (2012). Due to the age of the participants, the study was performed in the presence of the parents of the children involved, which may have partially influenced the willingness of the participants to share information regarding self-harm. Self-harm and its forms were observed through a structured clinical interview, SITBI (Self-Injurious Thoughts and Behaviours Interview), which identified a life-long prevalence, within this age group, of 8%. The prevalence was higher in girls and increased with age. As to forms of self-harm, the dominant form among girls was self-cutting, while self-hitting was typical of boys (Barrocas et al. 2012).

As part of a cross-sectional study on the health of Canadian youths, in the second wave of data collection (in 2005), the researchers included a set of questions related to self-harm into their relatively vast interview data. In the process of monitoring this behaviour, they used the CASE study[113] (Child and Adolescent Self-Harm in Europe) through which they analysed the lifetime prevalence of this phenomenon. Although they referred to the observed behaviour as non-suicidal self-injury, they observed the presence of not only self-cutting, scratching or self-hitting but also other forms such as medication overuse, ingestion of illicit drugs (with the intention to harm themselves) or the consumption of indigestible objects, while also providing space to add their own personal forms of self-harm (Nixon et. al 2008). The researchers obtained data related to self-harm through interviews with 568 adolescents aged 12–18 years old, with the total prevalence of self-harm reaching 16.9%. That being said, this figure also included adolescents who reported a single incident of self-harm – these made up 29% of the sample (ibid.).

---

113 CASE study was an international study that mapped the occurrence of self-harm in children and adolescents. The study was conducted in ten European countries in 2000. The complete report and further information relating to the project are available at: https://ec.europa.eu/justice/grants/results/daphne-toolkit/content/child-and-adolescent-self-harm-europe-study_en.

Latin and South America

The primary aim of the study carried out by Leiva Pereira and Concha Landeros (2019) in Chile was to analyse the correlation between self-harm and attachment style in adolescents. The data from the published study provides information regarding prevalence in a non-clinical population. The study sample was made up of 186 participants aged 14-18 (mean age 15.8), with a small majority of female subjects (57%). For the assessment of the presence of self-harm, the authors created an ad hoc scale based on the DSM criteria for non-suicidal self-injury. An NSSI occurred in 11% of the adolescents, mostly in female subjects (77.3%) (Leiva Pereira & Concha Landeros 2019).

Relatively recent data from Brazil has come from a study by Costa et al. published in 2021. The research involved 505 adolescents from 12 to 17 years of age (mean age = 14.32), and a Brazilian version of the FASM questionnaire (Functional Assessment of Self-Mutilation) was used to identify self-harming behaviour. Based on the data obtained, the authors classified the adolescents into three groups: those without any occurrence of self-harming behaviour, those with at least one episode of self-harm over the last twelve months and those whose self-harm met the criteria proposed by DSM-5. The prevalence of self-harm that met the DSM-5 criteria was around 6.5%, but when using the broader definition of self-harm (at least one episode over the past year), the prevalence increased to 38.8% (Costa et al. 2021).

The team led by L. Albores-Gallo also selected the proposed definition of self-harm within DSM-5 as their criterion. They collected data from 533 adolescents in Mexico aged between 11 and 17 (mean age 13.37), and in addition to the fulfilment of the diagnostic criteria, they also observed the time period and the frequency in which the individual performed self-harm. In the light of the above-mentioned data, they report a total prevalence of self-harm of 5.6%, with self-harm having most commonly occurred over the past year and having five episodes. The mean age at the onset of self-harm in the observed sample was 11.9, and self-harming activities occurred more commonly in girls than boys (Albores-Gallo et al. 2014).

Africa

A study by D. Boduszek et al. presents the results of observations on the prevalence of self-harm in children and adolescents in Uganda and Jamaica. In Uganda, 11,518 participants from 9 to 17 years of age were included in the study, 52.4% of the participants were female. The prevalence of self-harm in this extensive study was examined through a single question ("Have you ever harmed yourself on purpose in a way that was not intended to take your life?") with two possible answers: yes or no. The lifelong prevalence was average in comparison to other studies, but what was unusual was that the prevalence was higher in boys (25.5%) than in girls (23.2%) (Boduszek et al. 2021).

A large-scale overview of articles published in African scientific journals on the topic of self-harm is provided by the study of Quarshie et al., in which the authors analysed data from seventy-four articles published between 1950 and 2019, bringing together data from sixteen Sub-Saharan African countries[114]. The data on the prevalence of self-harm originates from various study samples and forms of data collection. The authors report an average lifelong prevalence of self-harm of 10.3%, the prevalence of self-harm over the past year of 16.9%, over the past six months of 18.2% and over the past month of 3.2% (Quarshie et al. 2020).

In his next study, Emmanuel N-B Quarshie specifically focused on the population of adolescents. He observed self-harm in Ghana through a sample of pupils and students (n = 1,723) and a sample of 384 young people living on the streets (total n = 2,107). The participants were between 13 and 21 years old. For the analysis of the prevalence of self-harm, the authors used their own self-reporting questionnaire; however, they stated that their questions were mostly inspired by the methods: Child and Adolescent Self-Harm in Europe (CASE), Self-Injurious Thoughts and Behaviour Interview (SITBI) and Suicide Attempt Self-Injury Interview (SA-SII). The lifelong prevalence of self-harm in this sample was 20.2%, and the authors state a prevalence of 16.6% for the past year and

---

[114] This included: Benin, Ghana, Mauritania, Nigeria, Togo, Ethiopia, Malawi, Rwanda, Seychelles, Tanzania, Uganda, Eswatini, Mozambique, Namibia, South Africa and Zambia (Quarshie et al. 2020).

3.1% for the past month. A total of 26% of the adolescents stated that they used several methods of self-harm. A positive aspect of the findings in this study was the relatively high prevalence of indirect forms of self-harm (e.g., use of alcohol, medications, etc.) (Quarshie et al. 2021).

Northern Europe

Over the course of two weeks, Ose et al. (2021) monitored the prevalence of self-harm in a specific sample of adult psychiatric patients hospitalised in Norwegian clinics. The data was obtained from 23,124 patients over the age of 18, and the data regarding self-harm over the previous four weeks was provided by their physician in collaboration with the patient (if possible). They monitored the presence of non-suicidal self-injury (NSSI). The highest prevalence was found in those patients being treated for personality disorders (14.4%) and the lowest prevalence in those patients suffering from substance use disorders (6.8%). On average, the prevalence of self-harm was 8.1% and decreased with age (Ose et al. 2021).

In 2007 and 2008, a cross-sectional study involving adolescents was conducted in Sweden, which included the monitoring of self-harming behaviour. Ten years after the second round of investigations (2017), the authors of the study (Daukantaité et al. 2021) contacted the participants and repeated the measurements in 50.2% of the young adults. To identify self-harming behaviour, they used a shortened (9-item) version of the DSHI (Deliberate Self-Harm Inventory) (Gratz 2001). In this inventory, the respondents reported the occurrence of several forms of self-harm[115] on a seven-point Likert scale (from "0" = never to "6" = more than five times). In 2007, the reported prevalence of NSSI was 41.5%, and in 2008, it had risen to 42.8%. Although the prevalence of this high-risk behaviour decreases with age (in 2017, only 18.7% of the participants monitored in 2007 and 2008 reported it), based on other analyses, the authors concluded that high-intensity self-harm in adolescence is a strong risk factor for the presence of mental health problems in young

---

115 But all of them only monitor visible damage to tissues, which means that this behaviour (in terms of its forms) is identical to NSSI.

adulthood, and the occasional occurrence of NSSI in adolescence is an indicator of vulnerability to poorer mental health in young adulthood (Daukantaité et al. 2021).

In their current study, Steeg et al. describe an unusual phenomenon in the adolescent population of Denmark. Over the period 2000–2016, they observed the development of self-harm in adolescents aged 10–19, which was registered via the interconnected national registers of health reports of the population. They included those episodes of self-harm that led to treatment in a hospital or to hospitalisation. Over the period observed, these criteria were met by 26,950 adolescents, and the prevalence of the identified type of self-harm showed a gradual increase, that peaked in 2007 (a prevalence of 25.1%); after that, the prevalence decreased year after year (to 13.8% in 2016), in all age groups and in both sexes (Steeg et al. 2020).

Data from the Baltic states regarding the prevalence of self-harm are hard to find in the available[116] scientific literature – they are mostly published in the local language[117], or they may be included in international studies that the countries participated in. For instance, Brunner et al. report that Estonia, France, Germany and Israel have the highest prevalence of life-long self-harm in adolescents (mean age of the sample of 12,608 adolescents = 14.9 years of age) out of the eleven countries observed[118], with a prevalence of 32.9%. They studied the prevalence of self-harm through a modified 6-item version of the Deliberate Self-Harm Inventory questionnaire (DSHI), and in addition to the life-long prevalence, they also observed the frequency of occasional or repetitive[119] deliberate self-injury. In these categories, the prevalence among Estonian adolescents was 23.8% (occasional) and 9.1% (repetitive) (Brunner et al. 2013).

---

116 Full texts published in English in standard databases.
117 Such as a study which suggested in its abstract that the prevalence of self-harm among Lithuanian adolescents aged 15–17 is 7.3% (Laskyte & Zemaitiene 2009).
118 The research was conducted in the following countries: Austria, Estonia, France, Germany, Hungary, Ireland, Italy, Romania, Slovenia, Spain, Sweden and Israel.
119 Occasional self-injurious behaviour referred to 1–4 episodes of the behaviour over a lifetime; repetitive self-injurious behaviour referred to 5 or more episodes (Brunner et al. 2013).

Western Europe

A long-term study and subsequent data analysis was carried out in Ireland by a team of authors led by Ewe Griffin. They obtained data on self-harm from the records of urgent admissions to hospitals that treated patients who had self-harmed. The prevalence of self-harm was relatively high – on average 3.2%, between 2007 and 2016, for the 10 to 24-year-old age group (Griffin et al. 2018) – partly due to the highly specific nature of the sample (individuals who sought urgent medical treatment as a result of self-harm that was reported as such).

A cross-sectional study of the prevalence of self-harm in 2000, 2007 and 2014 in the British population between the ages 16–74 was performed by the research team of McManus et al. (2018). Self-harm was detected through a self-reporting questionnaire (as part of a broader set of questions), and the authors attempted to interpret the data in line with the definition of non-suicidal self-injury. Owing to the cross-sectional character of data collection, the authors were able to observe the development of the prevalence, which according to the published data increased from 2.4% (in 2000) to 6.4% (in 2014), with the highest increase identified in women aged 16–24 (in 2014, the prevalence of self-harm in this group was 19.7%) (McManus et al. 2018).

Another relatively extensive study analysed the electronic health data held by almost 700 general practitioners and observed the prevalence of self-harm in the United Kingdom within the population of adolescents in the 10–19 age group over the period from 2001 to 2014. It defines self-harm in relatively broad terms as "an act of self-poisoning or self-injury, irrespective of motivation" (Morgan et al. 2017, 2). In spite of the non-specific criteria, the prevalence of self-harm identified was not high – it was an average of 3.7% in girls and 1.2% in boys over the observed period. As regards the forms of self-harm, the electronic records report that 84.1% of the cases were identified as drug overdoses, 12.3% as self-cutting, 2.5% as other self-poisonings, and the rest of the cases were various non-specified methods (Morgan et al. 2017).

The figures were considerably higher in a study by O'Connor et al. (2018) that mapped out self-harm in Scotland. In their definition of self-harm, they used the diagnostic criteria within DSM-5 (meaning they mapped non-suicidal self-injury), and the analysis was carried out on a representative sample of 3,508 young adults aged between 18 and 34. The presence of self-harm, identified through an interview with questions taken from the APMS (McManus et al. 2016) and the Child and Adolescent Self-Harm in Europe study (Madge et al. 2008), was 16.2%. Again, it was higher in women, and the authors discovered that the earlier self-harm starts in an individual's development, the higher the intensity and risk of attempted suicide (O'Connor et al. 2018).

Self-harm in the adult population in Belgium in the age group from 19 to 64 years (mean age of 39.4) was examined by Raemen et al. (2020). To identify self-harm, they used selected items from the SHI (Self-Harm Inventory) (Sansone et al. 1998); specifically, they only examined the occurrence of cutting, burning, scratching and self-hitting, which are activities that essentially correspond to the forms of self-harming behaviour identified by the NSSI definition. The research sample consisted of 254 adults and included a representative selection in terms of the age, sex and education of the Flemish adult population. The prevalence of non-suicidal self-injury (NSSI) in the non-clinical population was 13.8% (Raemen et al. 2020).

Central Europe

To observe the prevalence of self-harming behaviour in Germany, a scientific team lead by A. Müller used a translation of the Self-Harm Inventory (SHI). Their research identified a wide range of self-harming behaviours in a sample of 2,507 participants from 14 to 94 years old (mean age = 48.79). The prevalence data is only available for the sample as a whole; the data is not broken down into individual age groups. The lifetime prevalence of at least a single action of deliberate self-harm in an individual's history was 49%, and interestingly they found that there was a higher prevalence in men than women and the most common forms of self-harm reported were indirect forms (Müller et al. 2016). P. L. Plener et al. (2016) suggest that the prevalence of self-harm in German youths is one of the highest and indicates a lifetime prevalence in the range of 25–35%.

Joint research carried out in three German-speaking countries (Austria, Germany and Switzerland) focused on a mutual comparison of the prevalence of self-harm using the self-report questionnaire, the Ottawa Self-Injury Inventory (OSI). The study focused on the adolescent population (students) with 1,339 participants (mean age 14.99). The prevalence of self-harm in the individual countries is presented in Table 6, with the results suggesting stark differences between the countries (Plener et al. 2013).

Table 6. The prevalence of self-harm in Austria, Germany and Switzerland in a sample of adolescents

Participants	Austria	Germany	Switzerland	Total
	n (%)	n (%)	n (%)	n (%)
Male	54 (23.8)	285 (42.9)	234 (52.3)	573 (42.8)
Female	173 (76.2)	380 (57.1)	213 (47.7)	766 (57.2)
Total	227	665	447	1,339
Of which admitted to self-harm				
	n (prevalence)	n (prevalence)	n (prevalence)	n (prevalence)
Male	3 (5.6%)	55 (19.3%)	8 (3.4%)	66 (11.52%)
Female	25 (14.5%)	129 (33.9%)	32 (15.0)	186 (24.3%)
Total	28 (12.3%)	184 (27.7%)	40 (9.0%)	252 (18.8%)

Source : Plener et al. (2013, p. 1441)

Research carried out in Poland studied the prevalence of non-suicidal self-injury over the previous year, determining frequency through a 5-point scale. In total, 2,220 adolescents from 13 to 19 years of age participated in the study (mean age 16.8). The study used self-assessment based on an anonymous questionnaire, and the criterion used for the identification of a self-harming individual was in line with DSM-5. The prevalence of this type of self-harm in adolescents was 4.8%, with the highest prevalence identified in 15-year-old participants (Kądziela-Olech et al. 2015).

Data related to self-harm in the Czech Republic is presented in a study by Rozsívalová et al. – it found a prevalence of 4% in the general adult population and 21% among psychiatric patients, and the lifetime prevalence in adolescent psychiatric patients was as high as 60% (Rozsívalová et al. 2010).

Research into the prevalence of self-harm among adolescents in Hungary was carried out by Horváth et al. The data collection focused on students in the age group of 13–18 (mean age = 15.4). The researchers employed the DHSI (Deliberate Self-Harm Inventory) (Gratz 2001), which identifies sixteen forms of self-harm. All of these forms represent direct forms of physical self-harm; however, the questionnaire also allows respondents to add other (not mentioned) forms. The research sample consisted of 161 participants, 50% of whom were female, and the prevalence of self-harm was 23.6%.

Southern Europe

The prevalence of self-harm in 1,864 adolescents aged between 12 and 19 (mean age = 15.32) was investigated by a Spanish team led by E. Calvete. The presence of self-harm was assessed using a modified self-harm inventory, FASM – Functional Assessment of Self-Mutilation (Lloyd et al. 1997), which only included self-harm that had taken place over the last year. The authors reported a high prevalence – more than 50% of the sample had performed self-harm, with 32.2% exhibiting signs of severe self-harm (Calvete et al. 2015). A more specific study in Spain was published in the same year by Rebeca García-Nieto et al. (2015). They focused on the prevalence of self-harm in adolescents who had previously been hospitalised in psychiatric facilities. They used data from 2011 and 2012 which they acquired through the Spanish version of the SITBI (Self-Injurious Thoughts and Behaviors Interview). Based on the results, 21.7% of the adolescents stated they had performed self-harm at least once in their lives (García-Nieto et al. 2015).

A relatively high prevalence of self-harm was reported in the study by R. Cerutti et al., which was conducted in Italy on a sample of 365 young adults with a mean age of 23. The prevalence of self-harm was observed using the self-reporting Deliberate Self-Harm Inventory questionnaire (DSHI), with a reported prevalence of 39%.

Information on the occurrence of self-harm in Spanish adolescents was provided in the study by Ferreira Gonçalves et al. They observed self-injurious behaviour (SIB) using a questionnaire on a sample of 569 participants aged from 12 to 20 years old. The lifetime prevalence of self-injurious behaviour was 28%, and as many as 10% of adolescents stated that they had self-injured in the past month (Ferreira Gonçalves 2012).

A specific research sample in terms of the prevalence of self-harm was studied by the authors of a study led by V. Boričević Maršanić in Croatia. They studied the children (adolescents) of war veterans who had suffered from post-traumatic stress disorder. They built their hypothesis on the assumption that the condition suffered by the parent may have an impact on parenting methods and attitudes to their children, especially in terms of emotionality, which is the key aspect of self-harm. The research involved adolescents from 12 to 18 years of age, and the presence of self-harm was identified through the use of the Deliberate Self-Harm Inventory (DSHI). The lifetime prevalence of self-harm in this sample was 52.7%.

Eastern Europe

Data regarding the prevalence of self-harm in the countries of Eastern Europe is less readily available. A. M. Stoica et al. in their study carried out in Ukraine only focused on a specific part of the spectrum of self-harm – which they called "oral self-harm", which involves deliberate injuries to the lips or oral cavity. They established the prevalence in a sample of children between 10 and 14 years in institutional care (through the analysis of dental records). The prevalence of this specific form was 18.1% and was more than three times as high in girls compared to boys (Stoica et al. 2020).

A study by Koposov et al. reported the prevalence of self-harm in Russian adolescents using a very specific study sample. They focused on imprisoned individuals[120]; the research sample consisted of n = 368 inmates in juvenile detention centres between the ages of 14 and 19 (mean age = 16.4). The participants reported their life-

---

120 Studies of self-harm in prisons were especially popular in the past when this type of behaviour (as well as mental disorders and a history of sexual abuse in childhood) was particularly associated with the prison population.

time prevalence of self-harm; the researchers did not use any of the standard measurement methods, but the nature of the questions was aimed at non-suicidal self-injury. Using a self-reporting questionnaire administered to the inmates of juvenile detention centres, they revealed a prevalence of non-suicidal self-injury of 18.2% (Koposov et al. 2021).

Pan-European Research

A team led by R. Bunner conducted a survey through a questionnaire to establish the prevalence of self-harm in a sample of 12,068 adolescents (mean age = 14.9) from eleven countries (see Table 7). The prevalence of self-harm was investigated using a modified 6-item version of the Deliberate Self-Harm Inventory (DSHI). At the same time, the team also explored the frequency of self-harm using three different categories: lifetime (at least one episode of self-harm over their life), occasional (up to four episodes of self-harm over their life) and repeated (more than five episodes) (Brunner et al. 2013).

Table 7. The prevalence of self-harm in selected countries

	Lifetime		Occasional		Repeated	
Country	n	%	n	%	n	%
Austria	253	26.9	188	20.0	65	6.9
Estonia	339	32.9	245	23.8	94	9.1
France	387	38.5	257	25.6	130	13.0
Germany	502	35.1	327	22.9	175	12.3
Hungary	171	17.1	125	12.5	46	4.6
Ireland	215	20.4	160	15.2	55	5.2
Israel	379	32.6	262	22.5	117	10.1
Italy	249	20.9	103	16.2	56	4.7
Romania	230	20.6	200	17.9	30	2.7
Slovakia	306	27.3	206	18.4	100	8.9
Spain	295	28.9	218	21.4	77	7.6
Total	3,326	27.6	2,381	19.7	945	7.8

Source: Brunner et al. (2013, p. 5)

One of the most complex surveys in Europe that focuses on a wide range of high-risk behaviours is the European School Survey Project on Alcohol and Other Drugs (ESPAD). It focuses on students between 15 and 16 years of age (ESPAD) and is repeated at regular intervals. The project also monitors self-harming behaviour, and the self-reporting questionnaire included in the research battery monitors its lifetime prevalence. Several European countries regularly participate in the project, and the results are processed by a number of research teams from several different scientific domains, including psychology. One overview of the prevalence of self-harm (see Table 8) was published in 2013 by a Greek team led by A. Kokkevi. They presented the results of the

Table 8. An overview of the prevalence of self-harm in 15 and 16-year-old adolescents in selected European countries

Country	n	At least once in their life (%)	More than once in their life (%)
Hungary	2,817	23.5	13.4
Cyprus	6,340	14.9	7.4
Latvia	2,275	14.2	6.7
Isle of Man	740	13.6	6.2
Greece	3,060	12.5	6.2
Slovenia	3,085	12.5	5.5
Austria	2,571	11.1	4.8
Faroe Islands	552	10.5	5.5
Iceland	3,510	10.5	4.8
Romania	2,289	10.1	4.2
Bulgaria	2,353	10.0	4.2
United Kingdom	2,179	9.2	4.0
Croatia	3,008	8.4	4.2
Ukraine	2,447	7.5	2.7
Slovakia	2,468	7.4	3.2
Belgium	1,889	6.4	2.6
Armenia[121]	4,055	4.1	1.4

Source: Kokkevi et al. (2011, p. 383)

---

[121] Armenia was included in the research as a transcontinental country on the border between Europe and Asia.

2007 ESPAD survey. In that year, thirty-five countries participated in the project; however, that being said, only seventeen countries completed the optional psychosocial module, which included questions related to the prevalence of self-harm. Hence, the analysis of the prevalence of self-harm was only conducted on a sample of 45,806 secondary school students aged 15 and 16 (Kokkevi et al. 2013).

The results from ESPAD demonstrate that the highest level of self-harm in adolescents (lifetime and repeated) was recorded in Hungary. During this period, the lifetime prevalence in Slovakia was 7.4%; although it should be noted that there are more recent studies that will be presented separately in the following section.

The preceding text makes it clear that the data regarding the prevalence of self-harm differs between individual countries. The reasons for the disparities include:
- different definitions of the range of activities included under the term of self-harm (from the broadest definition, any self-injury regardless of motivation (Morgan et al. 2017), through to the narrower understanding of the term, taking motivation into consideration, but not limiting the forms of self-harm (Jahari et al. 2017), the determination of a specific range of self-harming behaviours (De Leo & Heller 2004) or all the way to what is probably the narrowest definition, that of DSM-5 (Barrocas et al. 2012), which is limited to deliberate self-inflicted damage to the surface of the body that leads to minor or moderate physical harm (without suicidal intent);
- different understandings of self-harm in terms of the reported frequency of the phenomenon (certain studies report self-harm even for individuals where there is only a single lifetime occurrence (Nixon et al. 2008), while others require the behaviour be repeated (Leiva Pereira & Concha Landeros 2019));
- the diversity of the study samples in terms of age (it is apparent that self-harm is most common in late adolescence and in early adulthood, meaning that the data from samples of children (Barrocas et al. 2012) will differ from that of the adolescent (Morgan et al. 2017) and adult (Ose et al. 2021) population, or from samples which are not age-specific (McManus et al. 2018));
- gender differences in the study samples (self-harm tends to be more prevalent in women, which means that research samples

that mainly consist of men (Jarahi et al. 2021) will provide different results to gender-balanced samples (Horváth et al. 2020) or those that primarily include women (Nixon et al. 2008);
- differences between the study samples as to the source of the participants (a randomised selection from the general public (Leiva Pereira et al. 2019) should demonstrate a different prevalence of self-harm to that observed at the in-patient departments of psychiatric clinics (Ose et al. 2021) or for samples made up of the official reports of the urgent treatment of individuals (Jung et al. 2018), who sought medical help after an injury);
- differences in the methods used in terms of the scope of the observed types of self-harming behaviours (methods that limit the possible range of monitored behaviours by explicitly listing certain forms of self-harm, without the possibility of adding other individual forms as opposed to questionnaires or interviews that allow the participant to add other specific forms to the offered list of forms of self-harm (Nixon et al. 2008), thus making the data on prevalence more accurate)[122];
- the diversity of the methodologies used in terms of the method used for the collection of data (anonymous self-reporting questionnaires (such as Watanabe et al. 2012) usually provides a higher level of subjective comfort for the participant in reporting self-harming as opposed to a confrontational interview (e.g., Barrocas et al. 2012), in which the reported prevalence tends to be lower);
- differences in the period of time over which self-harm is considered (lifetime prevalence that identifies the presence of self-harm at any point in the past, such as that used by Lim et al.

---

[122] In this context, further differences were pointed out by Muehlenkamp et al. (2012), who analysed the available studies on the prevalence of non-suicidal self-injury in adolescents. They discovered that if questionnaires only used the option of a dichotomous answer (yes/no) to questions related to the occurrence of self-harm, the mean lifetime prevalence of self-harm was 12.5%. However, if the researchers used methods which allowed the participants to choose a response from several items, the mean prevalence was 23.6%, which is almost double. Hence, it is clear that in order to map out the specific occurrence of this phenomenon, it is crucial to explain what the term self-harm encompasses to the participants – for example, by confronting the variability of forms of self-harm directly within the questionnaire (interview).

(2019) as opposed to limiting the considered period of time to the past year (APA 2013) or the past four months – Jarahi et al. 2021).

In the scientific literature, we can find efforts to integrate the findings from several studies and approaches – one of the first studies to do so is the work of J. J. Muehlenkamp et al. (2012), who analysed scientific studies related to the prevalence of self-harm in terms of two "types" of behaviour: non-suicidal self-injury (NSSI) and deliberate self-harm (DSH). Interestingly they found that while the mean lifetime prevalence of self-harm (in its broader definition of deliberate self-harm) in adolescents aged 11–18 was 16.1%, in the narrower meaning of non-suicidal self-injury, it had a mean lifetime prevalence of 18%. This paradox may be interpreted in the context of a further research finding from the authors of this study – they state that when more detailed questionnaires were used for the data collection, the prevalence of self-harming behaviour, reported by the participants, was almost twice as high as was reported with the use of simple questions that observed the lifetime prevalence of self-harm with a "yes/no" option (Muehlenkamp et al. 2012). Thus, it appears that mainly children and adolescents need clarification of what is actually meant by self-harm and need to understand the range of behaviours that are included in this phenomenon in order to be able to identify such behaviour in their lives. A similar interpretation may be made with regard to the higher result of the prevalence of non-suicidal self-injury, which is specifically defined, as opposed to the more general term "deliberate self-harm" – while the definition of non-suicidal self-injury stems from the DSM-5 diagnostic criteria, which set out, in detail, all the forms that are included under this term, "deliberate self-harm" is more vague and ambiguous and it is possible that when this term was used in the studies assessed, it was not entirely clear which forms of behaviour it was intended to cover.

An analysis of the existing scientific studies was also conducted by Donna Gilles et al. (2018). The authors collected data from 172 databases that were available, covering the period 1990–2015 and mapping the prevalence of self-harm in more than half a million participants in forty-one countries. The mean lifetime prevalence was 16.9%, and the maximum value was identified in the data from the last year they analysed (2015). Another interesting finding was observed in the data regarding the mean age of the onset of self-harm (13 years) as well as information on the higher prevalence of self-harm in female subjects (Gilles et al. 2018).

A similar approach was applied in the work of Lim et al. (2019). The authors analysed data from 66 studies from the period 1989–2018, with a total of 686,672 children and adolescents. First, they observed the prevalence of deliberate self-harm, which they defined as "self-injurious behaviour, both with and without suicidal intent that has a non-fatal outcome" (Lim et al. 2019, 3) as well as the prevalence of non-suicidal self-injury, defined as "deliberate, self-inflicted destruction of body tissue without suicidal intent and for purposes not socially sanctioned, such as cutting, burning, and biting" – ibid. The researchers identified stark differences in the prevalence of the two types of behaviour: the heterogeneity of data for deliberate self-harm was $I^2 = 99.63$, $p < 0.001$ and for non-suicidal self-injury $I^2 = 99.22$, $p < 0.001$; the lifetime prevalence of deliberate self-harm was 13.7%, and in the case of non-suicidal self-injury, the value was 22.1% (Lim et al. 2019).

3.2 The Prevalence of Self-Harm in Slovakia

Data related to the prevalence of self-harm in Slovakia is rather scarce. Slovakia has participated in several pan-European studies (such as ESPAD, which found that the prevalence, from the data collection in 2007, was 7.4% for lifetime self-harm and 3.2% for repeated self-harm – see previous chapter) which have investigated (among others) this high-risk behaviour. Specialised studies that have exclusively observed self-harm during adolescence, published in the available scientific literature, are quite rare.

In 2012, Širilová and Kasová published the results of research into both the total prevalence of self-harm as well as the prevalence of individual forms of self-harm. The research sample was made up of ninety-two pupils from primary schools in the Košice region (46 boys, 46 girls) from 12–16 years of age with a mean age of 13.84. In order to measure the prevalence of self-harm, they used the Self-Harm Inventory (Sansone et al. 1998), in particular,

3 The Occurrence of Self-Harm

14 of its 22 items that are dedicated to the "disturbance of bodily integrity". These included items (see Table 9), which considered physical self-harm, in both its direct (such as self-cutting) and indirect (overdose of medication) forms. It is a self-reporting questionnaire (see the following section) in which adolescents were invited to state their frequency of self-harm (1 – never, 2 – once a year, 3 – once a month, 4 – once a week), allowing the authors to observe the prevalence over three periods (the past year, the past months and the past week). According to the findings, self-harm occurred in forty-three adolescents, which is a total prevalence of 46.7%. The prevalence of self-harm over the specific periods monitored and the forms of self-harm are presented in Table 9.

Table 9. The prevalence of selected forms of self-harm among Slovak adolescents in 2012

Forms of Self-Harm	Frequency			
	Never n (%)*	Once a year n (%)	Once a month n (%)	Once a week n (%)
Medication overdose	36	5	1	1
Self-cutting	28	8	6	1
Skin-burning	40	2	0	1
Skin-piercing	35	5	2	1
Self-tattooing	31	3	2	7
Biting nails until they bleed	28	3	5	7
Self-hitting	36	1	2	4
Hair pulling	39	1	1	2
Scratching until one bleeds	35	4	1	3
Preventing wounds from healing	32	4	1	6
Suicide attempts	35	5	1	2
Deliberate self-injury	29	6	5	3
Starvation	36	3	3	1
Use of laxatives	41	2	0	0

Note: *Data regarding the percentages were added to the original table
Source: Širilová & Kasová (2012, 118)

A study that focused on self-harming behaviour in adolescents from orphanages was conducted in Slovakia in 2013 (Širilová & Radoňáková 2013). The study sample was made up of seventy-two children between 13 and 18 (mean age = 16.4), 73.6% of whom were boys. In order to identify self-harm, the study employed an abbreviated version of the Questionnaire of Self-Harm Forms by Širilová & Lovaš (2012), which monitored twelve forms of self-harm – self-cutting, skin-burning, skin-piercing, self-hitting, scratching, hair pulling, self-tattooing, biting nails, excessive use of medication, excessive use of alcohol, excessive smoking and preventing wounds from healing (Širilová & Radoňáková 2013). All of these are physical forms of self-harm, and the frequency of occurrence of each form was described by the participants on a five-point scale (from 1 = never to 5 = daily). Based on the results, the prevalence of self-harm in this sample of adolescents was 50%.

A study by a school psychologist published in 2015 presented the findings of the prevalence of self-harm in a class[123] of a primary school in the capital of Slovakia. The author of the paper mentions the presence of recent cuts, as well as older cuts on the forearms of seven out of thirty-four pupils (20.6%) (Ferková 2015), which is a high rate considering the method of inquiry into self-harm[124]. We assume that if the area of observation was extended beyond the forearm and visible wounds from cuts, with, in particular, the inclusion of forms of self-harm other than "self-cutting", the result would be a much higher prevalence.

In the same year, the results of another study by Z. K. Širilová were published. She observed the occurrence of self-harm in a sample of ninety-nine adolescents living at home and eighty-three adolescents living in social care facilities. The method used was the Self-Harm Inventory, but the author only used eight out

---

123 The survey was initiated after it was discovered that one of the pupils self-harmed and that this behaviour was not unusual in the class (see Ferková 2015).
124 It is not a scientific study, but only an isolated empirical piece of data about the prevalence on a small sample. The study fails to include information on the method used to obtain information regarding the cut wounds. It appears that other forms of self-harm were not investigated and the period over which the self-harm was observed is also not clear (i.e. how "old" could the scars be and how much time might have passed after the act of self-harm so that the author was still able to identify them), since the only criterion for labelling a pupil as a self-harmer was (probably) only the presence of visible cut wounds on forearms.

of the original twenty-two forms of behaviour (e.g., deliberate self-cutting, skin-burning) with the option to only respond either yes or no. The study focused on lifetime prevalence, and those adolescents who listed at least a single form of self-harm over their lifetime were considered to be self-harmers. It was discovered that the prevalence among adolescents living at home was 40.4%, but the figure was even higher for adolescents living in social care facilities (54.2%) (Širilová 2015). When compared to the lifetime prevalence of self-harm in Slovakia presented in the results of the ESPAD survey from 2007 (7.4%), the increase of this high-risk behaviour in adolescence is rather stark.

A more extensive study was published in 2018[125], the aim of which was to map out the prevalence of self-harm among adolescents in Slovakia. A modified version of the Self-Harm Inventory (SHI) (Sansone & Sansone, 2010) was used for monitoring self-harming behaviour. It is a self-reporting questionnaire that includes twenty-two questions that observe the presence of individual forms of self-harming behaviour. The translation, back-translation and translation quality evaluation were conducted by independent evaluators. The individual items of the questionnaire were preceded by the phrase: "Have you ever intentionally, or on purpose, done any of the following to hurt yourself?", followed by various forms of self-harm, such as: "Cut yourself on purpose", "Burned yourself on purpose", "Made medical situations worse on purpose (e.g. skipped medications)", "Tortured yourself with self-defeating thoughts", etc. Three items from the original questionnaire were omitted ("Engaged in sexually abusive relationships", "Lost a job on purpose" and "Driven recklessly on purpose"), since the target sample included adolescents aged 11 to 18, for whom these items were inappropriate. On the other hand, two items were added to the questionnaire: "Did not sleep enough to hurt myself" and "Overexercised on purpose". The resulting questionnaire consisted of twenty-one items with

---

[125] For detailed information regarding the research, see: Démuthová, S., & Doktorová, D. (2019). Interpohlavné rozdiely v prevalencii jednotlivých foriem sebapoškodzovania u adolescentov. [Gender differences in the prevalence of individual forms of self-harm in adolescents]. In A. Baranovská (ed.), Kondášove dni 2018. [Kondas´ Days 2018] (19–32). Univerzita sv. Cyrila a Metoda.

good internal consistency (Cronbach's α = 0.809). Those adolescents that reported at least one occurrence of any of the listed forms of self-harm were considered to be self-harmers (meaning that the questionnaire monitored the life-time prevalence, and the occurrence of only one self-harming act was sufficient). The prevalence was measured using a sample of 1,831 participants, with 11.4% (n = 209) excluded from the analyses due to incorrectly completed questionnaires or missing data. The final sample consisted of 1,622 respondents in the age range 12–18 (mean age = 15.27, standard deviation = 1.79), 62.9% of whom were female (n = 1,020). At least one form of self-harm was reported by 29.9% of the sample (n = 485) (Démuthová & Doktorová 2019).

Following on from this the data collection continued – in 2020, the data set was made up of 2,280 participants[126]. The methods used for the analyses of the prevalence of self-harm were identical – they used a modified version of the self-report questionnaire SHI, and they monitored the lifetime prevalence of self-harm. Out of a total number of 2,280 questionnaires, 61 (0,27%) were excluded due to incomplete data. The final study sample was made up of 2,219 adolescents (63.1% were female) in the age range 11–19 (mean age = 15.34). The prevalence of self-harm, with the occurrence of at least one form of self-harm, increased in comparison to the 2019 results, to 56%. This study (see Démuthová & Démuth 2020) also monitored the repeated[127] occurrence of self-harm. In this SHI questionnaire, the participants were asked to express how often they performed the individual forms of self-harm on a four-point scale (ranging from 0 = never to 3 = often). In order to classify a participant into the group of repeatedly self-harming individuals, it was necessary to score at least one form of self-harming behaviour with a frequency of 2 or 3, or to report several forms of self-harming behaviour with a frequency of 1 or above. Using these criteria, the prevalence of repeated self-harm was 45.2%; thus Slo-

---

[126] The results of the study are available in: Démuthová, S., & Démuth, A. (2020). Self-harm in adolescence as maladaptive coping. Brain : broad research in artificial intelligence and neuroscience, 11(2), 37-47, https://doi.org/10.18662/brain/11.2Sup1/92.

[127] In line with the definition proposed in the conclusion of chapter "1.4 The Definition of Self-Harm", which suggests that the term "self-harm" should be understood as the repeated act of harming oneself.

vakia should be included among countries that have a high prevalence of this form of high-risk behaviour.

3.3 Methods Used for the Study of the Prevalence of Self-Harm

As a result of differences in the understanding of self-harm and other (cultural, age...) differences, several methods have been established to try to identify the prevalence of this phenomenon as well as its intensity and nature. Scientific studies have employed several kinds of scales and questionnaires – self-reporting (where the answers are provided by the individual, who also evaluates their own behaviour), such as the Deliberate Self-Harm Inventory (Gratz 2001), the Non-suicidal Self-Injury Assessment Tool (Whitlock et al. 2014); "clinical" (in which the self-harming behaviour is evaluated by a clinician – psychiatrist, physician, psychologist, etc.), such as the Self-Injury Trauma Scale (Iwata et al. 1990), the Self-Injurious Behaviour Questionnaire (Paivio & McCulloch 2004); or combined (partially evaluated by the patient/client and partially by another person, usually a physician or a psychologist), such as the Alexian Brothers Assessment of Self-Injury (Washburn et al. 2015). In addition to (self-)assessment scales and questionnaires, there are also some interview methods – these may be strictly structured, such as the Self-Injurious Thoughts and Behaviours Interview (Nock et al. 2007), but there are also some that involve open (non-structured) interviews. The following paragraphs will present[128] the most common methods.

---

128 The full text of the methods is intentionally not presented (to preserve their validity, which would be threatened if they were published) – only their descriptions are used, and parts of them are presented as examples. The methods are listed in the alphabetical order; they are not categorised by type (self-report/assessment, questionnaire/interview).

The Alexian Brothers Assessment of Self-Injury

The Alexian Brothers Assessment of Self-Injury (ABASI) was developed by Washburn et al. (2015). It includes key items from the specific criteria for NSSI (non-suicidal self-injury) as formulated in the fifth revision of the Diagnostic and Statistical Manual of Mental Disorders (DSM-5), appendix Conditions for Further Study (APA 2013) (Table 10). It is a self-reporting scale, with the exception of sections E and F[129] of the criteria[130], which are assessed through diagnoses by psychiatrists and an evaluation of the total level of function of the individual (Victor et al. 2017). The remaining areas are assessed by the respondent themselves – making it a combined method – it is partially self-reporting and partially assessed by experts.

The authors verified the reliability and validity of the measurements of self-harming behaviour using ABASI on a sample of psychiatric patients aged 12–52 (mean age = 17.3), who had been treated for NSSI, limiting the validity of the study to the psychiatric population (Victor et al. 2017).

Washburn et al. also developed another method – the Alexian Brothers Urge to Self-Injure Scale (ABUSI), which specifically focuses on the severity of the urge to self-harm. This method was also tested on a sample of adolescents with excellent results in terms of its validity, reliability and internal consistency (Washburn et al. 2010).

---

129 These are the last two diagnostic criteria, i.e.: "E. The behavior or its consequences cause clinically significant distress or interference in interpersonal, academic, or other important areas of functioning; F. The behavior does not occur exclusively during psychotic episodes, delirium, substance intoxication, or substance withdrawal. In individuals with a neurodevelopmental disorder, the behavior is not part of a pattern of repetitive stereotypies. The behavior is not better explained by another mental disorder or medical condition (e.g., psychotic disorder, autism spectrum disorder, intellectual disability, Lesch-Nyhan syndrome, stereotypic movement disorder with self-injury, trichotillomania [hair-pulling disorder], excoriation [skin-picking] disorder)" (see: APA 2013, 803).

130 All the criteria were listed in the section "1.3 The Terminology of Self-Harm", sub-section Non-Suicidal Self-Injury.

Table 10. DSM-5 criteria for non-suicidal self-injury (NSSI) disorder and corresponding ABASI items

DSM-5 Criteria	ABASI Item(s)
A.	...*
B. The individual engages in the self-injurious behaviour with one or more of the following expectations: 1. To obtain relief from a negative feeling or cognitive state. 2. To resolve an interpersonal difficulty. 3. To induce a positive feeling state.	Met Criterion B if responded with Agree or Strongly agree to at least one of the following items: "When I self-injure, I expect that it will..." 1. Provide relief from negative feelings or thoughts. 2. Fix or resolve problems with other people. 3. Create or increase positive feelings (happy, joyful, excited, cheerful, etc.)
C.	...*
D. The behaviour is not socially sanctioned (e.g., body piercing, tattooing, part of a religious or cultural ritual) and is not restricted to picking a scab or nail biting.	Picking scabs and nail biting were excluded as NSI behaviours, and the phrase "to hurt yourself or cause pain" was added to clarify any behaviour that may be used for purposes other than self-injury,
E.	...*
F.	...*

Note: Criteria are drawn from the Diagnostic and Statistical Manual of Mental Disorders, 5th edition, copyright 2013, American Psychiatric Association
*These parts were intentionally left out.
Source: Washburn et al. (2015, 32)

The Clinician-Administered Non-suicidal Self-Injury Disorder Index

The Clinician-Administered Non-suicidal Self-Injury Disorder Index (CANDI) is another method that focuses on self-harm as understood in DSM-5 (as the Non-suicidal Self-Injury Disorder – NSSID). The authors of CANDI state that when constructing this method, they built upon the earlier Deliberate Self-Harm Inventory (DSHI)[131], adding items for the observation of the frequency

---

131 It is described in the following section.

and type of self-harming behaviour, as well as the number of days during which self-harm occurred. This adjustment allowed them to observe whether the criteria for NSSID in DSM-5 were met (especially criterion A). CANDI is a semi-structured clinical interview that was originally intended for the adult population (for which it was validated). Psychometric studies confirmed good internal consistency as well as good reliability of the measurement tool (Gratz et al. 2015). Several studies describe the successful use of CANDI on the population of adolescents, especially under clinical conditions (see Zetterqvist et al. 2020).

The Deliberate Self Harm Inventory

The Deliberate Self Harm Inventory (DSHI) is a 17-item self-reporting questionnaire used for monitoring behavioural expressions of self-harm. It was created by Kim L. Gratz (Gratz 2001), and in its early stages, it was validated on adults in the age group 18–64 (mean age 23.19). However, since it was created, it has also been

---

This questionnaire asks about a number of different things that people sometimes do to hurt themselves. Please be sure to read each question carefully and respond honestly. Often, people who...
...*
1. Have you ever intentionally (i.e., on purpose) cut your wrist, arms, or other area(s) of your body (without intending to kill yourself)? (circle one):
Yes   No
If yes,
How old were you when you first did this? _____
How many times have you done this? _____
...*
Have you ever intentionally (i.e., on purpose)
2. Burned yourself with a cigarette?
3. Burned yourself with a lighter or a match?
...*
16. Prevented wounds from healing?
17. Done anything else to hurt yourself that was not asked about in this questionnaire? If yes, what did you do to
hurt yourself? _____

*These parts were intentionally left out.

Figure 4. Examples of items from the DSHI questionnaire
Source: Gratz et al. (2001, 262)

successfully used on adolescents (see Brunner et al. 2013; Garish et al. 2015; Boričević Maršanić 2015); it was also confirmed that the inventory has good quality psychometric parameters (Fliege et al. 2006). DSHI considers self-harm to be deliberate, direct harm or a change to the tissue of the body without any suicidal intent; nonetheless, that leads to harm that is sufficiently severe that it results in visible damage to the tissue. This concept is almost identical to the definition presented by DSM. DSHI evaluates various aspects of deliberate self-harm including the frequency, severity, duration and type of self-harming behaviour (see Figure 4). The spectrum of behaviour monitored by DSHI is based on clinical observations, numerous testimonies of self-harming individuals and on various forms of behaviour described in the scientific literature (Gratz 2001).

The Functional Assessment of Self-Mutilation

The Functional Assessment of Self-Mutilation (FASM) was one of the first self-assessment scales used to monitor self-mutilation. It was developed in 1997 by Elisabeth Lloyd, and it monitors the frequency of self-harming behaviour, its function and other specific characteristics (see Figure 5), such as the degree of physical pain, the time during which participants contemplated self-harm, or the use of alcohol or drugs during self-harm. The author initially verified the method on a sample of 368 adolescents from 12 to 19 years old (Lloyd 1997), but since it was published, it has been used for various other samples (in terms of the age and nature of the sample) (e.g., Kaess et al. 2013; Andover 2014; Izadi-Mazidi et al. 2019).

The FASM is made up of two parts – the first monitors the occurrence of eleven types of self-harming behaviour over the past year, putting them into two categories that create independent factors: moderate/severe (such as cutting, burning) and mild (hair pulling, self-hitting…). The second part is only completed by those participants who reported at least one self-harming behaviour in their lifetimes. It includes twenty-two questions related to the reasons (motives) for self-harm (Lloyd-Richardson et al. 2007). These are evaluated by the respondent on the Likert scale: 0 – "never", 1 – "rarely", 2 – "some" to 3 "often" (Izadi-Mazidi et al. 2019).

> Have you ever engaged in the following behaviors within past year (check all that apply):
>
> No   Yes   Approx. how   Have you gotten
>   many times?   medical treatment?
>
> 1. cut or carved on your skin
> 2. hit yourself on purpose
> 3. pulled your hair out
> ...*
> 11. "erased" your skin
> 12. other: _____
> ...*
>
> Did you perform any of the above behaviors while you were taking drugs or alcohol?   Yes   No
> ...*
>
> Did you harm yourself for any of the reasons listed below?
> (check all reasons that apply):   0   1   2   3
>   Never   Rarely   Some   Often
>
> 1. to avoid school, work, or other activities
> 2. to relieve feeling "numb" or empty
> 3. to get attention
> 4. to feel something, even if it was pain
> ...*
> 21. to make others angry
> 22. to feel relaxed
> 23. other: _____
>
> *These parts were intentionally left out

Figure 5. Examples of items from the FASM questionnaire
Source: Lloyd (1997, 90-92)

The Inventory of Statements about Self-Injury

The Inventory of Statements about Self-Injury (ISAS) is a self-assessment method used for the complex assessment of the function of non-suicidal self-injury (NSSI). The ISAS consists of two parts – the first evaluates the lifetime frequency of twelve types of self-harming behaviour. The participants are asked to report whether they intentionally performed some of the listed forms of behaviour (i.e., on purpose) without any suicidal intent (examples are shown in Figure 6). The participants then report the frequency of the individual behaviours. The following five questions evaluate the descriptive and contextual factors of self-harm, such as the age of onset, the experience of pain during the NSSI, whether the

3 The Occurrence of Self-Harm

> SECTION I. BEHAVIOURS
> This questionnaire asks about a variety of self-harm behaviors. Please only endorse a behaviour if you have done it intentionally (i.e., on purpose) and without suicidal intent (i.e., not for suicidal reasons).
> 1. Please estimate the number of times in your life you have intentionally (i.e., on purpose) performed each type of non-suicidal self-harm (e.g., 0, 10, 100, 500):
> Cutting _____ Severe Scratching _____
> Biting _____ Banging or Hitting Self _____
> Burning _____ Carving _____
> ...*
> 5. When you self-harm, are you alone? Please circle a choice:
> YES – SOMETIMES – NO
> ...*
>
> SECTION II. FUNCTIONS
> This inventory was written to help us better understand the experience of non-suicidal self-harm. Below is a list of statements that may or may not be relevant to your experience of self-harm. Please identify the statements that are most relevant for you:
>   Circle 0 if the statement not relevant for you at all
>   Circle 1 if the statement is somewhat relevant for you
>   Circle 2 if the statement is very relevant for you
> "When I self-harm, I am ...
> 1. ... calming myself down   0   1   2
> 2. ... creating a boundary between myself and others   0   1   2
> 3. ... punishing myself   0   1   2
> ...*
> 11. ... creating a physical sign that I feel awful   0   1   2
> 12. ... getting back at someone   0   1   2
> ...*
> 38. ... trying to hurt someone close to me   0   1   2
> ...*
>
> *These parts were intentionally left out.

Figure 6. Examples of items from the ISAS questionnaire
Source: https://www2.psych.ubc.ca/~klonsky/publications/ISASmeasure.pdf

individual self-harms alone or in the presence of others, the time between the urge to self-harm and the act of self-harm and whether the individual wants to stop this behaviour. The second part of the questionnaire is completed by those respondents who reported at least one occurrence of self-harm in their lives. This part monitors thirteen potential functions of NSSI: affect-regulation, anti-dissociation, anti-suicide, autonomy, interpersonal boundaries, interpersonal influence, marking distress, peer-bonding, self-care, self-punishment, revenge, sensation seeking and toughness. Each function is assessed on a three-point scale (0, 1 and 2 points) depending on the intensity of the agreement with the statement (related to the corresponding function). In the second part of the ISAS, the participant may score 0–6 points for each of the thirteen functions (giving a total of 0–78 points) (Klonsky & Glenn 2009).

The Impulse, Self-Harm and Suicide Ideation Questionnaire for Adolescents

The Impulse, Self-Harm and Suicide Ideation Questionnaire for Adolescents (ISSIQ-A) is a self-reporting questionnaire specifically aimed at adolescents. It is made up of two parts – in the first part, which includes 25 items, the adolescent evaluates their impulsiveness, self-harming and risky behaviour as well as suicidal thoughts. In the second, 31-item section focuses on the evaluation of the motives/functions of self-harm. In this section, the adolescent describes the presence of "reinforcement" through self-harm by responding to 24 items – this function occurs in cases when the aim of self-harm is to induce a desirable emotional state or, on the contrary, to reduce or eliminate disturbing emotional states. The following seven items monitor "social reinforcement" as a motive/function of self-harm, in which self-harm is a way to manipulate social interactions – such as a call for help or self-harm performed as revenge on others. The adolescent marks the answers on a four-point Likert scale (from 0 – never to 3 – always), with the exception of the section dedicated to motives/functions, in which they respond yes/no. The validity and the reliability of the questionnaire were tested on a sample of 1,722 adolescents and provided satisfactory results (Caravalho et al. 2015).

The Non-suicidal Self-Injury-Assessment Tool

The Non-suicidal Self-Injury-Assessment Tool (NSSI-AT) was developed by Janis Whitlock and Amanda Purington (Whitlock et al. 2014) as part of the Cornell Research Program on Self-Injury and Recovery (www.selfinjury.bctr.cornell.edu), and it is one of the

A. Primary and secondary NSSI characteristics
1. Have you ever done any of the following with the purpose of intentionally hurting yourself?
   - Severely scratched or pinched with fingernails or other objects to the point that bleeding occurs or marks remain on the skin
   - Cut wrists, arms, legs, torso or other areas of the body
   ...*
   - Engaged in fighting or other aggressive activities with the intention of getting hurt
2. Are there any other ways that you have physically hurt or mutilated your body with the purpose of intentionally hurting yourself?
   - Yes; please specify
   - No

B. Functions
How true are the following statements about why you hurt yourself? Please select the most accurate response.
I hurt myself...   Strongly Disagree   Somewhat Disagree   Somewhat Agree   Strongly Agree
...to feel something
...because my friends hurt themselves
...*
...because of my self-hatred
...because I like the way it looks
...*
Other, please describe
...*

F. Initial Motivation
Which of the following descriptions best describes your motivations for first intentionally hurting yourself? (Please check all that apply)
- A friend suggested that I try it
- I read about it on the Internet and decided to try it
- I saw it in a movie / on television or read about it in a book and decided to try it
- It seemed to work for other people I know
...*
- I was drunk or high
- Other; please specify
- I cannot remember

G. Severity
Have you ever intentionally hurt yourself more severely than you expected?
...*

*These parts were intentionally left out.

Figure 7. Examples of items from the NSSI-AT questionnaire
Source: Whitlock et al. (2014; http://webcache.googleusercontent.com/search?q=cache:RB6-zlFhkWIJ:www.selfinjury.bctr.cornell.edu/perch/resources/bnssi-at-revised-final.pdf+&cd=1&hl=sk&ct=clnk&gl=sk)

more complex and extensive questionnaires in terms of its range and content. It is a self-reporting method that is made up of 12 parts (with a total of 39 questions) that observe: A/ forms of self-harm (all of the listed forms may be considered as physical self-harm), B/ functions of self-harm, C/ how recent and frequent is the self-harm, D/ the age of onset and possible disappearance/termination of self-harm, E/ the placement of wounds on the body, F/ the initial motivation, G/ the severity of self-harm, H/ habits in self-harm, I/ habituation and the perceived interference with life, J/ informing others of self-harm, K/ experiences with the treatment of self-harm, L/ personal reflections and advice (examples are provided in Figure 7).

The Non-suicidal Self-Injury Disorder Scale

The Non-suicidal Self-Injury Disorder Scale (NSSIDS) is based on the NSSI diagnostic criteria formulated in DSM-5 (just as is ABASI). Unlike ABASI, it does not monitor indirect physical forms of self-harm, such as deliberate starvation and does not include the option to add extra forms of self-harm. The NSSIDS is a self-assessment scale intended for older adolescents and adults; considering the fact that it requires a sufficient degree of introspection (in the self-assessment as well as the evaluation of motivation), it is not suitable for younger children (the individual items and corresponding questions are presented in Table 11). As to the description and analysis of the psychometric properties of this method, similar questionnaires were used: the ISAS (Inventory of Statements about Self-Injury), DSHI (Deliberate Self-Harm Inventory) and FASM (Functional Assessment of Self-Mutilation) (see Victor et al. 2017).

The Ottawa Self-Injury Inventory

The Ottawa Self-Injury Inventory (OSI) is a relatively extensive questionnaire that monitors self-harm in 26 areas. It monitors the frequency of self-harm over the past month/six months/year; attempted suicide; medical interventions; the onset of self-harm; feel-

3 The Occurrence of Self-Harm

Table 11. An example of the DSM 5 criteria for Non-suicidal Self-Injury Disorder (NSSID) and NSSIDS items

DSM-5 Criteria	NSSIDS Item(s)
A. Engagement in NSSI without suicidal intent on 5 or more days in the past year.	1. In the last year, on how many separate days have you engaged in any of these behaviours intentionally (i.e., on purpose) and without suicidal intent (i.e., not for suicidal reasons)? 2. In the past, prior to the last year, was there ever a time when you engaged in any of these behaviours on 5 or more separate days, over the course of 1 year? 2b. If so, how many separate days did you engage in these behaviours during that year? If there have been multiple years in which you have self-harmed on 5 or more days, please write down how many separate days during the year in which you harmed yourself most frequently.
B. C. D. E.	...* ...* ...* ...*
F. NSSI does not exclusively occur during psychosis, delirium (1), substance intoxication, withdrawal (2), or better explained by another disorder, such as stereotypes (3).	14. How often do you engage in these behaviours when under the influence of drugs or alcohol? 15. How often do you engage in these behaviours in response to odd experiences, like hearing or seeing things that other people can't hear or see (e.g., voices or visions)? 16. Have you been diagnosed with a mental health disorder? 16b. If so, please indicate which mental health disorders you have been diagnosed with

Note: Criteria are drawn from the Diagnostic and Statistical Manual of Mental Disorders, 5th edition, copyright 2013, American Psychiatric Association
*These parts were intentionally left out.
Source: Victor et al. (2017, 274)

ings whilst self-harming; disclosure of self-harm to others; the areas (body parts) and forms of self-harm in the first episode, at the present time and the most common; the reasons for self-harm at the beginning and at the present time; feelings after self-harm; the delay of self-harm; the perception of pain during self-harm; triggers of self-harm; resisting self-harm; efforts to stop self-harming and potential substitutional activities; changes in self-harming behaviour (towards behaviour that exhibits signs of addiction – for examples, see Figure 8); treatment undergone (if any), and it also provides the opportunity to freely add important supplementary information regarding self-harm (if it is not included in the questionnaire) (Nixon 2005).

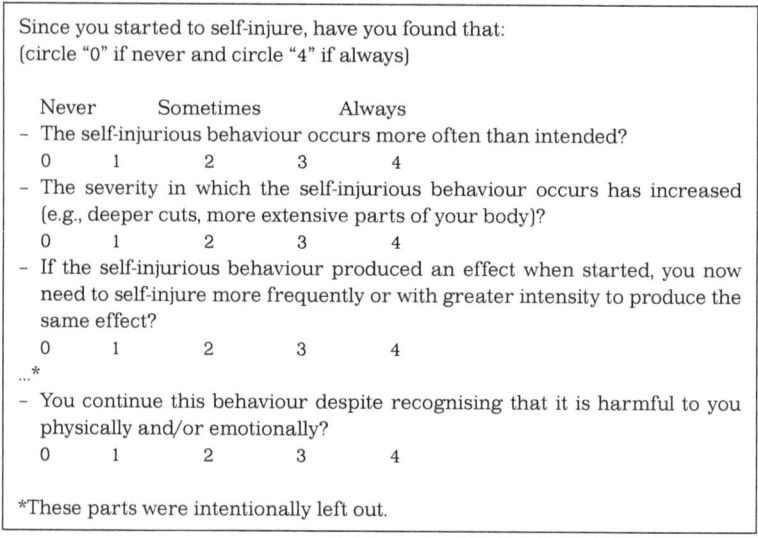

Figure 8. Examples of items from the OSI questionnaire
Source: Nixon (2005, 6; http://www.insync-group.ca/publications/OSI-2015-English-v3.1.pdf)

The OSI questionnaire is rather specific, in comparison to the other methods, in its potential to detect the addictive characteristics of self-harm. Ever since the OSI was first published, several studies have confirmed that it is a suitable method to use to identify self-harming behaviour in both the clinical (Matera et al. 2021) and non-clinical population (Brown et al. 2018), in both adolescents (Nixon et al. 2015) and young adults (Martin et al. 2013).

The Questionnaire for Non-suicidal Self-Injury

The Questionnaire for Non-suicidal Self-Injury (QNSSI) was developed by N. Kleindienst-om et al. in 2008. It was used on a sample of hospitalised patients with borderline personality disorder (Kleindienst et al. 2008). The QNSSI is a 34-item self-reporting questionnaire that monitors the frequency, forms and motives of self-harm. Its original (German) version was translated into English by B. Turner (Robillard 2018), which made it more widely available. Nevertheless, it is rarely used in studies.

The Risk-Taking and Self-Harm Inventory for Adolescents

Another self-reporting questionnaire, primarily developed for use with the adolescent population, is the Risk-Taking and Self-Harm Inventory for Adolescents (RTSHIA). This method is comprised of two factors – it assesses risky behaviour and self-harming behaviour (examples of the individual constituents are listed in Figure 9). It can be applied to both clinical and non-clinical samples of adolescents. The psychometric properties of the questionnaire were verified using a sample of 722 young people aged 11–18 (Vrouva et al. 2010).

The Self-Harm Behaviour Questionnaire

Apart from self-harm, the Self-Harm Behaviour Questionnaire (SHBQ) also observes suicidal behaviour. This self-reporting questionnaire was developed by P. M. Gutierrez, and the first psychometric data from this method was published in 2001 (Gutierrez et al. 2001), which was later confirmed by further measurements (Muehlenkamp et al. 2010). The SHBQ is not only used in English-speaking countries, but it has also been translated into German (Plener et al. 2009; 2012), extending its possible use. The questionnaire is mainly aimed at adolescents, but it has also been employed for young adults (see, for instance, Brausch et al. 2021). The SHBQ consists of 32 items divided into four sections (factors), which assess four different types of behaviour (the items under each of the individual factors are listed in Table 12).

The first part of the SHBQ questionnaire monitors self-harming behaviour, which is understood as deliberate, direct damage to bodily tissues without a conscious intent to commit suicide, that leads to an injury that is severe enough to cause damage to the tissue. In this part, the participant answers the question "Have you

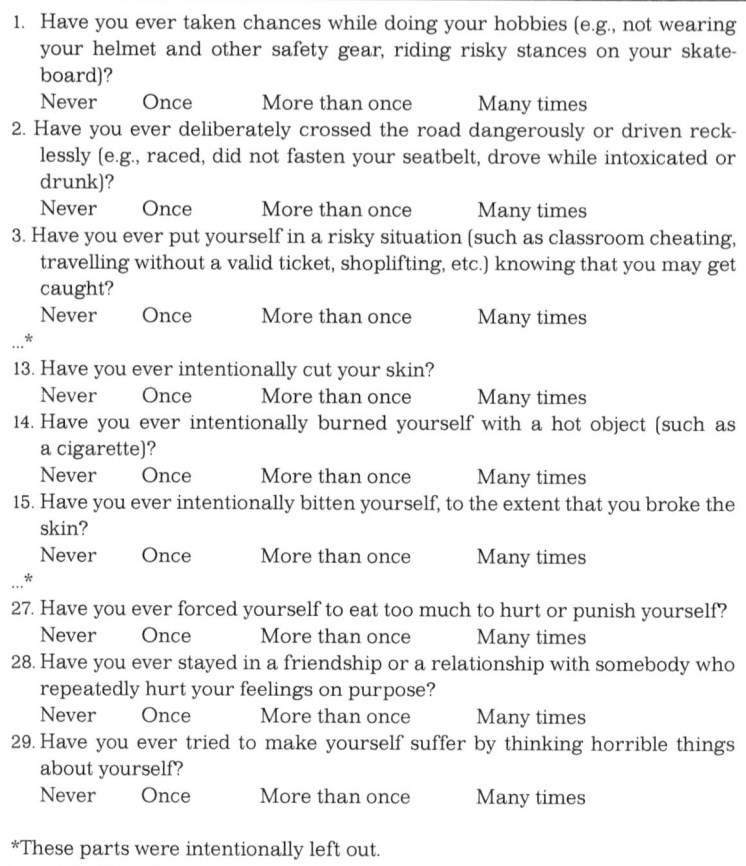

Figure 9. Examples of items from the questionnaire (RTSHIA)
Source: Vrouva et al. (2010, 863–865)

ever hurt yourself on purpose?" The following three parts deal with attempted suicide, threats to commit suicide and suicidal ideation. Each of these sections starts with the question of whether the behaviour has occurred before. The subsequent questions examine the specific characteristics of the behaviour including the methods, frequency, the first/last occurrence of the behaviour, the disclosure of the behaviour to others, the need for medical treatment and in those sections that assess suicidal behaviour, there are also questions concerning related events, intent, and preparations (Fliege et al. 2006).

Table 12. Items included in the factors of the SHBQ

Name of the Factor	Self-Harm	Suicide Ideation	Suicide Threat	Past Suicide Attempts
Items	Frequency	Method	Method	Method
	History	Related event	Frequency	Frequency
	Risk	Plan	History	Risk
	Disclosure	Reaction of others	Risk	Medical treatment
	Treatment	Preparation	Related event	Related event
			Intent	Intent

Source: Gutierrez et al. (2001, 481)

The Self-Injurious Behaviour Questionnaire

The Self-Injurious Behaviour Questionnaire[132] (SIBQ) was developed for a research study into alexithymia as a mediator between childhood trauma and self-injurious behaviour by S. C. Paivio and C. R. McCulloch (2004). In the process of developing the questionnaire, the authors built upon the method used to assess the occurrence of surface-level injuries caused by self-harming behaviour, developed by Weilderman et al. (1999). The questionnaire is completed by the participants themselves (it is a self-reporting method), who are asked to evaluate their lifetime frequency of self-cutting, burning, head hitting, scratching, self-hitting and pulling the hair on a 4-point Likert scale (ranging from 0 = never to 3 = often/many times). The reason the authors selected these specific forms of self-harm is that they are the most frequent types of surface-level self-harm. By adding the scores of the individual items, the method expresses the total involvement of the individual in self-harming behaviour. In their study (on a sample of 100 par-

---

[132] A questionnaire with the same name (Self-Injurious Behaviour Questionnaire) but a different acronym (SIB-Q) was developed earlier in 1997 by Schroeder et al. It is a clinically assessed (by an expert) 25-item scale with the possibility of assessing intensity on the Likert scale. However, since this method is mainly used to measure self-harming behaviour, especially in individuals with developmental disorders (Schroeder et al. 1997), it is not listed in the extensive overview of methods for general population (adolescents).

ticipants), the authors report a good level of internal consistency from this measurement tool (alpha coefficient = 0.84) (Paivio & McCulloch 2004).

The Self-Injury Trauma Scale

The Self-Injury Trauma Scale (SIT) is a "method for quantifying surface tissue damage caused by self-injurious behaviour" (Iwata et al. 1990, 99). The injuries are assessed by an expert and the scale allows for a highly precise assessment of several aspects of self-harm – its topography, the position of injuries on the body, types of injuries, and the number and estimated severity of the injuries (Figure 10).

PART II. MEASUREMENT OF SURFACE TRAUMA

For each area of the body containing a current (unhealed) injury, identify the location and number of wounds, and note the type and the severity of the worst wound at that particular location.

Number: Score: 1 One wound
                 2 Two-four wounds
                 3 Five or more wounds

Type: Abrasion or Laceration (AL): A break in the skin, either superficial or deep, caused by tearing, biting, excessive rubbing, or contact with a sharp object.
         Contusion (CT): A distinct area marked by abnormal discoloration or swelling, with or without tissue rupture, caused by forceful contact.

Severity: Score AL as: 1 Area is red or irritated, with only spotted breaks in the skin.
                       2 Break in the skin is distinct but superficial; no avulsion.
                       3 Break in the skin is deep or extensive, or avulsion is present.
          Score CT as: 1 Local swelling only or discoloration without swelling
                       2 Extensive swelling
                       3 Disfigurement or tissue rupture

Figure 10. An example of the assessment of injuries caused by self-harm on the SIT scale
Source: Iwata et al. (1990, 102)

In addition to the total score, the scale also works with three partial indexes – the number index (the number of injuries), the severity index (the severity of injuries) and the estimate of current risk. It can be applied to various age groups and since its development, it has been not only been used in clinical practice but also in several scientific studies (such as Symons et al. 2009; Kurtz et al. 2012; Fodstad et al. 2018).

The Self-Injury Questionnaire

The Self-Injury Questionnaire (SIQ) exists in two versions. According to Sansone and Sansone (2010), in addition to the Self-Injury Questionnaire developed by Alexander in 1999, there is also an older Self-Injury Questionnaire developed by Vanderlinden and Vandereycken used since 1997. The (older) questionnaire includes 54 items and exclusively captures self-harm (it does not consider suicidal behaviour). It monitors behaviours such as cutting, scratching, hair-pulling, bruising, burning, etc. The more recent questionnaire is made up of 30 items and investigates the total extent of self-harm. It evaluates self-harming behaviour from the perspective of its frequency, function and possible association with a history of childhood trauma.

The Self-Harm Inventory

The Self-Harm Inventory (SHI) was developed as a self-reporting scale that identifies self-harm. Originally, it was intended to be used as a screening method for borderline personality disorder (Sansone et al. 1998); however, after some time, it was also used in the monitoring of self-harm in other patients as well as the non-clinical population. In its pilot version, the questionnaire was made up of 41 items, and after some time, it settled on 22 items (Sansone & Sansone 2010) (Figure 11) with sufficient psychometric properties (Latimer et al. 2009).

SELF-HARM INVENTORY

Instructions:
Please answer the following questions by checking either, "Yes," or "No." Check "yes" only to those items that you have done intentionally, or on purpose, to hurt yourself.

Yes No Have you ever intentionally, or on purpose, done any of the following:
__ __ 1. Overdosed? (If yes, number of times ____)
__ __ 2. Cut yourself on purpose? (If yes, number of times ____)
__ __ 3. Burned yourself on purpose? (If yes, number of times ____)
__ __ 4. Hit yourself? (If yes, number of times ____)
...*
__ __ 21. Starved yourself to hurt yourself?
__ __ 22. Abused laxatives to hurt yourself? (If yes, number of times ____)

*These parts were intentionally left out.

Figure 11. Examples of items from the SHI questionnaire
Source: Sansone & Sansone (2010, 18)

The Self-Injurious Thoughts and Behaviours Interview

The Self-Injurious Thoughts and Behaviours Interview (SITBI) is a structured interview which evaluates the presence, frequency and characteristics of a wide range of self-injurious thoughts and behaviours, including suicidal ideation, suicidal plans, suicidal gestures, attempted suicide and self-injury (NSSI) (Nock et al. 2007). This method is thus primarily concerned with suicidal behaviour, but due to its broad scope, one of its (five) parts, that deals with self-harm, may be suitable for research into self-harm. The intent to cause death is excluded from the definition of self-harm, which follows the NSSI concept. The Self-Injurious Thoughts and Behaviours Interview is a relatively widely used form of a clinical interview – it has also been used outside of English-speaking countries (a German version was published in 2014) (Fischer et al. 2014) and gradually, updated versions have followed: The Self-Injurious Thoughts and Behaviours Interview-Short Form-Self-Report"(SITBI-SF-SR) and the more recent, revised Self-Injurious Thoughts and Behaviours Interview-Revised (SITBI - R) (Fox et al. 2020). The method was initially tested with adolescents, and it consists of 169 items divided into five sections that assess the pres-

Model:	Example of questions:
1/ Suicidal ideation	Have you ever had thoughts of killing yourself?
2/ Suicide plans	Have you ever actually made a plan to kill yourself?
3/ Suicide gestures	Have you ever done something to lead others to believe you wanted to kill yourself when you really had no intention of doing so?
4/ Suicide attempts	Have you ever made an actual attempt to kill yourself in which you had at least some intent to die?
5/ Non-suicidal self-injury	Have you ever done something to purposely hurt yourself without intending to die?

Figure 12. Examples of items in the individual SITBI modules
Source: Nock et al. (2007, 310)

ence, frequency and characteristics of the five types of SITB (Figure 12) (Nock et al. 2007).

The Suicidal Attempt Self-Injury Interview

The Suicidal Attempt Self-Injury Interview (SASII) is a structured interview intended to evaluate the factors that contribute to non-fatal attempted suicide and deliberate self-harm. Just as the previous method, this interview also primarily focuses on behaviour associated with suicidal tendencies – the lethality and impulsivity of the act, the likelihood of rescue, suicidal intent, motivations and consequences, and habitual self-injury. In terms of self-harm, it assesses, for instance, cutting, scratching, stabbing and burning as well as more severe forms, such as hanging, drowning, suffocating or the use of a gun. An interesting feature of the interview is that it also addresses indirect forms of self-harm – such as alcohol abuse for the purposes of self-harm (see Figure 13) or early termination of treatment. The validity and reliability of the method were examined through various samples of adult patients (Linehan et al. 2006), but in further studies, it was also used for the adolescent population (see, for instance, You et al. 2015).

To conclude, we have presented a practical overview of the basic areas and assessment methods used in the study of self-harm,

```
S1_____    At any time in the last year [your life, since last assessment, etc.]
           have you deliberately harmed or injured yourself or attempted
           suicide? (0 = No, 1 = Yes).
S2_____    How many times have you deliberately harmed or injured your-
           self or attempted suicide in the last year [your life, since last as-
           sessment, etc.]?
...*
FOR EACH OF THE FOLLOWING METHODS, CODE 0 = Not used, 1 = Used.
7.1_____   = Alcohol (used with direct intent to self-harm):
71a _____  What were you drinking?
           (1 = BEER, 2 = WINE, 3 = LIQUOR, 4 = COMBINATION OF 1 & 2, 5 =
           COMBINATION OF 1 & 3, 6 = COMBINATION OF 2 & 3, 7 = COM-
           BINATION OF 1, 2, & 3,  6 = OTHER, 71ao _____ )
71b _____  How much did you drink? (CODE SEC's) _____
...*
7.14_____  = Stopped required medical treatments or medications (with direct
           intent to self-harm):
714a What did you stop doing?
           _____ (1= STOPPED NEEDED MEDICAL TREATMENTS,
              2= STOPPED MEDICATIONS, 3=OTHER
714ao_____, 714b For how long was the treatment/medication stopped
           (hours)? _____
714c What was the treatment for? _____
714d What were expected consequences of stopping treatment: _____

*These parts were intentionally left out.
```

Figure 13. Examples of items from the SASII interview
Source: OSF | SASII-Standard-Short-Form-with-Supplemental-Questions.pdf (https://osf.io/zstnj/)

intended (among others) to be used for adolescents, as provided by E. Drzał-Fiałkiewcz et al. (2017). The author added this overview to the previous overview by Kubiak (2012). Both overviews are presented in[133] Table 13.

---

[133] Considering that Drzał-Fiałkiewcz et al. translated Kubiak's overview from the original language (Polish), it will only be listed as a secondary source; it is referred to in this way on page 349 of the work by Drzał-Fiałkiewcz et al. (2017).

3 The Occurrence of Self-Harm

Table 13. Methods used to monitor self-harming behaviour and their measurement goals

Methods	Scope of the Construct Definition							Goals and Application				
	Suicidal plans	Suicidal attempts	Suicide gestures	Suicidal thoughts	Non-suicidal self-injury	Culturally sanctioned	Indirect self-destructiveness	Frequency	Type	Severity	Reasons	Duration
Overview by Kubiak (2012):												
Self-Injury Self-Report Inventory (SISRI)		+			+		+	+	+	+	+	+
Deliberate Self-Harm Inventory (DSHI)					+			+	+	+		+
Self-Injurious Thought and Behaviour Interview (SITBI)	+	+	+	+	+			+	+	+	+	+
Inventory Statements about Self-Injury (ISAS)					+			+	+		+	
Self-Injury Motivation Scale II (SIMS)	+				+						+	
Functional Assessment of Self-Mutilation (FASM)					+			+	+		+	+
Self-Harm Behaviour Questionnaire (SHBQ)		+	+	+	+			+		+		
Ottawa Self-Injury Inventory (OSI)		+		+	+			+	+		+	
Self-Harm Inventory (SHI)		+			+		+					
Self-Injurious Behaviour Questionnaire (SIB-Q)					+							
Suicide Attempt Self-Injury Interview (SASII)		+	+	+	+			+		+	+	
Self-Harm Survey (SHS) I Motivations Underlying Self-Harm Questionnaire (HUSHQ)		+		+	+		+	+			+	

Tool										
Self-Injury Questionnaire (SIQ)			+	+	+	+	+		+	
Self-Injury Inventory (SII)			+		+	+	+			+
Self-Injury Questionnaire (SIQ)			+	+						
Overview by Drzał-Fiałkiewcz et al. (2017):										
Alexian Brothers Assessment of Self-Injury (ABASI)			+		+	+	+		+	
The Non-suicidal Self-Injury Assessment Tool (NSSI-AT)			+			+	+	+	+	+
Self-Injury Trauma Scale (SITS)			+				+	+		
Motivational Assessment Scale (MAS)			+						+	
Behaviour Problems Inventory (BPI)			+	+						
Overt Aggression Scale (OAS)			+	+			+			
Self-Injurious Thoughts and Behaviours Interview (SITB)	+	+	+	+	+					
Alexian Brothers Urge to Self-Injury Scale (ABUSI)			+			+				+

Source: Drzał-Fiałkiewcz et al. (2017, 349)

3.4 The Demographic Specificities of the Prevalence of Self-Harm

The data from published studies, presented in the previous sections, suggests that although self-harming behaviour is rather widespread in adolescents, its prevalence is higher in specific groups of individuals. These include patients with autism spectrum disorders (Maddox et al. 2017), mental retardation (van den Bogaard et al. 2018), borderline personality disorder (Glenn & Klonsky 2013), dissociative identity disorder (Webermann et al. 2016), post-traumatic stress disorder (Alharbi et al. 2020), eating disorders (Islam et al. 2015), depression (Nitkowski & Petermann 2011), obsessive-compulsive disorder (Bolognini et al. 2003) or individuals that suffer from anxiety disorders (Kiekens et al.

2018).¹³⁴ In the non-clinical population, these are individuals who use specific methods to process information that take the form of several cognitive distortions¹³⁵ and have an increased tendency to depressive moods (Andover et al. 2005), distorted self-image and low self-esteem (Forrester et al. 2017) or pronounced specific personality traits – such as an increased degree of impulsivity (Mitchell & Potenza 2014), or sensation seeking (Guérin-Marion et al. 2018).¹³⁶ In addition to the above-mentioned characteristics, many studies have observed correlations between the prevalence of self-harm and age or gender.

Age

Adolescence is believed to be the most vulnerable age for the initiation and the subsequent continuation of self-harming behaviour (Klemera et al. 2017). That being said, some studies suggest there is a peak intensity of self-harm at a certain age (e.g., Steinhoff et al. (2021) proposed age of 13), followed by a reduced tendency.¹³⁷

However, analyses carried out on a study sample of Slovak adolescents show that the prevalence, as well as the intensity, of self-harm during adolescence is probably not related to a specific age. This is the conclusion of a study from 2019, where an analysis of the prevalence of self-harm was conducted based on the age of participants on a sample of 966 adolescents from 12 to 18 years of age (mean age = 15.04), 59.9% of whom were females (n = 579) (Démuthová & Démuth 2019a). The study used a modified version of the Self-Harm Inventory (SHI – Sansone & Sansone 2010) to measure the prevalence. It includes a wide range of various forms of

---

134 Since the primary aim of this monograph is to analyse self-harming behaviour in the non-clinical population of adolescents, these cases will not be described in greater detail.
135 Such as dichotomous thinking, catastrophisation, etc. (Allen & Hooley 2015; Hasking et al. 2017).
136 These specific areas are discussed in Chapter 5.
137 However, more detailed analyses have demonstrated that where the authors took the gender and age of the adolescents into consideration, they obtained different data.

self-harm. It is a self-assessment questionnaire with 22 questions that establishes the presence (13 of the questions also attempt to establish frequency) of individual forms of self-harming behaviour. Three items included in the original questionnaire were deleted as the survey was conducted among children from the age of 11, namely: "Engaged in sexually abusive relationships", "Lost a job on purpose" (due to their inappropriateness for younger age groups) and "Driven recklessly on purpose" (since only individuals over the age of 18 may drive vehicles unsupervised in Slovakia). On the other hand, two additional items were added to the questionnaire, which tend to occur as forms of self-harm in the adolescent population: "Not slept enough on purpose to hurt myself" and "Overexercised on purpose". Thus, the modified form of the questionnaire was made up of 21 items. In order for self-harm to be present, an individual only needed to report a single form of self-harm in their lifetime.

An analysis of age versus the prevalence of self-harm found no significant trends. Chart 1 indicates that from the age of 12, there is a moderate rise in the prevalence of self-harming behaviour, but from 14 onwards there are fluctuations in the rise of the curve. At 18, the prevalence (63.8%) is almost the same as the maximum level that was reported at the age of 14 (64.4%) (Démuthová & Démuth 2019a).

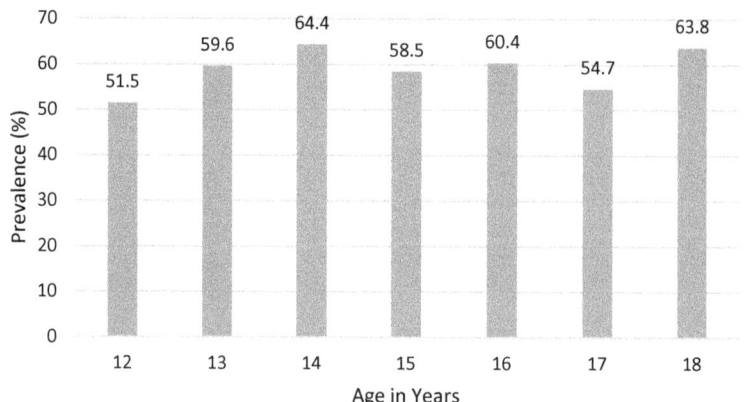

Chart 1. The prevalence of self-harm by age in the observed sample
Source: Démuthová & Démuth (2019a, 47)

Statistical analyses of links between age and the number of forms of self-harming behaviour also found no correlation between these variables (sig. = .678). The number of forms of self-harming behaviour in adolescents did not rise (they did not include new forms in their inventory) or fall (there is no tendency for the variability of self-harm to become more limited over time and develop into a preference for a smaller number of forms of self-harming behaviour) as age increased (Démuthová & Démuth 2019a).

Further analyses monitored the correlation between age and the intensity of self-harm for the individual forms of self-harm.[138] The individual forms of self-harm identified by the modified version of the self-reporting questionnaire SHI were classified into three groups depending on the method of causing harm and the intent – direct physical self-harm (corresponding to the criteria defined in DSM-5, including deliberate self-harm with visible damage to tissue), indirect physical self-harm (affecting the body but without any directly visible consequences) and mental self-harm (self-harm which causes damage to an individual's mental health). Of the 22 items in the questionnaire, 7 were included in the category of direct physical self-harm: hitting, scratching, cutting, exercising an injury, banging head, preventing wounds from healing and burning; indirect physical self-harm included 8 items: abusing alcohol, not sleeping enough, over-exercising, starving, making medical situations worse, abusing prescription medication, overdosing, and abusing laxatives; finally, the category of mental-self-harm included 5 items: torturing with self-defeating thoughts, engaging in emotionally abusive relationships, distancing from God, being promiscuous and setting up in a relationship to be rejected (Démuth & Démuthová 2019).[139]

As presented in Chart 2, the prevalence of direct physical self-harm at the individual ages does not suggest an unambiguous trend – from the age of 12, it slightly increases, and after that point,

---

138 For detailed information, see Démuth & Démuthová (2019).
139 The specific definition of the individual forms of self-harm is available in: Démuth, A., & Démuthová, S. (2019). Forms of Deliberate Delf-Harm and Their Prevalence in Adolescence. International Conference on Research in Psychology, 23-38, Diamond Scientific Publication. https://www.doi.org/10.33422/icrp-conf.2019.03.140

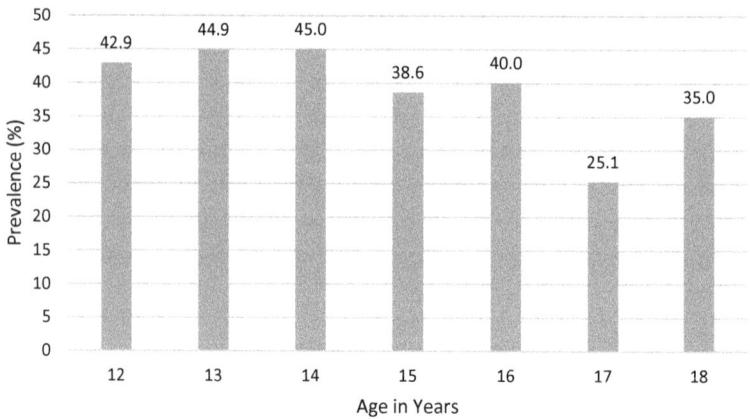

Chart 2. The prevalence of direct physical self-harm by age in the observed sample
Source: Démuth & Démuthová (2019, 29)

it has a falling, yet fluctuating, tendency. It reaches its maximum at 14 (45%) and minimum at 17 (25.1%) (Démuth & Démuthová 2019).

The distribution of the prevalence of the indirect physical forms of self-harm in the individual age categories is presented in Chart 3. As opposed to the previously discussed forms of direct physical self-harm, it appears that the prevalence increases as

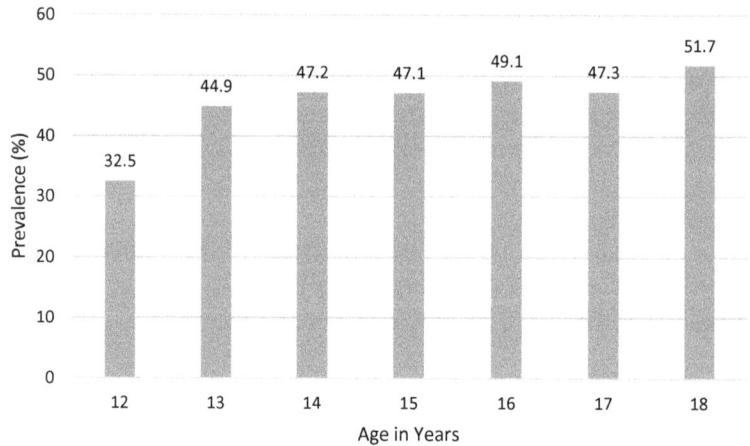

Chart 3. The prevalence of indirect physical self-harm by age in the observed sample
Source: Démuth & Démuthová (2019, 31)

3 The Occurrence of Self-Harm

age increases. But there is not a smooth upward trend, at the ages of 15 and 17 the prevalence decreased in comparison to the previous age group (by 0.1% between 14 and 15 and by 1.8% between 16 and 17).

The analysis of the occurrence of mental forms of self-harm in the individual age groups (Chart 4) did not show (as was the case for direct physical forms of self-harm) any clear trend – it increased slightly from the age of 12, with a first peak at the age of 16 (prevalence of 30.9%), then it decreased to the age of 18 before reaching its maximum value of 38.3% at the age of 18.

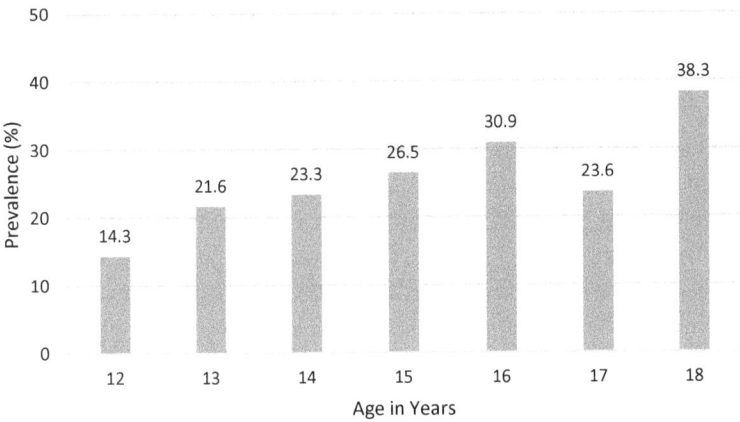

Chart 4. The prevalence of mental self-harm by age in the observed sample
Source: Démuth & Démuthová (2019, 33)

The ambiguity in the curve of the prevalence of self-harm may stem from the fact that the above-mentioned analyses were conducted on a sample of adolescents regardless of their gender. However, it turns out that the prevalence, as well as the intensity of self-harm, may differ between female and male adolescents (Moran et al. 2012; Steinhoff et al. 2021).[140]

Another area of interest in the study of self-harm, apart from monitoring the age of self-harmers, is their age at the onset of self-

---

[140] The results of research that analysed the prevalence of self-harm in the individual age categories separately for male and female subjects are presented in the following section dedicated to gender.

harm and its correlation with the key characteristics of this high-risk behaviour. The results in this area are more straightforward and have produced a lot of important findings. The most commonly reported age for the onset of self-harm is from 12 (Cipriano et al. 2017) to 13 (Morey et al. 2017; Gillies et al. 2018) or the period between these ages (Stallard et al. 2013).[141] Age at the onset of self-harm is also linked to the intensity of self-harm later on. A. Brager-Larsen et al. conducted a study using a sample of 103 adolescents aged 12 to 18, who were patients at psychiatric clinics in Oslo treated for self-harm. They discovered that the age at the onset of self-harm statistically significantly increases the frequency of the occurrence of subsequent episodes of non-suicidal self-harm (Brager-Larsen et al. 2022). Thus, it appears that the earlier the onset of self-harm, the more intense and serious the self-harm is likely to be in later adolescence (Ammerman et al. 2017). Moreover, they also made an effort to determine the "critical age" – the age at which the onset of self-harm might lead to an expectation of subsequent high-risk self-harm, and the age of onset that might lead to an expectation of a less risky course of this behaviour. The most common age reported in this context was 12 (Ammerman et al. 2017; Muehlenkamp et al. 2019).

Another important element linked to the onset of self-harm is its link with overall mental health, for instance, with the presence of suicidal thoughts, plans and attempts. Those individuals who reported attempted suicide along with self-harm, started self-harming significantly earlier than self-harming individuals who never exhibited signs of suicidality (Bae et al. 2020). Non-suicidal self-harm with an earlier onset turned out to be a significant predictor of later suicidal intent (Groschwitz et al. 2015; Szewczuk-Bogusławska et al. 2021).

---

141 It should be pointed out that this piece of data primarily depends on the age cohort included in the individual studies. Only a small number of studies have included children below the age of 12 (or 11); therefore, it is questionable whether the studies would have come to the same conclusions if they had included younger age groups. That being said, self-harm is most prevalent during adolescence.

Gender

Another variable that affects the prevalence of self-harm is gender. The results of studies are not unified in this regard either – although most studies report a greater prevalence in women (e.g., Sornberger et al. 2012; Jeong & Kim 2021), there are also some which found no cross-gender differences (Yang & Xin 2018), and some which reported a greater prevalence in men (e.g., among university students – Yang & Feldman 2017).

This means that generally speaking, the effect of gender is not quite clear. The reasons for different findings with regard to the greater prevalence of self-harm in any of the genders may lie in the reasons mentioned above, in the analysis of the differences in the total prevalence of self-harm as reported in various scientific studies.[142] However, the issue of cross-gender differences in the prevalence of self-harm becomes clearer if we take the character of the sample, the behaviour studied (forms of self-harm) or age into consideration. For instance, in their meta-study that analysed the results of previous studies, K. Bresin & M. Schoenleber report that women had a significantly higher prevalence of self-harming behaviour than men. This difference was even greater in studies using clinical samples and those made up of younger participants (Bresin & Schoenleber 2015).

Furthermore, it appears to be viable to consider age as a variable when studying the prevalence of self-harm and its link with gender. A study carried out by Steinhoff et al. (2021) identified a relatively clear descending tendency in the prevalence of self-harm vs age, with a peak at 13 and a subsequence slow reduction in prevalence within the older age groups; however, this trend only applied to the combined sample of male and female adolescents. Once the curves of prevalence vs age were produced separately for each gender, disparities showed up in the data (see Chart 5). In female participants, the prevalence increased from the age of 13, reaching its peak at 14, followed by a gradual decline. On the other

---

142 These include the use of different definitions of the term "self-harm", differences in the monitored period, differences in the make-up of the study samples with respect to their age, gender or other characteristics (such as the co-morbidity or occurrence of specific characteristics), the various methods used, etc.

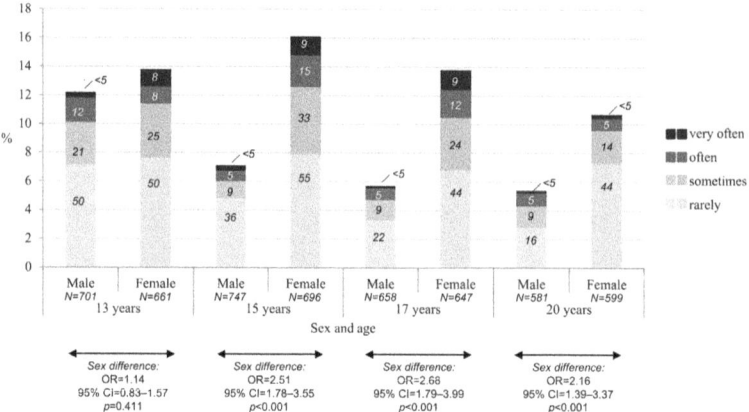

Chart 5. The cross-gender differences in the prevalence and frequency of self-harm by age category
Source: Steinhoff et al. (2021, 941)

hand, the prevalence of self-harm in male participants dropped after its peak at the age of 13. At the same time, the authors discovered that in addition to the age of onset (13), the prevalence of self-harm significantly differed between the two genders – it was statistically higher in female participants (Steinhoff et al. 2021).

This trend of a higher prevalence of self-harm in the female population was also demonstrated in a study[143] on a sample of Slovak adolescents (Démuthová & Doktorová 2019). The study sample consisted of 1,622 respondents between 12 and 18 (mean age = 15.27, standard deviation = 1.79), 62.9% of whom were female (n = 1020). Individuals (male and female) who reported at least one form of self-harm were 29.9% of the sample (n = 485). The prevalence in female participants was 32.1% (N = 327) and it was slightly lower in male participants (26.2%, n = 158). Thus, the link between

---

[143] More detailed results are available in: Démuthová, S., & Doktorová, D. (2019). Interpohlavné rozdiely v prevalencii jednotlivých foriem sebapoškodzovania u adolescentov [Gender Differences in the Prevalence of Individual Forms of Self-Harm in Adolescents]. In: A. Baranovská (ed.): In: Kondášove dni 2018: zborník vedeckých recenzovaných príspevkov z konferencie [Kondas' Days 2018: Proceedings of Scientific Peer-Reviewed Papers from the Conference], 19–32, Department of Psychology, Faculty of Arts of the University of Ss. Cyril and Methodius in Trnava.

gender and the prevalence of self-harm was shown to be statistically significant (the bidirectional significance of Fischer's exact test was 0.014); self-harming behaviour appears statistically significantly more often in female subjects than in male.

As was the case with age, our study of the prevalence of self-harm by gender included separate analyses for the individual types[144] of self-harm. These analyses were conducted as part of the study in 2019,[145] which was conducted in Slovakia on a sample of 1,020 adolescents between 12 and 18 (mean age = 14.96), 59.5% of whom were female (n = 607) (Démuth & Démuthová 2019). The individual forms of self-harm were classified into three groups depending on the method and intent in hurting themselves – direct physical self-harm (corresponding to the criteria defined in DSM-5, including deliberate self-harm with visible damage to tissue), indirect physical self-harm (affecting the body but without any directly visible consequences) and mental self-harm (self-harm that affects mental health). The classification of the individual forms of self-harm into the three areas as well as their prevalence in male and female participants are presented in Tables 14, 15, and 16.

The most frequent form of self-harm reported by female participants was hitting, whereas for male participants it was cutting. The order of the individual forms of self-harm determined based on the results of the prevalence in male and female participants is presented in Table 14. An analysis of the statistical significance of the difference in the prevalence of self-harm by gender, with a significance level of $p < .05$, identified those forms of self-harm, whose prevalence was statistically significantly correlated with gender – these include (sig. = .000) banging head (sig. = .021), preventing wounds from healing (sig. = .007) and exercising an injury (sig. = .000). All of these forms (except for banging head) had a statisti-

---

[144] Self-harm forms refer to the different variants of self-harming behaviour (such as cutting, abusing laxatives, etc.), which may be classified into groups (forms) based on various criteria (e.g., direct physical self-harm, indirect physical self-harm, etc.). The classification of the individual forms into types has already been described in the previous paragraphs discussing the age and may also be found in the following Chapter 4.

[145] The results were published in the following study: Démuth, A., & Démuthová, S. (2019). Forms of Deliberate Self-Harm and Their Prevalence in Adolescence. International Conference on Research in Psychology, 23–38, Diamond Scientific Publication. https://www.doi.org/10.33422/icrpconf.2019.03.140

Table 14. The prevalence of the individual forms of direct physical self-harm

Forms	The Whole Sample (n = 395)		Male Participants (n = 142)		Female Participants (n = 253)	
	Prevalence (%)	Order	Prevalence (%)	Order	Prevalence (%)	Order
Hitting	47.8	1	53.5	1	44.7	3-4
Scratching	46.3	2	40.1	3	49.8	2
Cutting	43.3	3	27.5	4	52.2	1
Exercising an injury	36.5	4	21.8	5	44.7	3-4
Banging head	34.2	5	41.5	2	30.0	5
Preventing wounds from healing	21.5	6	14.1	7	25.7	6
Burning	14.7	7	14.8	6	14.6	7

Source: Démuth & Démuthová (2019, 28–29)

cally significantly higher prevalence in female subjects (Démuth & Démuthová 2019).

As to indirect physical self-harm, the most frequent form was abusing alcohol (prevalence of 52.2%) for female subjects and not sleeping enough (prevalence of 58.30%) for male subjects (Table 15).

To describe the results of the statistical analyses, it appears that men tend to opt for three forms of indirect physical self-harm (abusing alcohol, not sleeping enough and over-exercising), while there is greater variability in the forms of indirect self-harm in female subjects. If we focus on the correlation between gender and the individual forms of indirect physical self-harm, in this group (of indirect physical self-harmers) gender only statistically significantly correlates with two variables: making medical situations worse (sig. = .001) and starving (sig. = .001). Both of these forms were more prevalent in the female participants (Démuth & Démuthová 2019).

As to mental self-harm, torturing with self-defeating thoughts was the dominant form for both genders (Table 16). Observations of the mutual relationship between gender and the prevalence of a specific form of mental self-harm in mentally self-harming in-

Table 15. The prevalence of the individual forms of indirect physical self-harm

Forms	The Whole Sample (n = 395)		Male Participants (n = 142)		Female Participants (n= 253)	
	Prevalence (%)	Order	Prevalence (%)	Order	Prevalence (%)	Order
Abusing alcohol	52.8	1	53.7	2	52.2	1
Not sleeping enough	52.5	2	58.3	1	49.2	2
Over-exercising	26.1	3	31.4	3	22.9	3
Starving	17.4	4	4.0	7	25.3	4
Making medical situations worse	15.3	5	6.9	4	20.5	5
Abusing prescription medication	6.6	6	6.3	5-6	6.7	6
Overdosing	5.1	7	6.3	5-6	4.4	7
Abusing laxatives	2.8	8	2.3	8	3.0	8

Source: Démuth & Démuthová (2019, 30–31)

dividuals revealed that this relationship is statistically significant for promiscuity (sig. = .000), engaging in emotionally abusive relationships (sig. = .007) and torturing with self-defeating thoughts (sig. = .01). For two of these the prevalence was higher in the female participants (Démuth & Démuthová 2019).

The prevalence of self-harm is intertwined with many variables that significantly influence the data reporting the presence of this behaviour in adolescents as well as other groups within the population. However, in order to observe the prevalence of self-harm in various groups of individuals and to monitor the way its occurrence or intensity develops over time, it appears that it is vital to make an effort to define this term clearly and unambiguously. This is an inevitable requirement to allow experts to minimise the impact of the various different views of the term self-harm and to share crucial and reliable information about this high-risk behaviour. It is equally necessary to put effort into the development of valid and reliable methods (or at least to initiate work into the validation and modification of existing methods) so that studies that

Table 16. The prevalence of the individual forms of mental self-harm

Forms	The Whole Sample (n = 395)		Male Participants (n = 142)		Female Participants (n = 253)	
	Prevalence (%)	Order	Prevalence (%)	Order	Prevalence (%)	Order
Torturing with self-defeating thoughts	75.0	1	63.9	1	79.3	1
Engaging in emotionally abusive relationships	22.7	2	15.3	4	25.5	2
Distancing from God	14.5	3	16.7	3	13.6	3
Being promiscuous	13.3	4	27.8	2	7.6	4
Setting up in a relationship to be rejected	7.0	5	13.9	5	4.3	5

Source: Démuth & Démuthová (2019, 32)

investigate this high-risk behaviour can deliver consistent data. Regardless of the specificities of the various studies that have been conducted, the data on prevalence has highlighted that self-harm is a serious problem which is gradually intensifying, especially in the adolescent population.

4 The Forms and Types of Self-Harm in Adolescence

The perception of self-harming behaviour within society is loaded with many stereotypes. This includes, for instance, the widespread belief that self-harm is only an attempt by adolescents to gain attention during a complicated period in their lives or that it only occurs in individuals with mental disorders. Another frequent stereotype concerns the forms of self-harm chosen – people generally believe it mostly consists of cutting or burning. Nevertheless, clinical practice has demonstrated that self-harm is often not only aimed at physical parts of the body but also at the psyche of an individual, which may be even more common than somatic self-harm (Démuthová & Démuth 2019; Jarahi et al. 2021a).

4.1 The Forms of Self-Harm

The reason that so many people believe that self-harm is made up of a small number of mostly physical forms may lie partially in the views presented in scientific literature. As mentioned in the previous chapters, the appendix Conditions for Further Study of the 5th (the most recent) revision of the Diagnostic and Statistical Manual of Mental Disorders (DSM-5) mentions behaviour that leads to damage to the body and refers to it as non-suicidal self-injury – NSSI. It is characterised as "self-inflicted damage to the surface of his or her body of a sort likely to induce bleeding, bruising, or pain (e.g., cutting, burning, stabbing, hitting, excessive rubbing), with the expectation that the injury will lead to only minor or moderate physical harm (i.e., there is no suicidal intent)" (DSM-5 2015, 845). Clearly, this approach fails to take other forms of self-harm into consideration; it only describes behaviour that exclusively leads to damage to the surface of the body (without any suicidal intent). DSM-5 does not mention any other diagnostic category that might include other forms of self-harm, neither in its main chapters nor in its appendices. In this regard, the European version of ICD-10 (International Statistical Classification of Diseases and Related Health Problems, 10th version) has a wider scope. The chapter External Causes of Morbidity and Mortality works with the term intentional self-harm, which covers a wide range of behaviours (X60 – X84). Therefore, it is not a diagnostic criterion in terms of mental disorders, but within intentional self-harm, it covers cases that are also mentioned by DSM-5 – such as intentional self-harm using a sharp (X78), blunt (X79) or a hot object (X77) or flames (X76), as well as many other forms, such as intentional self-harm by drowning (X71), poisoning, or through exposure to various substances (X60–69), it also includes attempted suicide (ICD-10, 2011). These forms not only include surface damage to tissues (as is the case of DSM-5) but also forms which may cause harm to the organism from the inside (poisoning) or in more complex ways (jumping from height or under a motor vehicle).

Nevertheless, ICD-10 clearly describes some forms of self-harm that only affect somatic health, just as does DSM-5. The truth is that both of these manuals are diagnostic manuals for disorders. Yet, self-harm may not necessarily have the intensity or nature of a mental disorder. In many cases, it is a maladaptive coping strategy, characteristic of adolescence, which is not primarily associated with mental disorders and neither does it predict them. Self-harm in the non-clinical population may therefore exhibit different signs than it does when accompanied by mental disorders. However, there is a lack of data on this maladaptive behaviour in Slovakia[146]. This is due to the lack of any nationwide representative study that maps out the forms of self-harm in the non-clinical population. Furthermore, since adolescents only rarely come into contact with experts, the latter may not always discover the hidden, less visible forms of self-harm. Adolescents try to keep their behaviour secret and even if they do seek professional help, it is considerably easier to detect the physical forms of self-harm that have visible consequences than the mental forms, which are hidden. As a result of these (and many other) facts, most people believe that self-harm, even in the non-clinical population, is physical.

Thus, experts differ in their approach to mapping out the individual forms of self-harming behaviour (depending on their theoretical frameworks). Results that have been published in the sci-

---

[146] And even in countries that have conducted more intense research into self-harm and for a longer time, it is still difficult to evaluate this data since there is no consensus in the definition, understanding and mapping of this problem (as previously stated above).

4 The Forms and Types of Self-Harm in Adolescence   163

entific literature suggest that self-harmers adopt many different forms of self-harm[147]. For a better picture, the following sections categorise[148] these forms in line with the definitions in DSM-5 and ICD-10.

DSM-5

This section mentions those forms of self-harm that are covered by the definition of non-suicidal self-injury (NSSI), as formulated in DSM-5, in terms of their nature[149]. These include forms of self-harm (Table 17) with visible consequences (most commonly in terms of damage to the skin or bodily tissues), with the injuries either caused using tools/objects or without them.

Table 17. Forms of self-harm that cause external, visible wounds

Self-hitting
Self-burning
Self-biting
Re-opening wounds
Self-hitting with objects
Preventing wounds from healing
Scratching
Skin-piercing
Stabbing
Extreme (painful) nail biting (with damaged nail folds)
Causing frostbite using ice

Source: author

ICD-10

The International Statistical Classification of Diseases and Related Health Problems, Version 10, lists a number of ways that an individual may intentionally harm themselves or inflict pain upon

---

147 The most frequent forms of self-harm, including their prevalence as measured by individual studies, are listed in the following section "4.2 The Prevalence of the Forms of Self-Harm".
148 In the following sections, they are categorised by "type".
149 Since this section deals exclusively with the forms of self-harm, other NSSI criteria (such as frequency, duration, etc.) are not included.

themselves (self-harm). In addition to those forms described in DSM-5, it mentions many others. Moreover, the "list" is left open with the inclusion of category X84: Intentional self-harm by unspecified means. However, considering the nature of the forms of self-harm described, there is no doubt that they are all forms of damage to physical health. For this reason, this section names all[150] those forms (Table 18) that are associated with damage to the body, without duplicating those which are included in the behaviour described within DSM-5 (as mentioned in the previous section).

Table 18. Forms of self-harm that cause hidden (less visible) damage to the body

Abusing harmful substances	Using substances in quantities that are harmful
Intentional falls	Ingesting indigestible objects
Suffocating	Provoking a fight with the intention to be beaten up
Self-poisoning	Staying outside without adequate protection (from the cold, from the heat)
Breaking bones	Intentional passivity and failing to reject sexual harassment
Hair pulling	Meeting "bad" people in order to be hurt by them
Holding breath	Slapping oneself, hitting oneself (without visible injuries)
Inducing vomiting	Walking barefoot on sharp objects
Strangulation	Jumping from high places with the intention to harm oneself
Not sleeping enough	Not following prescribed treatment with the intention to make a medical situation worse
Over-exercising	

Source: author

Other

Other common forms of self-harm may not be intended to cause physical harm, but rather mental self-torture, social isolation, etc. By doing so, adolescents make themselves suffer mentally and deliberately provoke a negative emotional mood, during which

---

[150] It also includes forms which are not explicitly mentioned by the ICD, but whose nature causes them fall into the category of forms of self-harm that cause damage to the physical health of the individual.

they feel unwell, lonely, excluded or even hated. These forms are closely linked to a common conviction within self-harming adolescents that they are less worthy, or unworthy of attention and love. Through their actions, they often aim to intentionally provoke others, in order to be considered as a bad person which causes their rejection. Through these forms they are hostile to their friends and close ones, they "push them away", which naturally makes their friends and close ones angry or causes a deterioration in their relationship with the individual. Generally, these actions cause harm to the mental health of the individual (examples are shown in Table 19).

Table 19. Forms of self-harm primarily aimed at mental health

Underestimating oneself	Playing sad music, watching sad videos in order to feel bad
Social isolation	Cutting hair to look awful
Worrying about the past	Treating people I like badly in order for them to get angry
Denying oneself favourite things	Self-deprecation in order for others to think I am bad/stupid
Distancing from a close person	Undermining own self-confidence

Source: author

4.2 The Prevalence of the Forms of Self-Harm

Research that focuses on the prevalence of the various forms of self-harm is a prerequisite for an overview of all the forms of self-harm that occur in the adolescent population. Currently, there are several non-standardised methodologies – questionnaires that map out the prevalence of the individual forms.[151] Their number and the different approaches make it difficult to compare the individual findings or to observe changes in the prevalence of self-harm over time. In this context, research into self-harm requires (in addition to the unification of the understanding of the term and

---

151 An overview of the most commonly used methods is presented in section 3.3 Methodologies Used for the Study of the Prevalence of Self-Harm.

an unambiguous definition of the forms of behaviour included) experts to agree on a smaller number of methods, which would need to be validated in various countries and used universally; as is the case for many other mental phenomena which are observed through psychometric methods. The absolute requirement in the establishment of a good quality methodology is its potential to identify various (but especially the characteristic) forms of the observed behaviour, even with the variability it exhibits in the studied groups. At the same time, the measurement tool must be efficient and should not include an excessive number of items. In order to meet these fundamental[152] requirements, it is necessary to not only know all the possible variants of self-harming behaviour but to also have an overview of how common they are within the adolescent population.

The Prevalence of Different Forms of Self-Harm Abroad

M. K. Nixon et al. conducted a study into the prevalence of different forms of self-harm on a sample of 568 adolescents between 14 and 21. Self-harming individuals accounted for 16.9% of the sample, with the most frequent forms being cutting, scratching and self-hitting (which was 83.2% of the cases of self-harm), ingesting a medication over the prescribed dosage (or harmful excessive use) (31.5%), using illicit drugs with the intent to cause self-harm (16.29%) (Nixon et al. 2008). Since the authors gathered several different forms of self-harm into groups, the prevalence of the individual forms is not entirely clear. A more detailed overview of the prevalence of different forms was provided by Raemen et al. In their study, involving 254 participants, they only observed the prevalence of non-suicidal self-injury (in the context of DSM-5). The most frequent form was head banging (present in 9.8% of the sample), followed by hitting (3.9%) and cutting (3.1%) (Raemen et al. 2020). A wider range of the forms of non-suicidal self-injury and their prevalence in adolescents (n = 519) was published by Somer et al. (Table 20).

---

152 However, in order for the method to be of good quality, these should not be the only requirements.

4 The Forms and Types of Self-Harm in Adolescence

Table 20. The prevalence of selected forms of self-harm in adolescents

Form of Self-Harm	Prevalence in %	Form of Self-Harm	Prevalence in %
Banging/hitting	50.9	Wound picking	46.9
Cutting	44.0	Carving*	38.4
Severe scratching	27.6	Pinching	26.7
Biting	25.3	Hair pulling	21.7
Swallowing chemicals	19.7	Needle sticking	14.6
Rubbing skin	14.6	Burning	10.2

Note: *carving signs (symbols, figures, words) into the skin
Source: Somer et al. (2015, 1167)

Lloyd-Richardson et al. also focused on non-suicidal self-injury, which means they only investigated those forms of self-harm that directly lead to damage to the surface of the body/to tissues. The ten forms with the highest prevalence are shown in Table 21.

A study that focused on the various forms of self-harm, using the Self-Harm Inventory (SHI – Sansone et al. 1998), was conducted by Müller et al. SHI not only works for the forms of self-harm covered by the non-suicidal self-injury classification (NSSI) but also with the indirect forms partially covered by the ICD-10 classification as well as with forms which do not primarily affect so-

Table 21. The prevalence of different forms of non-suicidal self-injury in adolescents

Form of Self-Harm	Prevalence in %	Form of Self-Harm	Prevalence in %
Bit self	16.1	Cut/carved on skin	13.9
Burned skin	12	Hit self on purpose	11.5
Picked at areas of body to draw blood	8.7	Gave self a tattoo	4.8
Inserted objects under nails or skin	6.4	Pulled out hair	4.6
Scraped skin	3.9	Erased skin	3.4

Source: Lloyd-Richardson et al. (2007, 1187)

Table 22. The prevalence of individual forms of self-harm in a sample of 2,507 participants

Form of Self-Harm	Prevalence N (%)
Overdosed	61 (2.4)
Cut yourself	61 (2.4)
Burned yourself	18 (0.7)
Hit yourself	37 (1.5)
Banged your head	74 (3.0)
Abused alcohol	339 (13.6)
Driven recklessly	237 (9.5)
Scratched yourself	87 (3.5)
Prevented wounds from healing	65 (2.6)
Made medical situations worse	104 (4.2)
Been promiscuous	125 (5.0)
Set yourself up in a relationship to be rejected	66 (2.6)
Abused prescription medication	73 (2.9)
Distanced yourself from God as punishment	34 (1.4)
Engaged in emotionally abusive relationship	145 (5.8)
Engaged in sexually abusive relationships	96 (3.8)
Lost a job on purpose	609 (24.4)
Attempted suicide	71 (2.8)
Exercised an injury	51 (2.0)
Tortured yourself with self-defeating thoughts	744 (29.8)
Starved yourself to hurt yourself	41 (1.6)
Abused laxatives to hurt yourself	14 (0.6)

Source: Müller et al. (2016, https://www.ncbi.nlm.nih.gov/pmc/articles/PMC4928828/)

matic health but rather mental health (see Table 22). Müller et al. carried out the study in 2016 on a large sample, 2,507 participants, and it included adolescents above the age of 14 and adults (mean age = 48.8 years) (Müller et al. 2016). In this case, it is difficult to estimate the prevalence in adolescents only, since it is influenced

4 The Forms and Types of Self-Harm in Adolescence

by two opposing mechanisms – on one hand, SHI monitors the lifetime prevalence of self-harm, thus we assume the prevalence of self-harm would be lower in adolescents alone. On the other hand, it is well-known that the prevalence has been on the rise within the adolescent population over the last few decades, thus the prevalence of this high-risk behaviour may be considerably higher in adolescents than in adults.

The study by Müller et al. (2016) highlighted that the indirect and mental forms of self-harm should not be omitted from research into this high-risk behaviour. The forms of self-harm which had the highest prevalence included: "Tortured yourself with self-defeating thoughts" (29.8%), "Lost a job on purpose" (24.4%), "Abused alcohol" (13.6%), "Driven recklessly" (9.5%), "Engaged in an emotionally abusive relationship" (5.8%). All of these are forms that are not mentioned under the non-suicidal self-injury (NSSI) classification of DSM-5. Similar conclusions have been drawn by studies that focused on the prevalence of self-harm in the Slovak adolescent population.

The Prevalence of Different Forms of Self-Harm in Slovakia

One of the first studies that focused on this problem was conducted in 2012. Širilová and Lovaš (2012) created the Questionnaire of Self-Harm Forms, in which they monitored the prevalence of the individual forms of self-harm, self-harming tendencies and the perceived severity of the individual forms of self-harm, both by participants as well as psychologists. The first part included nineteen forms of self-harm, the participants evaluated their occurrence on a four-point scale (from 1 = never to 4 = often/daily). The list of forms of self-harm was preceded by the phrase: "Does this occur in my life?"[153] Cronbach's alpha for this data was 0.846. The tendency to perform self-harm was observed by answering the

---

[153] In the case of this formulation, it is debatable whether the primary motive was to hurt oneself. It is not entirely certain whether adolescents made a distinction between, for example, biting nails painfully due to nervousness as a maladaptive strategy to cope with strain, in spite of its harm/painfulness, and choosing the strategy due to its harmful/painful nature (which is the condition for the behaviour to be considered as self-harming). This uncertainty should be reflected in the interpretation of the results.

question: "Would I ever try this?", to which the participants could respond and evaluate their tendency to try each of the nineteen forms of self-harm on a five-point scale (from 1 = no to 5 = yes). In the last section, the participants (both adolescents and teachers) evaluated the extent to which each of the 19 forms of self-harm is harmful to an individual (again, on a five-point scale from 1 = no to 5 = yes). These parts of the questionnaire also exhibited good internal consistency (Cronbach's alpha = 0.866 and 0.957) (Širilová & Lovaš 2012). The prevalence of the individual forms of self-harm is presented in Table 23. The Questionnaire of Self-Harm Forms includes several specific[154] forms of self-harming behaviour – such as piercing or tattooing, which tend to be excluded from the list of self-harming behaviours (mainly due to their decorative or social importance). However, the forms that were listed as the most common by the authors have also been found to be the most common in other studies (see the preceding paragraphs).

Table 23. The frequency of occurrence of the individual forms of self-harm

Form of Self-Harm	%[155]	Form of Self-Harm	%
Preventing wounds from healing	47.50	Holding breath	13.13
Abusing alcohol	41.20	Cutting	11.88
Scratching	32.50	Tattooing	11.88
Extreme nail biting	32.50	Using dangerous chemicals	8.13
Piercing	23.13	Pulling out hair	6.88
Excessive smoking	20.63	Skin-burning	6.88
Drug abuse	20.00	Breaking bones	5.63
Skin-piercing	19.38	Stabbing	4.38
Hit self on purpose	18.75	Swallowing metal objects	2.50
Medication overdose	16.25		

Source: Širilová & Lovaš (2012, 265)

---

154 Specific in terms of the usual areas of the monitoring of self-harm.
155 The published study does not clearly state whether the percentage refers to the prevalence of the self-harm form among self-harming individuals or whether it is the prevalence of the self-harm form in the whole study sample. Given the absence of this information, the results only show the most preferred forms of self-harm and do not provide any reliable data on the prevalence of the forms.

This study was carried out on a relatively small sample of adolescents (n = 160). In an effort to identify the widest possible range of forms of self-harm on a larger sample of Slovak adolescents, data was collected in 2018–2020 from individuals aged 11–19.[156] To allow, as a minimum, a partial comparison of the findings, the analysis of self-harm used one of the best-known methods – the self-report questionnaire SHI (Self-Harm Inventory) developed by R. A. Sansone and L. A. Sansone (2010), in its modified form. At the same time, the researchers attempted to identify the widest possible range of self-harming behaviours, thus the participants were allowed to include their own forms of self-harm. The modified SHI questionnaire included questions that attempt to establish the presence of 20 forms of self-harm (as listed in Table 24). Previous studies (see e.g., Démuthová & Doktorová 2019) have confirmed the relatively high quality of the internal consistency of this methodology (Cronbach's = 0.809). In addition to the explicitly formulated forms, respondents were allowed to add any other forms they had performed that were not mentioned. An analysis of the prevalence of forms of self-harm was conducted using a sample of 2,219 participants. They had a mean age of 15.34 and 63% of the participants were females. Considering the sensitive nature of the research topic, the participants did not respond to all the questions, which is why the prevalence of each of the forms is based on the number of questionnaires available.

The data shows that the most common form of self-harm was an action that primarily affected the mental health of the individual. It was "torturing with self-defeating thoughts", which is very similar to other forms of "mental" self-harm (such as underestimating, denying oneself favourite things, self-humiliation) and it is not included in the category of direct damage to bodily tissues (as per DSM-5) or damage to the body (as per ICD-10). In the order of the prevalence of the individual forms of self-harm, it was followed by forms which produced direct and visible harm ("Scratched yourself on purpose", "Hit yourself", "Cut yourself on

---

[156] For detailed information regarding the conducted research, see: Démuthová, S., & Démuth, A. (2020). Self-Harm in Adolescence as Maladaptive Coping. Brain: broad research in artificial intelligence and neuroscience, 11(2), 37-47, https://doi.org/10.18662/brain/11.2Sup1/92.

Table 24. Forms of self-harm and their prevalence in a group of self-harming Slovak adolescents

Form of Self-Harm	%*	N
Tortured yourself with self-defeating thoughts	26.8	2,056
Scratched yourself on purpose	25.2	2,012
Hit yourself	24.6	2,025
Cut yourself on purpose	21.6	2,046
Exercised an injury on purpose	20.1	2,057
Banged your head on purpose	18.3	2,040
Abused alcohol to hurt yourself	17.6	2,062
Not slept enough to hurt yourself	14.7	1,992
Starved yourself to hurt yourself	13.8	2,060
Over-exercised to hurt yourself	11.5	2,060
Engaged in emotionally abusive relationships	9.9	2,038
Made medical situations worse on purpose	9.2	2,063
Prevented wounds from healing	8.8	2,051
Burned yourself on purpose	8.1	2,065
Attempted suicide	8.1	2,053
Distanced yourself from God as punishment	6.8	2,038
Overdosed	3.9	2,064
Abused prescription medication	3.8	2,064
Set yourself up in a relationship to be rejected	3.8	2,061
Abused laxatives to hurt yourself	2.2	2,055

Note: *Each participant could mark several forms of self-harm (i.e., the total % does not equal 100).
Source: Démuthová & Démuth (2020, 41)

purpose", "Exercised an injury on purpose", "Banged your head on purpose"). However, these were followed by four other forms ("Abused alcohol to hurt yourself", "Not slept enough to hurt yourself", "Starved yourself to hurt yourself", "Over-exercised to hurt yourself"), which suggest that indirect (hidden) forms are equally common in the repertoire of self-harming behaviours. Another form of "mental" self-harm was next – "Engaged in emotionally abusive relationships". Clearly, forms that have a high prevalence are not necessarily visible to others.

The participants were asked to report the occurrence of specific forms of self-harm that were explicitly listed in the SHI questionnaire; however, the adolescents (n = 1,291) were also given the opportunity to add their own forms of self-harm in a free-form section (Kalivodová 2021). The most frequent additions are listed in Table 25.

Table 25. The prevalence of forms of self-harm not included in the SHI questionnaire

Form of Self-Harm	Prevalence
Convincing myself I do not belong to this world	1.60%
Self-biting	1.20%
Undermining own self-confidence	0.80%
Distancing from a close person	0.60%
Jumping from high places with the intention to harm myself	0.40%
Strangulation	0.20%
Vomiting on purpose	0.20%
Smoking with the intention to harm myself	0.20%
Pulling out hair	0.20%
Hitting stomach with the intention to induce nausea	0.20%
Drowning	0.20%

Source: Kalivodová (2021, 71)

When we look at the prevalence, none of these freely reported forms of self-harm was comparable to the forms of self-harm listed in the SHI questionnaire. Thus, it may be assumed that the range of self-harming behaviours offered by the SHI questionnaire is sufficient and is capable of detecting the majority of forms of self-harm.

4.3 The Types of Self-Harm

The prevalence of individual forms of self-harm proves that adolescents opt for various different ways of hurting themselves on purpose. To characterise and define self-harm, it appears vital to identify the types of self-harming behaviour that occur in adolescents. Tsirigotis (2016) defined two "types" of self-harm: direct self-destructiveness and indirect self-destructiveness. By direct self-destructiveness, he refers to auto-mutilation, self-harm and suicidal actions. Indirect self-destructiveness covers a wide range of behaviours (intentionally getting into dangerous situations, poor maintenance of health, personal and social neglect, intentional helplessness and passivity when facing problems/difficulties, etc.), and these behaviours may be classified as active (seeking hazards and risk) or passive (neglecting safety and health) forms of indirect self-destructiveness.

Müller et al. (2016) also describe (apart from direct self-harm in the context of NSSI) "cognitive forms" (such as torture with self-defeating thoughts), "interpersonal forms" (such as engaging in emotionally abusive relationships) and "other forms of indirect self-harm" including alcohol abuse with the intention to hurt oneself.

In their study from 2007, Lloyd-Richardson et al. reported a slightly different categorisation of forms of self-harm in adolescents (n = 633, of which 46.5% were self-harmers). They only considered forms covered by the non-suicidal self-injury (NSSI) classification from DSM-5, but they distinguished between severe and mild forms – severe forms included cutting, burning, self-tattooing, skin friction and scratching, and mild forms were biting, self-hitting, exercising an injury with the purpose of bleeding, piercing objects under skin or nails, pulling out hair. This categorisation was carried out through a principal component analysis of the monitored forms of behaviour (Lloyd-Richardson et al. 2007).

Hooley et al. make a distinction between direct and indirect self-harm. Their differentiation is based on the effect of the behaviour – while direct self-harm requires the behaviour to lead to immediate damage/disturbance to the tissues (such as cutting), indirect self-harm harms the body through a mediator (such as poisoning) (Hooley et al. 2020).

4 The Forms and Types of Self-Harm in Adolescence

Based on the differences between the concepts of self-harm defined by DSM-5 (exclusively direct forms of self-harm) and ICD-10 (which also includes indirect forms of self-harm), along with a large group of other frequent forms of self-harm they do not cover (as Müller et al. (2016) point out), it is possible to classify the individual forms of self-harm into three basic types based on their intent[157] (Démuthová et al. 2020): direct physical self-harm, indirect physical self-harm and mental self-harm. Direct physical self-harm could include the forms of behaviour that lead to direct damage to the surface of the body (such as cutting, burning, scratching, stabbing, hitting…). Indirect physical self-harm would cover behaviour which leads to indirect damage inflicted to the body, in a hidden way (through the abuse of substances, by neglecting treatment, poisoning, risky behaviours, starvation, etc.). Mental forms of self-harm would include forms of behaviour that cause a deterioration in the mental health of the individual (self-deprecation, engaging in abusive relationships, inducing negative emotional states or mental suffering).

In order to establish whether these three types of self-harm could work as separate "categories" of self-harm, a factor analysis (the results are presented in Table 26) was conducted for the categorisation of the individual forms of self-harm (Kalivodová 2021). The analysis included data from 1,291 Slovak adolescents who formed a representative selection[158] of the total of 1,492 respondents. Forms of self-harm were investigated using a modified SHI questionnaire[159], which, apart from the occurrence of a form of self-harm in the history of the individual, also established the intensity of the self-harm form through reporting of the frequency of this behaviour on a four-point scale (from "never" to "often").

---

157 From the perspective of what the self-harm focuses on.
158 The selection from the original sample was carried out based on quota reflecting age, gender and type of school for the representative selection of the adolescent population in the age of 12–19 years in Slovakia.
159 The modifications of the questionnaire are described in more detail in the section 3.2 The Prevalence of Self-Harm in Slovakia.

Table 26. A factor analysis of the forms of self-harm

Form of Self-Harm	Factors				
	1	2	3	4	5
Exercised an injury on purpose	.746				
Tortured yourself with self-defeating thoughts*	.599		.372		
Cut yourself on purpose	.561	.426			
Prevented wounds from healing	.543			.377	
Attempted suicide	.540	.420			
Not slept enough to hurt yourself*	.509				.337
Overdosed		.768			
Abused alcohol to hurt yourself		.676			
Burned yourself on purpose*		.577			
Abused prescription medication		.575			.482
Made medical situations worse on purpose (e.g., by not using the prescribed medications)	.301	.490	.354		
Over-exercised to hurt yourself			.808		
Starved yourself to hurt yourself	.476		.655		
Abused laxatives to hurt yourself		.306	.593		.425
Banged your head on purpose				.768	
Hit yourself				.705	
Scratched yourself on purpose	.302	.315		.542	
Set yourself up in a relationship to be rejected					.735
Engaged in emotionally abusive relationships	.437				.525
Distanced yourself from God as punishment	.360				.445

Note: *Items with content not fitting the scope of the factor
Source: Kalivodová (2021, 72)

The factor analysis identified five factors. After content analysis, these factors (with certain modifications[160]) can be characterised by the following names: visible direct physical self-harm (Factor 1), indirect physical self-harm (Factor 2), self-harm associated with eating disorders (Factor 3), hidden (discrete) direct physical self-harm (Factor 4) and mental self-harm (Factor 5).

Visible direct physical self-harm is made up of the forms of self-harm that cause visible wounds on external parts of the body (exercised an injury on purpose, cut yourself on purpose, prevented wounds from healing, attempted suicide, etc.) and can be observed. However, this factor is not identical to the concept of non-suicidal self-injury (NSSI) formulated in DSM-5 (although its signs might suggest it is), since this factor also includes the most extreme forms of efforts to damage one's body – attempted suicide – which is strictly excluded by DSM-5.

The next factor, indirect physical self-harm, represents the hidden forms of self-harm that specifically have an impact on the somatic health of an individual (overdosed, abused alcohol, abused prescription medication, made medical situations worse). Even though the proposed definition of self-harm in DSM-5 does not take this type of self-harm into consideration, it includes frequently occurring forms of self-harm, if they were eliminated, the understanding of self-harm would be substantially limited and there would be a risk that a proportion of self-harming adolescents[161] (with the use of the DSM-5 criteria) would not be identified.

The third factor covered the following forms: "Over-exercised to hurt yourself", "Starved yourself to hurt yourself", and "Abused laxatives to hurt yourself" and was characterised as self-harm associated with eating disorders, since these types of behaviour are typical of anorexia or bulimia. Separating this type of self-harm is supported by the existence of a close link between the prevalence of self-harm and eating disorders, which has been confirmed by

---

160 Factors 1 and 2 included forms whose content does not fit their characteristics. These are marked with an asterisk (*) in Table 26. This is further reflected in the interpretation of the results of the factor analysis.
161 The number of self-harming adolescents concerned is calculated in the following section "4.4 The Prevalence of the Types of Self-Harm".

several local and international studies (such as Doktorová & Démuthová 2021; Claes et al. 2001; Smithuis et al. 2018).

Possibly the most consistent factor is the fourth (hidden (discrete) direct physical self-harm), which was populated by three forms of self-harm: "Banged your head on purpose", "Hit yourself" and "Scratched yourself on purpose". The factor analysis revealed that it is a compact factor in which all of the contents of the individual items correspond to the overall scope (characteristic) of the factor, unlike factor 1 and 2. At the same time, an analysis of the relevant correlations shows that there is another form similar to factor 4: "Prevented wounds from healing". Although it was primarily classified under factor 1 (direct visible physical self-harm), parts of its content could allow us to classify it under factor 4 (depending on the way in which wounds are prevented from healing). Factor 4 represents a type of self-harm in which direct damage to the body does occur (hitting, banging), but the consequences of this behaviour may not be visible.

The final factor, number 5, is mental self-harm which several authors believe to be a specific type of self-harm (among international studies, see Müller et al. (2016); among domestic (Slovakia) studies, see Démuthová & Démuth (2020)). This factor was populated with forms, such as: "Set yourself up in a relationship to be rejected", "Engaged in emotionally abusive relationships" or "Distanced yourself from God as punishment", which allows us to characterise it as a type of self-harming behaviour that primarily affects the mental health of an individual.

In addition to the forms of self-harm that were listed under the individual factors, the factor analysis classified items that did not fully correspond with the focus of factor 1 (visible direct physical self-harm) and 2 (indirect physical self-harm) (see Table 27). Within factor 1 (visible direct physical self-harm), these were: "Tortured yourself with self-defeating thoughts" (the content of which is closer to mental self-harm – factor 5) and "Not slept enough to hurt yourself" (which could be covered by indirect physical self-harm – factor 2). Within factor 2 (indirect physical self-harm), the non-corresponding form was: "Burned yourself on purpose", the nature of which is closer to visible direct forms of self-harm. The correlation matrix also suggests that although several forms of self-harm could be attributed to one of the five factors, they are

4 The Forms and Types of Self-Harm in Adolescence

related to other factors too.[162] This means that some forms of self-harm occur in various combinations among adolescents, and although it is formally possible to identify "types" of self-harm, real self-harming adolescents use several forms of self-harm from various factors at the same time.

These conclusions are supported by the findings of Germain and Hooley (2012), who compared selected psychological characteristics of individuals who opt for direct forms of self-harm (meeting the definition of non-suicidal self-injury – NSSI) and those who opt for indirect forms of self-harm (indirect physical and/or mental forms). The study sample was made up of 156 individuals, 50 of whom met the criteria for NSSI, an additional 38 had only used indirect forms of self-harm (such as engaging in an abusive relationship, abusing addictive substances, risky behaviour or self-harming behaviour with regard to eating habits), and finally, 68 of them had not committed any forms of self-harm. A comparison of the NSSI group of self-harmers to the group of indirect self-harmers did not reveal any significant differences in the rates of dissociation, aggressiveness, impulsiveness, self-respect, negative temperament, nor in the presence of depressive symptoms or symptoms of borderline personality disorder (Germain & Hooley 2012). Different forms of self-harm are not associated with different types of individuals – they are merely different variants of behaviour that occur in various combinations.

These analyses prove that self-harming adolescents choose a variety of forms of self-harm and freely combine them. Hence, it is impossible to isolate pure "types" of self-harm in the history of self-harm which would represent a specific approach to harming oneself. This is not to say that the study of the types of self-harm (as categories that are used to detect groups made up of various forms of self-harm) is unimportant. This type of data emphasises an important fact – the understanding of self-harm cannot be limited to a certain way of hurting oneself[163]; self-harming behaviour

---

162 This is shown in the values of correlation coefficients. Table 27 indicates the correlation coefficients with value of over 0.3 with the given number of participants (in this case N %1,492) (for the process of determining the value, see: Mareš et al. 2015).
163 Just as it is proposed by the above-mentioned DSM-5.

is expressed through a wide range of forms and ignoring a part of its spectrum could substantially limit our understanding of this phenomenon and lead to the detection of fewer cases among adolescents.

4.4 The Prevalence of the Types of Self-Harm

Despite the fact that scientific literature does not categorise the forms of self-harm into generally accepted valid categories, that could be universally employed, it is obvious that several experts who study forms of self-harm and their prevalence point to the existence of various categories of self-harming behaviour (e.g. Lloyd-Richardson et al. 2007; Müller et al. 2016; Hooley et al. 2020). The fact that the prevalence of the forms of self-harm in their various categories is not negligible is proven by an analysis of the prevalence of the individual types of self-harm.

One such example is the analysis of data collected using the SHI questionnaire[164], which monitors a broader spectrum of forms of self-harm and is able to detect both direct and indirect forms of physical self-harm as well as mental forms of self-harm. Table 27 presents the prevalence of self-harm in terms of the individual types identified in a sample of 1,020 adolescents aged 12–18 (mean age = 14,96). A total of 59.5% of the samples were females.

The results allow us to conclude that when describing self-harming behaviour, it is necessary to not only consider direct physical forms of self-harm (i.e. the forms which represent the key components of the definition of non-suicidal self-injury, as found in DSM-5) but also indirect physical forms (mentioned by ICD-10 with regard to the concept of intentional self-harm together with direct forms) as well as mental forms (the high prevalence of which has been highlighted by several experts, e.g., Müller et al. 2016; Jarahi et al. 2021). The average prevalence of the forms of the three types

---

[164] The questionnaire was used in a form modified for the purposes of collecting data from individuals aged 11–19 (the modifications are described in more detail in the section "3.2 The Prevalence of Self-Harm in Slovakia").

4 The Forms and Types of Self-Harm in Adolescence

Table 27. The prevalence of forms of self-harm and their average prevalence in the individual categories of self-harm

	Prevalence in %
Direct physical self-harm (average)	34.9
Hit yourself	47.8
Scratched yourself on purpose	46.3
Cut yourself on purpose	43.3
Exercised an injury on purpose	36.5
Banged your head on purpose	34.2
Prevented wounds from healing	21.5
Burned yourself on purpose	14.7
Indirect physical self-harm (average):	22.3
Abused alcohol to hurt yourself	52.8
Not slept enough to hurt yourself	52.5
Over-exercised to hurt yourself	26.1
Starved yourself to hurt yourself	17.4
Made medical situations worse on purpose	15.3
Abused prescription medication	6.6
Overdosed	5.1
Abused laxatives to hurt yourself	2.8
Mental self-harm (average):	26.5
Tortured yourself with self-defeating thoughts	75.0
Engaged in emotionally abusive relationships	22.7
Distanced yourself from God as punishment	14.5
Been promiscuous (i.e., had many sexual partners)	13.3
Set yourself up in a relationship to be rejected	7.0

Source: author

of self-harm suggests that although direct physical forms are the most common (an average prevalence of 34.9%), other types of self-harm (indirect physical self-harm had an average prevalence of 22.3% and mental self-harm had an average prevalence of 26.5%)

Table 28. The forms of self-harm classified into types and their inclusion in "diagnostic" systems

Types and Forms of Self-Harm	Systems		
	DSM-5	ICD-10	SHI
Direct physical self-harm			
Hit yourself	x	x	x
Scratched yourself on purpose	x	x	x
Cut yourself on purpose	x	x	x
Exercised an injury on purpose	x	x	x
Banged your head on purpose	x	x	x
Prevented wounds from healing	x	x	x
Burned yourself on purpose	x	x	x
Attempted suicide		x	x
Indirect physical self-harm (average):			
Abused alcohol to hurt yourself		x	x
Not slept enough to hurt yourself		x	x
Over-exercised to hurt yourself		x	x
Starved yourself to hurt yourself		x	x
Made medical situations worse on purpose		x	x
Abused prescription medication		x	x
Overdosed		x	x
Abused laxatives to hurt yourself		x	x
Mental self-harm (average):			
Tortured yourself with self-defeating thoughts			x
Engaged in emotionally abusive relationships			x
Distanced yourself from God as punishment			x
Been promiscuous (i.e., had many sexual partners)			x
Set yourself up in a relationship to be rejected			x

*Note: Although attempted suicide is a direct and physical form of self-harm, it is strictly excluded from DSM-5 – for this reason, it was included in the ICD-10 and SHI systems (Self-Harm Inventory). Source: author

are also fairly frequently found among adolescents. Although the analyses in the previous section, 4.3, showed that forms of self-harm are mutually combined within the individual categories and that the occurrence of a certain form of self-harm from one category may well be associated with the presence of self-harm from another category, it is not necessarily sufficient to focus on a single category of self-harm in order to describe and identify self-harming behaviour as such. After all, this has already been confirmed (in section 1. 4, The Definition of Self-Harm) by the analysis of the impact of accepting the definition of self-harm as proposed by DSM-5[165]. Self-harm clearly encompasses various forms that may be classified as indirect or mental self-harm. An illustration of the spectrum of behaviours that is covered by the diagnostic systems DSM-5 and ICD-10, as opposed to the broader definition of self-harm including its mental forms, is presented in Table 28.

Self-harm is a high-risk phenomenon that is highly prevalent, especially during adolescence. It has many different forms, and it does not necessarily only target the body of an individual but may also impact their mental health. Self-harming individuals tend to mutually combine both various forms of self-harm and also various types of self-harm. Even less-known forms of self-harm (such as not sleeping enough to hurt yourself, torturing with self-defeating thoughts or setting up in a relationship to be rejected) occur relatively frequently among adolescents and quite a substantial number of adolescents (around 15%) exclusively use indirect or mental forms of self-harm to harm themselves. Although efforts to distinguish and categorise the various forms of self-harming behaviour into types (e.g., cognitive, interpersonal, direct, indirect...) are still mostly theoretical (in practice, the various forms appear in different combinations with the types), it is apparent that self-harm should be observed over its whole range of expression.

---

[165] This analysis was incorporated in the analysis of the aims (targets) of self-harm, and it showed that if the DSM-5 criteria were used to identify self-harming adolescents, 15.5% of the cases of self-harming adolescents would be "lost", meaning that 34,369 adolescents would not be identified as self-harmers, and consequently they would not receive treatment or help/intervention. For a more detailed analysis, see: Démuthová & Spasovski (2020).

5 The Characteristics of Self-Harming Adolescents

As of today, self-harm has still not been defined as a separate clinical category, and there is no consistent summary of the typical psychological characteristics of self-harmers. Nevertheless, the topic is frequently subjected to scrutiny, and we already have significant outputs from empirical studies, which suggest, for example, certain patterns in the behaviour or personality traits of self-harming individuals. Mental disorders and illnesses are the most relevant in this regard – self-harm commonly appears as a typical symptom or a frequent indication of many conditions. However, this publication aims to address self-harm as a phenomenon whose prevalence is on the increase, mainly in psycho-pathologically intact population. Thus, this chapter briefly discusses mental disorders, and the majority of attention is paid to the non-pathological characteristics of self-harming individuals, such as personality traits, characteristics of motivation, cognition or the tendency to lean towards specific emotions.

5.1 Mental Disorders

As has already been explained in the introductory chapter, dedicated to the history of the study of self-harm[166], in the past, self-harm was mostly studied within the psychology and psychiatry fields as a symptom of several mental disorders. Nowadays, as experts are considering whether self-harm should be classified as a separate syndrome, it is crucial to observe its presence not only within the existing diagnoses but also its co-morbidity with other disorders. The comparison of groups of individuals without an associated diagnosis versus those with a related diagnosis (including the percentage of self-harming individuals within any group with a specific diagnosis) provides essential information for the decision of whether it is more useful to define self-harm as a separate nosological unit (diagnosis), or whether it should be understood as a typical symptom of several mental disorders or illnesses.

---

166 Section "1.1 The History of Research into Self-Harm".

Neurodevelopmental Disorders

Self-harm is often mentioned in the context of neurodevelopmental disorders – such as mental retardation[167] (van den Bogaard et al. 2018) or autism. When connected to intellectual disabilities, self-harm tends to be present in various degrees of severity, even leading to an increased risk of suicidal actions (APA 2013). Self-harm as a repetitive auto-aggressive behaviour frequently appears in autism[168], especially in adults and women, but as it turns out, the age of onset and the forms and functions of self-harm do not differ between those individuals who have been diagnosed as autistic and those who have not (Maddox et al. 2017). Considering the lower intellectual level typical of intellectual disabilities and autism, it is necessary to estimate the level of self-recognition and controllability of this behaviour with regard to the individual's motivation/intent when studying self-harm. If we characterise self-harm as "the repeated infliction of harm on our health (in its physical/psychological/social domain) with the intention to harm oneself directly or indirectly, or to provoke pain" (see the end of Chapter 1), the motivation/intent to cause harm or to provoke pain, which might not be apparent in an individual with a reduced level of intellect, is highly important[169]. That being said, this factor also needs to be taken into consideration in other mental disorders.

Since self-harming behaviour shows signs of a limited degree of control of impulses, it also occurs in attention deficit hyperactivity disorders (ADHD) (Swanson et al. 2014; Balázs et al. 2018). Studies of the relationship between ADHD and self-harm have shown that a major factor that has an impact on this link is the additional presence of affective disorders or dependency disorders (Balázs et al. 2018).

---

[167] Today, scientific literature and diagnostic manuals prefer the term "intellectual disabilities" since the term "mental retardation" has acquired a derogatory connotation due to its use in non-professional contexts.

[168] In the case of autistic spectrum disorders.

[169] In both, intellectual disabilities and autism, auto-aggressive behaviour may not be conscious, or its primary intent might not be to intentionally and purposefully hurt oneself/provoke pain.

Schizophrenia Spectrum Disorders

Another group mentioned with self-harm includes schizophrenia spectrum disorders and other psychotic disorders, which can, at the same time, be classified as personality disorders (schizoid and schizotypal disorders – Claes et al. 2018). The prevalence of self-harm in patients suffering from schizophrenia is relatively high – non-suicidal self-injury[170] is present in almost 44% of patients, with the most common form being cutting and the most frequent motive being the regulation of emotion (just as in other – non-clinical – groups). Individuals with schizoid or schizotypal personality disorders are characterised by the avoidance of social relationships, by a limited range of emotional expression, by cognitive distortions and they experience discomfort in close social relationships (APA 2013). The prevalence of self-harm in patients suffering from schizophrenia spectrum disorders is significantly increased by the use of addictive substances (Güney et al. 2020).

Disorders Associated with the Use of Addictive Substances and Addictive Disorders

The link between the (ab)use of addictive substances and self-harm is not rare – according to the available literature, self-harming behaviour occurs fairly frequently in individuals who are addicted to substances (see e.g., Baer et al. 2020, Serra et al. 2022), and may even represent a direct correlation. Studies point out the link between NSSI and alcohol abuse (Dahlgre et al. 2018; Westlund Schreiner et al. 2020) or the abuse of other types of drugs (Osuch et al. 2014). The reason for this link might be mechanisms that contribute to the development and preservation of both high-risk forms of behaviour (self-harm and addiction) – in this context, self-harm is believed to be a highly addictive behaviour[171] (Tantam

---

170 I.e., self-harming behaviour as defined in DSM-5.
171 The concept of self-harm as addictive behaviour was already introduced in scientific literature in the 1990s (see: Tantam & Whittaker 1992 or Faye 1995); since then, the relevance of this view has been supported by several studies (see e.g., Victor et al. 2012, Himelein-Wachowiak et al. 2022).

& Whittaker 1992; Faye 1995; Washburn et al. 2010). An intensive study that focused on this was carried out by Nixon et al. (2002), who observed the presence of seven signs of addiction in self-harmers: 1/ the behaviour occurs more often and/or the severity of SI increases; 2/ SI continues despite having recognised it as harmful; 3/ if the behaviour is stopped, an increase in the level of tension occurs; 4/ SI urges are upsetting, but not enough to cause the individual to stop; 5/ SI causes social problems; 6/ the frequency and/or intensity has to increase to achieve the same effect; 7/ the behaviour is time-consuming. The results revealed that 97.6% of self-harming individuals exhibited three or more signs of addiction, and 81% exhibited five or more signs of addiction (ibid.). In this context, it is interesting that a large proportion of the patients treated by doctors for the consequences of self-harm abused alcohol immediately before or during the self-harming episode (Merrill et al. 1992; Horrocks et al. 2003), with approximately a quarter of them meeting the criteria for a diagnosis of harmful alcohol use (Haw et al. 2001).

Personality Disorders

Another group of disorders that co-occur with self-harm are personality disorders (Hauber et al. 2019). Extensive research on a group of students conducted in Belgium showed that up to 80.7% of self-harming individuals met the criteria for the diagnosis of at least one personality disorder in the previous 12 months, with more than a half suffering from two or more co-morbid disorders (Kiekens et al. 2018).

In addition to the schizophrenia spectrum disorders mentioned above, this group also includes several other disorders, most commonly borderline personality disorder (Brickman et al. 2014; Guénolé et al. 2021). The link between borderline personality disorder and self-harm is so common that self-harm is actually one of the diagnostic criteria of this disorder (APA 2013). Borderline personality disorder typically exhibits patterns of behaviour that are characterised by instability in various domains – such as emotions or interpersonal relationships; it manifests in unstable impulse control and distorted self-image (ibid.). While international literature

5 The Characteristics of Self-Harming Adolescents

reports an average prevalence of self-harm of 17% among adolescents and 6% for the adult population, its prevalence in individuals with a borderline personality disorder is 95% for adolescents and 90% for adults (Reichl & Kaess 2021). It is obvious that a diagnosis of borderline personality disorder is closely linked to self-harm; Figure 14 demonstrates the overlap and the relationship between the prevalence of self-harm and bipolar personality disorder.

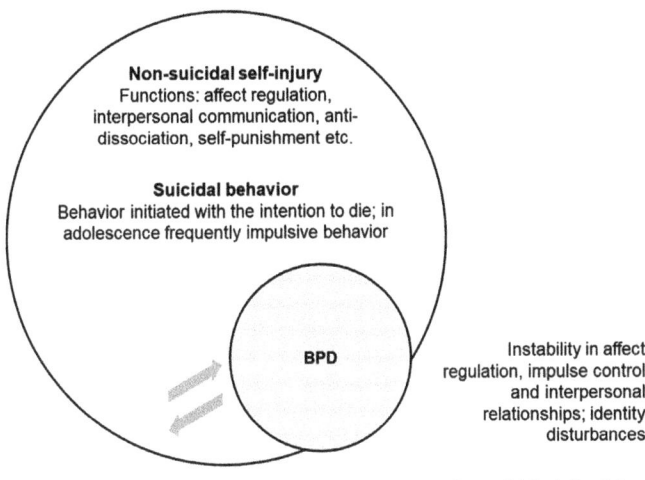

Figure 14. Core features of borderline personality disorder and self-harm in adolescence. The various-sized circles demonstrate the differences in the rate of prevalence between borderline personality disorder and self-harm in terms of overlapping populations
Note: BDP = Borderline Personality Disorder
Source: Reichl & Kaess (2021, 140)

On the other hand, it is well known that self-harm also occurs in individuals who do not suffer from a borderline personality disorder, and not every patient with borderline personality disorder performs self-harm (In-Albon et al. 2013). The differences between the group of self-harmers and the group diagnosed with borderline personality disorder suggest that it could be appropriate to classify self-harm as a separate syndrome (Selby et al. 2012; Turner et al. 2015).

There are also other personality disorders that may be accompanied by self-harm (although not as often as a borderline personality disorder). Obsessive-compulsive disorders (Claes et al. 2007), which are characterised by limited impulse control, suggest a possible background of both problems, where a self-harming individual cannot suppress the urge to cope with a problematic situation through an inappropriate method (hurting oneself) or cannot resist the urge to continue with this behaviour (repeated self-harm). The co-occurrence of self-harm and avoidant personality disorder (characterised by feelings of inadequacy and hypersensitivity to negative social evaluation) (APA 2013) has been confirmed by several studies (see e.g., Nock et al. 2006; Snir et al. 2015). Avoidance (as a behavioural strategy) is present in the context of self-harm as one possible method to retain this behaviour in the repertoire of maladaptive forms of coping. According to the avoidance model[172], self-harming behaviour is primarily retained by negative reinforcement through the escape or avoidance of unwanted emotional experiences (Chapman et al. 2006). Avoidance in the context of avoidant personality disorder rather means avoiding social interactions and is based on a massive feeling of inadequacy, worry about how they are judged by others, rejection by others and low self-esteem. These feelings are often linked to cognitive distortions related to the self-image of the individual (see section "2.4 Cognitivist Concepts"), which lead them to the conviction that they are worthless, incapable, not loved by others and unworthy of love and affection. It was also discovered that avoidant personality disorder has a moderating effect in relation to post-traumatic stress disorder (described below) and self-harm – the results of studies have revealed heightened levels of deliberate self-harm only among patients with post-traumatic stress disorder and co-occurrent avoidant personality disorder (Gratz & Tull 2012). In terms of the prevalence of personality disorders in self-harming individuals, there are also reports of the following personality disorders: histrionic (Ferrara et al. (2012) report its prevalence among self-harmers at 13.5%), passive-aggressive (prevalence: 17.3%) or narcissistic (5.7%). Like the commonly diagnosed borderline personality disorder, these often have anxiety-related or dysphoric characteristics (Ferrara et al. 2012).

---

[172] Experiential Avoidance Model (EAM) (Chapman et al. 2006).

Affective Disorders

In addition to personality disorders, self-harm also tends to occur in affective (mood) disorders. These include depressive and bipolar disorders, as well as their more persistent variants (dysthymia and cyclothymia). The depressive mood of various degrees of severity[173] occurs in a large number of self-harming individuals and has long been documented by numerous scientific studies (see e.g., Ennis et al. 1989; Mullick et al. 1994; Chibanda et al. 2002; Zubrick et al. 2017). Moreover, the presence of depression is associated with a greater degree of intensity of self-harm along with the occurrence of more severe forms; it significantly increases the likelihood of attempted suicide (Muehlenkamp & Gutierrez 2007; Knorr et al. 2016). A close link between self-harming behaviour and another disorder that affects the mood of the individual – bipolar affective disorder – has been reported by several authors who conducted their studies on both the adult population (Singhal et al. 2014; Esaki et al. 2020) and on groups of young people (Masi et al. 2018; Llamocca et al. 2022). As is the case with depression, other specific correlations with self-harm were also identified with bipolar disorder – for instance, the presence of bipolar disorder and its acute course (an ongoing episode) increase the intensity and severity of self-harm (Esposito-Smythers et al. 2010), as well as the probability of repeated occurrences in the future (Clements et al. 2015).

Anxiety Disorders

Several studies into the link between self-harm and psychiatric conditions have identified an increased prevalence of self-harm with anxiety disorders – especially with generalised anxiety disorder, social anxicty disorder (social phobia), agoraphobia, and others. G. Kiekens et al. (2018) suggest that up to 54.1% of self-harming students meet the diagnosis criteria for generalised anxiety disorder. A detailed analysis of the prevalence of individual anxiety

---

173 Ranging from the presence of only a few depressive symptoms to the unambiguous diagnosis of, for example, depressive disorder.

disorders in self-harming adolescents (in comparison with a non-clinical sample[174]) was conducted by a team of authors in Hungary, led by G. Mészáros (2020). The most frequent condition within the group of self-harmers was social anxiety disorder (social phobia) (see Table 29).

Table 29. The prevalence of anxiety disorders in a clinical and non-clinical sample of self-harming adolescents

Diagnosis	Prevalence in Self-Harmers (%)		
	The whole sample (n = 145)	The clinical sample (n = 107)	The non-clinical sample (n= 38)
Panic disorder (lifetime)	29.9	36.4	10.8
Panic disorder (current)	21.5	27.1	5.4
Agoraphobia (current)	35.9	43.0	15.8
Separation anxiety disorder	16.7	21.5	2.7
Social anxiety disorder	32.6	37.4	18.9
Specific phobia	14.6	15.9	10.8

Source: Kiekens et al. (2018, 214)

Traumatic Disorders and Stress Disorders

Self-harm also occurs in the clinical picture of reactions to trauma, stress or life crises. The most common disorder in this regard is post-traumatic stress disorder (see e.g., Dixon-Gordon et al. 2014; Webermann et al. 2016; Alharbi et al. 2020). The large body of literature dedicated to the link between this and self-harming behaviour stems, inter alia, from the outdated concept that self-harm is a consequence of sexual abuse in childhood (van der Kolk et al. 1991; Romans et al. 1995). Nowadays, scientists reject the existence of a direct link between self-harm and sexual abuse (Klonsky & Moyer 2008), but research still addresses the impact of the distal factors (Nock 2009), including poor treatment in childhood

---

[174] The clinical sample was made up of former (currently stable) patients of psychiatric clinics, and the non-clinical sample came from ordinary schools.

or a hostile/overly critical attitude in the family[175]. We have evidence that stressful events in someone's personal history (Lan et al. 2019), bad experiences from childhood or bullying (Wang et al. 2022) correlate with an increased prevalence of self-harm. More recent studies have also expanded our knowledge of the moderating factors that affect the relationship between traumatic events and the prevalence of self-harm, such as the presence of borderline personality disorder (Dixon-Gordon et al. 2014), a lack of resilience (Baralla et al. 2021) or affect dysregulation (Raudales et al. 2020).

Dissociative Disorders

The occurrence of dissociations in self-harming individuals is very common (Saxe et al. 2002; Nester et al. 2022). Discontinuities in the experiences of the self-harming individual are exhibited in several phases and areas – it may affect not only conscious thoughts but also memory, emotions and physical impulses (APA 2013). Dissociation frequently occurs as a reaction to trauma or stress (these circumstances are quite common in self-harming individuals), and self-harm is intended to bring an end to these unpleasant states of dissociation (Nock and Prinstein 2004). The presence of "anti-dissociation" as motivation for self-harm has been reported in a large number of studies (see e.g., Paul et al. 2015; Burke et al. 2018; Case et al. 2020). But case studies point out that dissociative states (such as depersonalisation, feelings of emptiness, numbness, derealisation, etc.) may not only be halted through self-harm[176] but also induced by it. As stated by Nester et al. (2022), self-harm allows individuals to dissociate, which helps them to avoid or escape from undesirable or averse internal states. By doing so, they reduce (or eliminate) emotional stress, excessive excitement or internal conflicts. The correlations and mechanisms between

---

175 See Figure 3 in section "2.6 Integrative Concepts".
176 These include cases in which adolescents describe their motivation to self-harm with reasons such as: "causing pain so I will stop feeling numb", "trying to feel something even if it is physical pain" or "making sure I am still alive when I don't feel real" (Klonsky & Glenn 2009).

dissociation, self-harm and mental disorders are still being studied, with several new (and sometimes contradictory) findings coming to the surface. Nevertheless, the prevalence of dissociations and depersonalisation in self-harming individuals is significantly higher than in non-self-harming individuals (Cerutti et al. 2012).

Eating Disorders

Common indirect forms of self-harm (see the overview in the section "4.1 The Forms of Self-Harm") include starvation to hurt yourself or over-exercising. Although these forms of self-harming behaviour overlap with the symptoms of certain eating disorders, it might not necessarily imply their presence. That being said, it is possible that if these patterns of behaviour are reinforced and become more permanent, they may eventually evolve into an eating disorder. But it is more common for self-harm (regardless of its manifested forms) to co-occur with eating disorders (especially among adolescent girls) (Muehlenkamp et al. 2009; Peebles et al. 2011). The common background for both (self-harm and eating disorders) may be seen in mechanisms that produce a lack of control and in regaining control in alternative areas. Self-harm may be understood as a maladaptive coping strategy, a reaction to a mishandled situation, and self-harming individuals often report that only through self-harm do they feel in control of their lives. Since they are incapable of controlling the situation around them (or within themselves[177]), they try to conceal their problems, tension or emotional pain through intense physical pain, which, in contrast, they are able to control. It helps them to compensate for the loss of control over the aspects that are causing their psychological distress (Démuthová & Démuth 2019a; Petermann & Nitkowski 2015). Similarly, the obsession with controlling body weight or food intake found within eating disorders often compensates

---

[177] Self-harmers often try to cope with tension and emotional pain, which they cannot regulate, by "turning them into" physical pain. Through this transformation, self-harming individuals get their pain (in its physical form) "under control" – they can determine its extent and length, and they can decide when to end it – which is certainly not true for mental or emotional pain.

for an inability to regulate and control what is happening in the individual's life (Froreich et al. 2016). Both of these conditions (eating disorders and self-harm) help to regulate emotions, thus they are used as coping mechanisms in stressful situations (Smithuis et al. 2018). Self-harm and eating disorders also have other common characteristics – they share distorted interoceptive awareness[178] (Clausen et al. 2011; Doktorová & Démuthová 2021), a distorted relationship with one's own body (Black et al. 2019; Benzel 2019) and a lower level of self-protection (Cerutti et al. 2012). Just like individuals with eating disorders, self-harmers frequently use maladaptive and ineffective coping strategies and more often fail in the solution of their problems (Wenzel & Spokas 2014; Liu et al. 2016).

It is evident that, in many cases, the occurrence of self-harm as well as other mental disorders stem from a similar and specific function of our mental mechanisms (emotionality, cognition, coping...). The previous paragraphs confirm that self-harm appears in the symptomatology of several disorders (since it frequently occurs as part of them). But it is questionable, whether it is correct to identify it as a symptom (i.e., as a part of the disorder) or if there is just (as in many other conditions) co-morbidity between the disorder and self-harm. Since, as yet, self-harm has not been defined as a separate clinical category, it cannot be understood as a nosological unit and thus, be reported as a co-morbid illness. However, it is possible that once the symptoms, areas and characteristics of self-harm have a unified (and well-defined) description, research will show whether it is possible (based on outputs that point out the etiopathogenesis, prevalence, course, prognosis and typical symp-

---

178 Interoceptive awareness means the ability to perceive and integrate visceral signals of physical states (such as hunger, intestinal tension, heartbeat, breathing, pain...) (Khalsa & Lapidus 2016). The experience and resultant interpretation of these impulses provides the individual with feelings related to their physical self and plays a key role in processing emotions and the subsequent regulation of behaviour (Craig 2002). Individuals with eating disorders have distorted interoceptive awareness, both on the perceptive (e.g., the inability to clearly distinguish a feeling of fullness or other physical states) and behavioural (such as ignoring feelings of hunger or fullness) levels (Khalsa & Lapidus 2016). A similar distortion can also be observed in self-harming individuals – they ignore the warning signs from the body (pain) when self-harming, and in the clinical picture, they often show deficits in the perception, processing and regulation of emotions (Andover & Morris 2014).

toms and characteristics of the affected persons) to identify self-harm as a separate nosological unit or if it is better understood as a symptom of other disorders. In this regard, we should ask what data we should collect[179] in order to say whether it is (not) viable to define self-harm as an independent nosological unit and whether its explicit classification can provide more reliable and valid data (on the causes, course and treatment) for use by psychologists and psychiatrists as opposed to studying this phenomenon within various other disorders.

It should also be noted that the existence of self-harm with individual disorders does not mean that if self-harm does occur, the individual must necessarily be diagnosed with one of the previously mentioned conditions. Self-harm is a possible symptom, but it is not always present. It does not always appear as a part of a given disorder (the patient can be diagnosed without the presence of self-harm); and vice versa, although an individual may self-harm, they do not necessarily have to suffer from a specific mental disorder. Several authors have pointed out that the existence of these differences (i.e., the fact that there are individuals diagnosed with self-harm and other individuals with the same diagnoses, but without self-harm) implies that self-harm should be considered as a separate clinical category (see e.g., Selby et al. 2012). Defining self-harm as a separate unit raises another issue: the prevalence of self-harm in the non-clinical population, that means, in individuals who do not suffer from any other mental

---

[179] It might not be necessary to collect new data, since there is quite a rich amount of data from research into self-harm. What prevents us from reaching any conclusions is the fact that different studies have a different definition for self-harm, this leads to various views and conclusions. Once again, it shows that it is crucial to reach a consensus in the definition of self-harm. The consensus would allow us to carry out meta-studies that would evaluate the data from the studies conducted to date, and within new studies no data would be produced which could not be compared to other studies. When we contemplate if we should (or not) coin a new nosological unit, the need to set a clear definition also arises in other serious circumstances – for instance, if a study works with the concept of self-harm in the context of NSSI, it does not take threats of suicide into consideration (since suicidal behaviour is automatically excluded from the definition of non-suicidal self-injury). The view of the "disorder", its impacts or prognosis will, therefore, be considerably different than when using a definition that classifies the severity of self-harm through its tendency to eventually lead to suicidal behaviour.

problems[180]. Again, it is not clear (as a result of the varied definitions of self-harm) what percentage of the total number of self-harmers make up this group; however, it is apparent that these individuals do exist[181] and that they not only do not currently suffer from any mental illness, but long-term studies have also shown that they are not expected to develop any mental disorder in the future.

In the introductory chapters[182], we presented several mechanisms that contribute to the formation, development and retention of self-harm in the behavioural repertoire of an individual. The worldview or self-image of an individual (especially in the context of numerous cognitive distortions), their reactions to stressful situations (maladaptive strategies) and the way they process experiences (e.g., in the form of memory pessimism), all of which are typical of self-harmers, can be related to several personality traits of the individual. A description of motivational, cognitive or temperamental characteristics, together with the emotionality of the individual, can substantially contribute to our understanding of why certain, even mentally healthy (in the sense of an absence of a mental disorder), individuals exhibit self-harming behaviour.

5.2 Personality

The Big Five Concept

Possibly the most extensively studied aspect of the personality traits related to self-harm is the prevalence of the individual Big Five personality traits – openness, conscientiousness, extraversion, agreeableness and neuroticism[183]. Research suggests that

---

180 In such cases, there is no disorder that self-harm could be considered to be included in as a symptom.
181 There are many studies into self-harm in the non-clinical population (see e.g., Klonsky et al. 2003; Swannell et al. 2014; Horváth et al. 2020).
182 For more information, see Chapter 2 "Theoretical Bases".
183 In Slovak literature, this is also referred to as "negative emotionality" (See: Halama et al. 2020).

self-harming individuals typically have high levels of neuroticism and openness, and low levels of agreeableness, conscientiousness and extraversion (Mullins-Sweatt et al. 2013; Allroggen et al. 2014; Jiao et al. 2022). These characteristics are among the main personality traits. They are within the higher levels of the hierarchy of personality traits and are further saturated by other traits, which inhabit the lower levels of the hierarchy. In order to understand the specificities of the personality of self-harming individuals, it is vital to be familiar with not only the main traits but also to analyse their components, their lower-level traits or "facets" – see Table 30). These traits provide more specific information on the basic affective, cognitive and behavioural tendencies of the higher-order traits (Perlman et al. 2018).

Table 30. Facets that correspond to the individual Big Five personality traits

Big Five Trait	Corresponding Facets[184]
Openness	Intellectual curiosity, aesthetic sensitivity, creative imagination
Conscientiousness	Organisation, productiveness, responsibility
Extroversion	Sociability, assertiveness, energy level
Agreeableness	Compassion, respectfulness, trust
Neuroticism	Anxiety, depression, emotional volatility

Source: Halama et al. (2020)

The importance of observing the individual facets is the same for all higher-order personality traits which represent several lower-level traits. For instance, an individual who typically scores low in conscientiousness can be characterised as someone who does not tend to comply with social norms, lacks ambition, is not

---

[184] In international studies, the range of lower-level traits of the 2nd order is wider, and the facets of Big Five traits include: facets of neuroticism: anxiety, angry hostility, depression, self-consciousness, impulsivity, vulnerability; facets of extroversion: warmth, gregariousness, assertiveness, activity, excitement-seeking, positive emotion; facets of conscientiousness: competence, order, dutifulness, achievement striving, self-discipline, deliberation; facets of agreeableness: trust, straightforwardness, altruism, compliance, modesty, tendermindedness; facets of openness: fantasy, aesthetics, feelings, actions, ideas, values (see e.g., Cox et al. (2000), Jourdy & Petot (2017), Lyon et al. (2020)).

methodical, cannot postpone rewards and does not respect rules (Roberts et al. 2009). The above-mentioned facets clearly show that conscientiousness is mainly saturated by individuals who are organised, productive, and responsible. That being said, self-harming individuals are also often characterised by depressive moods[185] or they may even suffer from depression (Mullick et al. 1994; Chibanda et al. 2002; Zubrick et al. 2017). The symptoms of depression often include lower levels of productivity or limited self-organisation, which are the key characteristics of conscientiousness. Thus, a self-harming individual may score low in conscientiousness, mainly due to affective disorder (or at least due to their negative emotional mood), but the trait "not conscientious" may not describe them well, quite the opposite – the individual might normally be responsible and complies with norms and rules, but as a result of a negative emotional mood and the presence of hypobulia, may perform less conscientiously, thus they are classified as part of the group that displays a low level of conscientiousness.[186] Although to refer to such an individual as "not conscientious" would be correct, based on any of the methodologies (especially questionnaires) that measure this variable, in terms of the internal mindset of an individual and the way they react it could lead to a partially misleading conclusion as a result of overgeneralisation (labelling the individual using the term "not conscientious"). It is unfortunate that there are few studies that describe the level of the sub-components (facets) when addressing the Big Five traits. A more detailed analysis of the components of conscientiousness (not at the level of facets, but of the individual items in the questionnaire) was also conducted by Agos et al. (2021). They discovered that self-harming individuals tend to score even higher in work-related conscientiousness (diligent, good employee/worker/student) than the general population (Agos et al. 2021).

Therefore, it is important to not only observe the Big Five traits but also to analyse the major facets and characteristics that satu-

---

185 For more details, see the following section "5.6 Emotionality".
186 The overall image of the hypobulic, depressed self-harming individual is also in line with the results of a study that investigated the differences in the personality traits of self-harming and non-self-harming adolescents. It showed that these two groups demonstrated significant differences in the "untidiness" trait (Soyyiğit Oktan et al. 2022).

rate them in self-harmers. Yet, most studies that observe the prevalence of personality traits in self-harmers have not analysed these facets (Perlman et al. 2018), and these studies are rather rare. For example, MacLaren and Best (2010) found that self-harming individuals who exhibit a higher frequency and variety of self-harm score higher in the individual aspects of neuroticism, they have high levels of depressive mood and vulnerability; in terms of conscientiousness, they have low levels of self-discipline, poor decision-making and obedience; in terms of low agreeableness, they exhibited low levels of trust, straightforwardness and altruism. At the same time, higher levels of openness to experience were only related to feelings, and out of the several aspects of the low level of extraversion, only assertiveness was found to be typical. Mullins-Sweatt et al. (2014) also reported that self-harming individuals had a considerably higher level of the aspects of neuroticism and its facets (i.e., anxiety, anger/hostility, depressive mood, self-confidence, impulsiveness, vulnerability), higher levels of openness and its facets (i.e., aesthetics, feelings and values) and significantly lower levels of conscientiousness and its facets (order, ambitiousness, self-discipline, deliberation) (Mullins-Sweatt et al. 2014).

The Psychobiological Model of Temperament from C. R. Cloninger

Another approach is represented by the psychobiological model of temperament and character from Robert C. Cloninger (1987, 1993). Within this concept, the personality is characterised by four dimensions of temperament and three dimensions of character. While temperament dimensions (novelty seeking, harm avoidance, reward dependence and persistence) are determined by genetics and are exhibited at an early age and contribute to the formation of habits[187], character dimensions mature in adulthood and have an impact on the effectiveness of the individual in their personal and social life. According to Cloninger, character dimensions are the product of learning and in their essence,

---

[187] Temperament characteristics are described in the following section "5.3 Temperament".

they reflect the self-image of the individual on three levels that are based on the extent to which the person identifies themselves as: 1/ an autonomous individual, 2/ an integral part of humanity, and 3/ an integral part of the "universe" as a whole. Each aspect of self-image corresponds to one of the three character dimensions: self-directness, cooperativeness or self-transcendence (Cloninger et al. 1993). Self-harming adolescents exhibit lower levels of self-directness and cooperativeness (as opposed to non-self-harming adolescents), and the difference increases as the severity of their mental health problems (if there is co-morbidity with a borderline personality disorder) increases (Tschan et al. 2017). This trend appears with several personality traits – the typical traits of self-harming individuals tend to be more accentuated (compared to the non-self-harming population), with the significance of the differences in extent increasing with the increasing prevalence of problematic self-harm (both quantitative (intensity, frequency) and qualitative (such as attempted suicide) aspects), and the rising tendency continues with the presence of co-morbidities in the form of mental disorders (Allroggen et al. 2014; Tschan et al. 2017; Démuthová & Rojková 2019).

Psychoticism

Apart from the Big Five, scientists also focus on other characteristics – for instance, the Big Five concept excludes psychoticism, which may be one of the key variables in the frequent co-morbidity of self-harm and mental disorders[188] (including psychoses). This view is also supported by studies in which psychoticism has been associated with a higher prevalence of self-harm (Carli et al. 2010) and self-harming individuals who report the more serious forms of self-harm (especially attempted suicide) (Liang et al. 2014). We reached similar conclusions through an analysis of the levels of psychoticism found in self-harming adolescents in Slovakia (n = 1151), and levels of psychoticism were statistically significantly higher (p = 0.000) in those who reported attempted suicide in their history of self-harm (Démuthová & Rojková 2019). The level of psychoticism

---

[188] See the previous section "5.1 Mental Disorders".

as a trait together with its facets was measured on a representative sample (in terms of age, gender, and education) of the Flemish population by L. Smets and L. Claes. They also observed the lifetime prevalence of self-harm of the respondents and compared the data related to psychoticism from individuals without self-harm and from the sample that self-reported self-harm (Table 31).

Table 31. Levels of psychoticism and its facets in individuals with and without non-suicidal self-injury (MANCOVA)

		NSSI		nNSSI		MANCOVA	
		M	SD	M	SD	F	p
Psychoticism		21.19	18.71	12.82	12.25	15.36	<0.001
Facets	Unusual beliefs and experiences	3.97	4.37	2.83	3.50	5.42	0.020
	Eccentricity	11.28	10.85	6.16	6.76	19.90	<0.001
	Perceptual dysregulation	5.94	5.76	3.84	3.94	6.51	0.011

Notes: NSSI = individuals with non-suicidal self-injury; nNSSI = individuals without non-suicidal self-injury
Source: Smets & Claes (2017, 98)

The results of this study clearly show that individuals who self-harm score statistically significantly higher in psychotism and all of its facets than the population who do not self-harm.

Antagonism

Another characteristic associated with self-harm is antagonism. This is not an area that is frequently studied, since the trait refers to behaviour that leads to conflict (incompatibility) with others. People with a high level of antagonism have strong feelings of their own importance, they are convinced that they should be treated differently than others and they do not understand, or do not want to understand, the needs of others (Riegel 2018). These characteristics are generally not considered to be typical of self-harming individuals. However, several studies (see Smets & Claes 2017; Evans & Simms 2019; Acosta et al. 2020), have found a link between antagonism (or its characteristics –facets) and self-harm.

L. Smets and L. Claes studied the lifetime prevalence of self-harm and compared the data on antagonism (as well as its individual facets) in a group of self-harmers with that from a control sample of non-self-harmers. Their results show (see Table 32) that self-harming individuals have higher levels of antagonism and most of its facets (with the exception of grandiosity and attention seeking) than the control sample (Smets & Claes 2017).

Table 32. Levels of antagonism and its facets in individuals with and without non-suicidal self-injury (MANCOVA)

		NSSI		nNSSI		MANCOVA	
		M	SD	M	SD	F	p
Antagonism		31.33	20.42	22.90	15.61	7.99	0.005
Facets	Manipulativeness	5.03	3.87	3.59	2.96	6.40	0.012
	Deceitfulness	8.33	6.03	5.33	4.37	9.92	0.002
	Grandiosity	2.86	3.04	2.53	2.78	0.38	0.537
	Attention seeking	8.14	5.18	5.98	4.67	2.68	0.102
	Callousness	6.97	7.21	5.49	4.71	7.18	0.008

Notes: NSSI = individuals with non-suicidal self-injury; nNSSI = individuals without non-suicidal self-injury
Source: Smets & Claes (2017, 98)

Grandiosity and attention-seeking are not typical traits found in self-harming individuals – the levels of these traits are not higher than in the sample of non-self-harming individuals. Although attention-seeking has been reported as a dominant motive for self-harm in the past, nowadays, this view is considered obsolete, and attention-seeking seldom appears as a motive for self-harm (Lewis & Heath 2013). These findings fit the overall image of a self-harming individual, who is better characterised by internalisation rather than externalisation. This is why external expressions are not typical; on the contrary, internalisation (especially depression, anxiety and eating disorders) have strong correlations with self-harm and are considered significant risk factors for self-harm (Fox et al. 2015). Although manipulativeness and deceitfulness were more frequently found in self-harming adolescents than in the control sample, we assume that they were a result of the effort to hide self-harm[189]; however, they may also represent characteristics that supplement the clinical picture of the associated personality disorders[190] that co-occur with self-harm – manipulativeness is more typically found in men who suffer from a borderline personality disorder[191] (Tragesser & Benfield 2012), while deceitfulness is more typical of women with associated behavioural disorders (Szewczuk-Bogusławska et al. 2021). Antagonism may also occur in cases where the primary function (motive)[192] of self-harm is revenge (Acosta et al. 2020). However, there are also studies that found no significant correlation between self-harm and antagonism. An explanation is offered by the study of C. M. Evans and L. J. Simms, who found that expressions of antagonism differ depending on the nature of the self-harm. While self-harm with signs of suicidal intent is characterised by anhedonia, non-suicidal self-injury (NSSI) is rather associated with antagonism and obsessive-compulsive tendencies (Evans & Simms 2019).

Resilience

Resilience has a specific position in the personality traits of adolescents, since for the most part, it evolves together with other personal experience and through the solution of problems during our lifetime. It is not only the result of learning – in the formation of resilience, an important part is played by the mindset of the individual, depending on their personality – it determines, whether the individual will see obstacles as challenges and a way to gain skills or as a bitter blow that leads to even more problems. Generally, resilience is the ability of an individual to effectively adapt to adverse situations (Luthar 2003). As with other personality traits, resilience is also saturated by several lower-order characteristics (dimensions); these include characteristics used by the individual when facing adverse situations, for example, goal concentration,

---

189 Especially during adolescence, when the individual is still in the care of their parents.
190 See the previous section "5.1 Mental Disorders".
191 Nevertheless, borderline personality disorder occurs mostly (75%) in women (APA 2015).
192 See the following section "5.4 Motivation".

interpersonal assistance, emotion regulation, positive perception, or family support.[193] All these dimensions (as well as their overall level of resilience) significantly negatively correlate with the prevalence of self-harm – the higher the degree of resilience, the lower the levels of self-harming behaviour exhibited by the adolescent. Of all the domains, emotionality had the closest link with self-harm (Tian et al. 2020). The same results were confirmed by Zhang et al. (2021) with a sample of 875 young people – they also discovered a close negative correlation between resilience and self-harm. When it comes to the interaction between personality and temperament traits, an interesting study by Ran et al. observed links between impulsivity and resilience and the prevalence of self-harm in 4,552 adolescents. Not only did they confirm a link between resilience and self-harm, but they also discovered that resilience is a major moderator[194] of impulsivity and the prevalence of self-harm (Ran et al. 2022). Similar to Luthar (2003), the authors not only considered the overall level of resilience but also its subscales. They found that the domains that provide the greatest reduction in the prevalence of self-harm in adolescents are goal concentration and emotion regulation. Once again, emotion regulation appears to be a significant contributory element in the prevalence of self-harm, which fits into the overall clinical picture of a self-harming individual. The latter is characterised by significant emotional instability[195], and moreover, the motivation for this high-risk behaviour frequently involves emotion regulation[196]. If an individual is highly resilient in this area, they are more able to successfully resist the pressure that might otherwise lead them to self-harm.

---

193 These dimensions are identified using the method for the measurement of the level of resilience in adolescents: Resilience Scale for Chinese Adolescents (Hu & Gan 2008).
194 The study suggests that resilience is responsible for 42.90% of the total number of connections between impulsivity and self-harm (Ran et al. 2022).
195 See the following section "5.6 Emotionality".
196 See the following section "5.4 Motivation".

5.3 Temperament

To date, several studies have focused on the observation of the temperament traits of self-harming individuals. These characteristics describe the typical and relatively stable emotional reactivity of a person (Rettew & McKee 2005). However, when looking at research findings related to the temperament traits of self-harmers, there are certain characteristics that we have already encountered in the descriptions of the personality traits – these include impulsivity, emotion regulation and extraversion. Personality and temperament (as well as other) traits cannot be observed separately – they are united in the personality of the individual, they interact with, supplement and overlap with each other[197], and furthermore, there is no clear consensus in terms of the boundaries between temperament and personality. Many scientists who study personality traits argue that both temperament and personality are related to the basic internal tendencies that affect thought, emotions and behaviour and that any differences between these constructs are to a certain extent artificial (Rettew & McKee 2005).

Impulsivity

Impulsivity is often mentioned in the context of the temperament traits of self-harming individuals (Chamberlain et al. 2017; McHugh et al. 2019; Cassels et al. 2020). Impulsivity as a temperament trait represents the individual's predisposition to quick, unplanned reactions to both internal and external impulses, with limited regard to the negative consequences of these reactions, neither for the impulsive individual nor the people around them (Mitchell & Potenza 2014). The link between impulsivity and self-harm can be observed at several levels. It can be the underlying reason for the onset of self-harming behaviour, since individuals who have difficulty controlling their impulses are more likely to

---

[197] Therefore, dividing personality traits into sections is motivated more by the need for clarity in the text than any need to clearly differentiate them and process them separately.

use self-harm as a strategy to reduce the negative effects of critical or stressful situations (Allen et al. 2019). It may also contribute to the retention of self-harm in the repertoire of maladaptive responses – an impulsive individual does not consider the negative consequence of their actions when choosing a coping mechanism, but instead, they opt for the first available method that reduces their tension, often through self-harm due to its immediate availability (our bodies are always available). And last but not least, impulsivity may contribute to a higher frequency and intensity of self-harm, especially as a result of a lower ability to resist the impulse to repeatedly cause self-harm, which tends to occur after some time due to the high degree of the addictiveness of self-harm. Over the course of the history of the study of self-harm, many studies have attempted to clarify the role of impulsivity. Many studies have found a correlation – for instance, Lynam et al. found a link between the individual factors of impulsivity[198] (negative urgency, lack of premeditation, lack of perseverance and sensation seeking) and self-harm. All four factors were found to be major predictors of self-harm and suicidal behaviour (Lynam et al. 2011). Similar conclusions were also reached by Cassels et al., who observed the development of self-harm in adolescents. The study focused on impulsivity, attachment and distress levels of 1,686 young people aged 14–25 years. Through a self-reporting methodology with a follow-up after a year the authors discovered that impulsivity predicted the onset of NSSI, to a greater extent than other risk factors.

On the other hand, other studies have suggested only a moderate correlation between impulsivity and self-harm (the results of

---

198 The authors developed these four factors in 2001, when they unified all the personality models of impulsivity (that existed at that time) (see Whiteside & Lynam 2001). Their factor analysis included items from 20 subscales taken from 9 different models of impulsivity and 14 original items. Based on their analysis, they came up with four impulsivity factors, "negative urgency" (the tendency to act on impulse under the influence of negative emotions), "lack of premeditation" (the tendency to act without any prior consideration), "lack of perseverance" (the inability to focus on the task at hand) and "sensation seeking" (the tendency to seek intense, immediate and exciting experiences). After the initial four-factor model, they added another, a fifth factor – "positive urgency" because the individual may act also hastily under the influence of a positive impulse (e.g., when in a good mood – such as when gambling). Today, this model is known as UPPS-P, and although it is not in very wide-spread use in Slovakia, it is still considered to be the most complex, high-quality impulsivity model (Linhartová et al. 2017).

meta-analyses are available, for example, in Hamza et al. 2015), while some studies have also suggested that the predictive power of impulsivity in longitudinal studies was relatively weak (Fox et al. 2015). As already suggested in previous chapters, the different results that have come from the various studies are, to a large extent, caused by the lack of a clear definition of self-harming behaviour and the use of different methodologies. The roots of the inconsistencies can also be found in the method of operationalisation of impulsivity; some studies use it as a trait that covers several personality characteristics and behavioural expressions, while others focus on its components/facets. All of this contributes to a substantial degree of incompatibility, which is confirmed by some studies that studied the specificities of the link between impulsivity and self-harm. For example, Chamberlain et al. classified 3 subtypes of self-harm – self-injurious self-harm (such as cutting, burning and overdosing), interpersonal-related self-harm (engaging in emotionally or sexually abusive relationships) and reckless self-harm (losing one's job deliberately, driving recklessly). A correlation with impulsivity was only found with self-injurious and interpersonal-related self-harm (Chamberlain et al. 2017). Another study showed that an increased degree of impulsivity was present in those self-harming individuals who self-reported it. When laboratory measurements were used to measure impulsivity, self-harming adolescents did not exhibit any higher levels than non-self-harming individuals (Hamza et al. 2015; Tschan et al. 2017).

The Psychobiological Model of Temperament from C. R. Cloninger

The psychobiological model from R. C. Cloninger considers four dimensions of the typology of temperament – novelty seeking, harm avoidance, reward dependence and persistence (Cloninger 1987, 1993). These four dimensions represent four basic dynamics of temperament – behavioural activation (novelty seeking), behavioural inhibition (harm avoidance), maintenance (reward dependence) and perseverance (persistence) (Tomita et al. 2000). Novelty seeking is a characteristic defined by two opposites: impulsive vs deliberate action, which means that individuals with a higher score in this dimension are characterised by their reaction to new impulses with excitement (Moreira et al. 2015). In the context of self-harm, this characteristic is exhibited by a greater tendency to try new methods of self-harm (thus exhibiting several forms of self-harm) and by weaker resistance to impulses, thus the overall frequency of self-harm might be higher. It could be assumed that the extent of novelty seeking should positively correlate with the intensity (and thus frequency and the number of different forms) of self-harming behaviour. At the same time, novelty seeking is a characteristic which may allow us to distinguish self-harming individuals from non-self-harming individuals – in stressful situations, this may be a factor that will influence the method used to cope with the situation and this may lead the individual to opt for an impulsive solution or an unusual (new) solution (in this case, it is self-harm). These assumptions have been confirmed by several studies – for example, J. Lüdtke et al. confirmed a positive correlation between novelty seeking and repeated self-harm (Lüdtke et al. 2017). Novelty seeking is also a significant risk factor for the occurrence of suicide attempts in adolescence (Fergusson et al. 2000). A detailed study focusing on this was carried out by Tschan et al. – they compared the level of novelty seeking within three groups of female adolescents – adolescents without NSSI (control sample), adolescents with NSSI and adolescents with an associated borderline personality disorder. The results confirm trends that have already been identified in the personality traits – the more pathologies occur in adolescents, the more the specific personality traits are accentuated (at higher levels). In this case, it turned out that self-harming adolescents scored significantly higher in the temperament dimension, novelty seeking, than the control group (adolescents without NSSI), and furthermore, adolescents with borderline personality disorder had significantly higher levels of novelty seeking than self-harming adolescents without this disorder (Tschan et al. 2017).

Another dimension of temperament within R. C. Cloninger's model that is related to self-harm is reward dependence. Reward dependence is a characteristic that describes the extent to which an individual is willing to maintain a particular behaviour in their repertoire of reactions if it was (behaviour) rewarded in the past (Kose 2003). High reward dependence leads to a greater tendency to repeat behaviour that has been rewarded in the past. The reward may create either positive or negative reinforcement – it may bring benefits to the individual (such as: "...I am bonding with peers", "...I am creating signs of friendship or kinship with friends or loved ones"), or prevent loss/punishment (such as: "...I am avoiding the impulse to attempt suicide", "...I am causing myself pain so I will stop feeling numb"). If one of the primary motives/functions of self-harm is to induce the feeling the individual desires (relief from emotional pain, diversion of tension, etc.), it will probably be strongly reinforced as a reward, which will help it to be quickly retained in the repertoire of reactions. It can be assumed that individuals with higher reward dependence will succumb to repeated self-harm earlier and to a greater extent than individuals with a low level of this trait. So far studies have not yet confirmed this assumption – findings related to the level of reward dependence in self-harming individuals have tended to differ. Some studies (see e.g., Gómez-Expósito et al. 2016) suggest that the level of reward dependence is low in self-harming individuals, while others have found no link between self-harm and reward dependence (Ohmann et al. 2008; Hefti et al. 2013). However, more recent studies have revealed that the link between temperament traits and self-harm might not be a direct one. Often a combination of several characteristics (mutually interacting factors, mediators, etc.) is required to increase the risk of self-harm.[199] As to reward dependence, it was found that it is closely linked to the symptoms of internalisation, especially anxiety and depression (Kim et al. 2006). The consequent close link between these symptoms (or the clinical categories of anxiety and depression) was described in detail in the previous section "5.1 Mental Disorders"[200]. The ambiguity of the results may be due to the presence or absence of these contributing/mediating variables that may produce a correlation between reward dependence and self-harm.

---

[199] An example of this combination is impulsivity with a neurotic personality – individuals whose personality is susceptible to negative emotionality (neuroticism) cannot control their tendencies to opt for maladaptive responses in stressful situations (due to their high impulsivity) and repeatedly harm themselves (Valencia & Sinambela 2021).

[200] More specifically, these are sections dedicated to anxiety disorders and affective disorders as well as the following section "5.6 Emotionality".

Harm avoidance is yet another temperament trait found in C. R. Cloninger's model and it refers to behavioural inhibition when an individual anticipates negative events in the future and tries to avoid them. Logically, it might seem that since self-harming adolescents deliberately perform the behaviour that leads to the infliction of severe harm on themselves, you would expect their tendency to avoid harm to be very low. Yet, studies do not confirm this assumption – for instance, Tschan et al. found that self-harming adolescents score higher in harm avoidance than the control (non-self-harming) group (Tschan et al. 2017). Similar findings came from the study of Lüdtke et al., who measured the prevalence of self-harm and selected personality traits in a group of 447 students. They discovered that repeated self-harm occurred together with high levels of harm avoidance (Lüdtke et al. 2017). A possible explanation might be the excessively high levels of anxiety exhibited by self-harming individuals – it is rooted in the concept of harm avoidance, as the opposite of the typical characteristic of "risk-taking" (Moreira et al. 2015). Harm avoidance is a characteristic associated with high levels of anxiety (the individual worries excessively about what might happen) (Rettew et al. 2006; Chen et al. 2015), thus harm avoidance levels might be very high in self-harming individuals. Ironically (in this case), self-harm results from the fear of emotional pain that one experiences in difficult situations. Mental and emotional pain are so unbearable for these individuals and so harmful that they try to eliminate or avoid them "at any cost", even using forms of behaviour that cause them harm. The high level of harm avoidance as an expression of the mechanism of self-preservation in self-harming individuals[201] was partially confirmed by a study by Bae et al.[202] conducted on three groups of participants – individuals with non-suicidal self-injury (NSSI), individuals with self-injury and suicide attempts (NSSI + SA) and individuals who have attempted suicide (SA). As the risk of a fatal

---

201 In its essence, self-harm is considered to be a behaviour that leads to the preservation of the organism, in spite of the seemingly contrary actions that lead to injuries to the organism. One of its important functions is the prevention of suicide (see Klonsky 2007).
202 The differences in the extent of harm avoidance were visible on a descriptive level. The use of statistical methods did not reveal any statistically significant differences between these three groups.

injury increased (in the direction NSSI – NSSI + SA – SA), the level of harm avoidance decreased (Bae et al. 2020), which suggests that self-harming individuals (as opposed to individuals trying to end their lives) are primarily trying to protect themselves from harm, even though they opt for a highly maladaptive strategy (that leads to harm). The presence of self-harm with other disorders also increases the level of harm avoidance – individuals with eating disorders had higher levels of anxiety (they had a significantly higher score for harm avoidance) if they were also diagnosed with self-harm (Buelens et al. 2020).

The last temperament trait of the psycho-socio-biological model is persistence. Persistent individuals tend to be competitive and perfectionists. They show perseverance even despite repeated failures, frustration or fatigue (Buelens et al. 2020). Persistence is the resistance to adverse circumstances; it can be seen in an individual that tends to stick with their intentions. There are few scientific studies in this area – Lüdtke et al. suggested that the level of perseverance (as a temperament trait) is low in self-harming individuals (Lüdtke et al. 2017). However, another study found no link between self-harm and persistence (Buelens et al. 2020), although it should be noted that the research sample for this study was entirely made up of women hospitalised as a consequence of eating disorders.

5.4 Motivation

Establishing the motivation for self-harm is very important – the motivation behind the behaviour is what distinguishes it from similar activities; a behaviour may only be labelled as self-harm, if we know the motivation for it.[203] However, an analysis in this area is not only important to allow the behaviour to be correctly classified (i.e. differentiating self-harm from unintentional/undesired behaviour with similar consequences – but different motivations)

---

[203] A more detailed analysis of the significance of motivation and the role it plays in the definition of self-harm is provided in the introductory section "1.4 The Definition of Self-Harm".

but also to understand the circumstances behind self-harm and the functions that this behaviour might fulfil.

There are many different motivations for self-harm. Clinical practice as well as qualitative research, that examine the early stages of this high-risk behaviour, have highlighted many reasons for its appearance and retention in the repertoire of responses of individuals (see Šefarová 2019, 2020; Václavíková 2020; Shahwan et al. 2021). Quantitative research in this area has focused on the identification of the most common motivations; outputs from studies have included (among others) methodologies for the identification of the prevalence of the most common motivations/reasons for self-harm. One of the best-known methodologies is the ISAS (Inventory of Statements About Self-Injury – Klonsky 2007; Klonsky & Glenn 2009; Klonsky 2021). The questionnaire maps thirteen potential motives (functions) for self-harm (see Table 33). Each of

Table 33. Motivations and examples for 13 forms of self-harm measured by the ISAS

Area of motivation:	Example:
	When I self-harm, I am:
Affect Regulation	...calming myself down.
Anti-Dissociation	...causing pain so I will stop feeling numb.
Anti-Suicide	...putting a stop to suicidal thoughts.
Autonomy	...demonstrating that I do not need to rely on others for help.
Interpersonal Boundaries	...creating a boundary between myself and others.
Interpersonal Influence	...letting others know the extent of my physical pain.
Marking Distress	...creating a physical sign that I feel awful.
Peer Bonding	...fitting in with others.
Revenge	...getting back at someone.
Self-Care	...creating a physical injury that is easier to care for than my emotional distress.
Self-Punishment	...expressing anger towards myself for being worthless or stupid.
Sensation Seeking	...doing something to generate excitement or exhilaration.
Toughness	...seeing if I can stand the pain.

Source: (Démuthová & Václavíková, 2019, 25)

the thirteen areas includes a rating of three statements (items) on a three-degree scale of "not relevant – somewhat relevant – very relevant" (39 statements in total).

Using data obtained from a population of 323 Slovak adolescents who repeatedly self-harm, from 11 to 19 (mean age = 15.5, st. dev. = 1.475), it was found that the most common function/motivation for self-harm was emotional regulation (affect regulation) (see Table 34).

Table 34. The individual functions/motivations for self-harm in Slovak adolescents, in order of prevalence

Function/motivation	Mean Score (min./max. score)
Affect Regulation	2.6997 (0/7)
Self-Punishment	2.5373 (0/8)
Marking Distress	1.8607 (0/6)
Anti-Dissociation	1.6161 (0/6)
Anti-Suicide	1.4783 (0/6)
Toughness	1.2074 (0/8)
Interpersonal Boundaries	0.9907 (0/6)
Self-Care	0.9441 (0/6)
Interpersonal Influence	0.7864 (0/6)
Autonomy	0.7307 (0/6)
Sensation Seeking	0.5820 (0/6)
Revenge	0.5559 (0/6)
Peer Bonding	0.2601 (0/5)

Source: author

Many theoretical papers and study results have suggested that affect regulation has an important function in self-harm (for an overview, see Klonsky 2007). It is a result of the deficits that self-harming adolescents frequently exhibit in this area (Andover & Morris 2014). An inability to adequately (adaptively) cope with emotions may stem from several circumstances associated with self-harm. In a relatively healthy population[204], this might be a temporary imbalance between the rapid development of emotionality

---

204 That meets the required criteria, as suggested by clinical psychology, and lacks any risk factors in their history.

as a consequence of the developmental period[205] that adolescents are going through and a simultaneous lack of experience[206] that comes along with their relatively young age. In such cases, we assume that it is only a temporary maladaptive strategy that will eventually disappear (after the achievement of a certain level of emotional maturity along with the development of more adaptive patterns to cope with emotional stress). In more complex cases, problems with the regulation of emotions are caused by their contents. Some members of the population suffer from increased levels of tension, frustration, anxiety and depressive moods (Kumar et al. 2004; Laye-Gindhu & Schonert-Reichl 2005; Klonsky 2009). These negative emotions may overwhelm the individual's emotions and depress them to a level where the individual is unable to cope with them adaptively; thus, the individual will attempt to find alternative approaches that are, from a long-term and general perspective, considered to be maladaptive but are highly effective at that particular moment. The use of self-harm as a tool to hide from negative emotions or as a distraction has been confirmed by several studies (Nock & Prinstein 2005; Lloyd-Richardson et al. 2007; Matera et al. 2021). And last but not least, there are cases both in adolescence and young adulthood, where the emotionality of the individual is disturbed as a result of (developing) borderline personality disorder. The symptoms of borderline personality disorder include a substantial degree of affect instability and problems with affect regulation (APA 2013). In all three cases – from a relatively healthy individual up to an individual with a mental disorder – self-harm may be a way of venting tension (or another

---

[205] One of the specificities of adolescence is that it is the period when we reach a degree of cognitive maturity (level of formal operations) that allows an individual (among others) to work with metacognition and to think hypothetically. These new components of thought reveal new details (which were not available up to this point) – such as the ability to monitor their own thought processes and emotional experience, contemplation of the possible consequences of their reactions, regulation of behaviour based on the formation of hypothetical models of the consequences of their actions, etc. As a result of this shift, an adolescent will "discover" new dimensions, which pose greater demands on the way the individual deals with their experiences (such as the analysis of own emotions and their processing).
[206] The adolescent has not yet adapted, meaning he/she has not identified or developed effective coping mechanisms for emotional distress.

negative experience), or possibly a way to substitute a negative experience (that the individual is unable to cope with) with physical pain (which they are able to control, since they are causing it).

In addition to international studies, there is also a body of data that originates from Slovakia. A study into the motivation for self-harm, using a sample of the Slovak population, also included other variables, such as age, gender and attempted suicide for those who self-harm (Démuthová & Démuth 2019c; Démuthová & Václaviková 2019). The investigation of cross-gender differences revealed statistically significant differences in four areas of motivation, namely "Marking Distress" and "Self-Punishment" (dominant in girls) and "Toughness" and "Sensation Seeking" (dominant in boys) (Démuthová & Démuth 2019c). Marking Distress as a typical area of motivation in self-harming girls implies that, for the female gender, self-harm may be a maladaptive means of communicating problems. Self-Punishment also exhibits the characteristic signs of feminine self-harm, which is associated with a negative self-image and high demands on oneself, which leads to the conviction that the individual deserves the punishment. Since others do not perceive the individual in this light (in most cases, it does not reflect the objective reality) or evaluate them in the way that they expect (they do not scold/punish the individual), the individual feels the need to do so themselves. Kostić et al. (2019) came up with similar results, they identified self-punishment as the second most common function of self-harm in girls aged 13–18. There is also a further aspect typical of self-punishment – the history of self-harming individuals includes mistreatment in childhood or a cold/hostile family environment (Nock 2009). An inadequate degree of punishment of children during childhood (both direct and indirect – for example, the rejection of attention, affection, etc.) leads to a low level of self-confidence or even self-hatred ie adolescence. It also creates a pattern of behaviour, where even the slightest hint (feeling) of imperfection is followed by punishment. Adolescence also involves a progressive shift from the external regulation of behaviour (by parents, close ones) to internal control mechanisms (self-regulation). While going through puberty, parental control diminishes, but as the individual has developed a maladaptive scheme of experience and behaviour, punishment by adults is replaced by self-punishment. Whereas for boys, the dominance of Sensation Seeking and Toughness indicate that this might be a way to satisfy the desire for strong enough sensations or the enhancement of self-esteem by taking risks and overcoming pain. These differences reflect the natural differences in the behaviour of boys and girls during adolescence when boys are more impulsive and need stronger impulses to reach arousal than girls (Moir & Moir 1998). Furthermore, social pressures, during the period when they are reaching manhood, have a very strong influence on the ability to withstand pain and willingness to expose themselves to risk. Despite the fact that in both cases self-harming behaviour is an undesirable mechanism to solve problems or to satisfy needs, it is apparent that the mechanisms that underlie this high-risk behaviour may differ between the individual genders (Démuthová & Démuth 2019C).

An analysis of the motivations for self-harm only showed a statistically significant negative correlation with age in four areas: "Autonomy", "Interpersonal Influence", "Marking Distress" and "Self-Care". Hence, the reasons for self-harm are more significant at a younger age and diminish with time (Démuthová & Démuth 2019c). The dominance of Anatomy and Interpersonal Influence at a younger age may be interpreted through the pivotal importance of interpersonal contacts and the need to gain independence within early and middle adolescence. These are typical developmental roles at these ages (Shaffer & Kipp 2010), which is why the importance of these phenomena decreases once a mature identity has developed within late adolescence. Marking Distress is a way for adolescents to create physical evidence of their feelings of misery through self-harm. They express their emotional pain by creating an analogy between their mental and physical pain (Klonsky & Glenn 2009). The reduction in the occurrence of this motive as age increases may be related to two phenomena. The first is the tendency of younger adolescents to express mental pain and suffering in an effort to seek support or help from others. This may become less prevalent with age, since a greater degree of experience and improvements in their coping mechanisms help older individuals to become more reliant on themselves and their internal sources of support. This may equally indicate their abandonment of the effort to outwardly communicate their problems, as this strategy has failed (this may be assumed among older individuals, as they also continue to self-harm when they are older). The second phenomenon might be the previously mentioned change in forms of self-harm, which become more sophisticated and better concealed with age, thus it may lead to a change in the purpose of self-harm, which will no longer be of a "presentational" nature. In the case of Self-Care, it is perhaps that it is difficult for younger children to take care of their mental health. They are more knowledgeable about their physical health, how their bodies work, what causes diseases and how to treat them. This is certainly not the case for their mental health – adolescents lack knowledge of their mental mechanisms, of potential efficient coping mechanisms or "treatments" for their mental problems. Thus, it is easier for them to take care of their bodies than their psyche, and thus attention to and treatment of mental problems is substituted by care for their own bodies and treatment of injuries (Démuthová & Démuth 2019c).

A descriptive analysis[207] of the mean score in the individual areas of motivation for self-harm in individuals who have attempted suicide and those who have not showed that the main motivators for both groups are the same – "Affect Regulation" and "Self-Punishment". No significant differences were identified in the other areas of motivation based on their order of prevalence – thus, these groups do not differ in their typical motivators for self-harm. The only difference appeared to be in the intensity of the individual motives – an analysis of the statistically significant differences in the scores for the individual areas of motivation for self-harm in the group of adolescents who had attempted suicide compared to those who had not revealed that in all areas, the group who had attempted suicide had a statistically significantly higher score than those who had not. In the context of the study of the differences in the prevalence of the individual forms

---

[207] For more detailed information (and a full text of the scientific study) on differences in self-harm motivation among adolescents with or without a history of attempted suicide, see the following publication: Démuthová, S., & Václaviková, I. (2019). Rozdiely v motivácii k sebapoškodzovaniu u adolescentov so suicidálnymi pokusmi a bez nich. [The differences in the motivation for self-harm in adolescents who have attempted suicide and those who have not]. In S. Démuthová, & A.Baranovská (eds.), Kondášove dni 2019. [Kondas´ Days 2019] (26-34). Univerzita sv. Cyrila a Metoda.

(all areas of motivation can be found in both groups), the results highlight differences in the intensity, not in the topology of the motivators (Démuthová & Václaviková 2019). The higher intensity of the reported motivators is the obvious consequence of the significantly higher prevalence and frequency of various types of self-harm, which had been documented by previous studies that focused on the differences in the reported types and intensity of forms of self-harm in adolescents who had attempted suicide versus those who had not (Démuthová & Démuth 2019b). The results of this study and previous research suggest that attempted suicide is an extreme manifestation, but, nevertheless, it is still a part of the wide range of forms of self-harm. This view has also been presented by several international authors whose research identified close links between self-harm and attempted suicide (Muehlenkamp & Gutierrez 2007; Jacobson et al. 2008). Tormoen probably put it in the clearest possible way, arguing that non-suicidal self-injury (NSSI) and suicidal self-injury are parts of the same construct. The potential differences mostly only concern the degree, not the type (Tormoen et al. 2013).

5.5 Cognition

Several studies have emphasised that self-harming individuals process, interpret and retain information differently than their non-self-harming peers (Allen & Hooley 2015; Liu et al. 2016; Pollock & Williams 2001), especially if the information concerns them (Aizenman & Jensen 2007; Nelson & Muehlenkamp 2012; Smith et al. 2015). To a certain extent, this is the result of the more frequent overall negative emotional mood[208] of self-harming individuals, which leads them to, for example, an increased degree of self-criticism, a more pessimistic view of the future and feelings of helplessness. Other specificities in the form of perfectionism, maladaptive problem solving (a "black-and-white" view of the world), etc. imply

---

208 For more detailed information, see the following section "5.6 Emotionality".

that there are many other cognitive sources (cognitive distortions, mistakes, biases[209]) related to self-harm that either moderate it or have even been identified as causes.

A Negative Self-Image

As has already been suggested in section 2.4, self-harming individuals are often convinced that nobody likes them, that they are unworthy of love and affection, and they are a burden to others because of their lack of ability (Chu et al. 2016). As with other core convictions, in this case, it is also very difficult to convince an individual that this is not true. As a result of their mindset, an individual mainly notices the negative and hostile expressions of others and overlooks the positives or minimises their importance. This is why the individual reacts negatively to others, which minimises the possibility of positive feedback from others, which further convinces the individual that they correctly "read" the hostility and negative attitudes. These closed-cycle mechanisms are typical of most faulty cognitive schemes – in general, they are self-affirming. Moreover, self-harming adolescents may demonstrate a phenomenon where the hostile behaviour of the individual, and the subsequent reactions of others, is a form of self-harm[210]. Adolescents also display poor self-image in other areas – self-harmers are convinced that they are less intelligent and have poorer social skills than their peers (Case et al. 2020). This negative self-image does not only apply to the abilities and mental characteristics of self-harmers but also their physical traits (their appearance). Self-harming individuals report that they are significantly less satisfied by their appearance (Muehlenkamp & Brausch 2012; Black et al. 2019). In some cases, this may stem

---

209 Some examples were already listed in the section "2.4 Cognitivist Concepts".
210 In the study that focused on the forms of self-harm in Slovak adolescents (for more information, see Chapter 4 "The Forms and Types of Self-Harm in Adolescence"), the respondents were invited to add their own forms of self-harm. In this task, adolescents reported forms such as: "I was purposefully mean to others to make them hate me", "I lied to make my classmates hate me", "I mistreated my friends to make them stop talking to me", etc.

from an increased level of perfectionism[211], although for many other individuals, this comes from their core conviction that others consider them unattractive.

The correlation between a negative self-image and self-harm also appears on several other levels. The self-conviction that the individual is bad, ugly and unworthy of others can lead to self-disgust or even self-hatred, which may consequently lead to self-destructive tendencies, which undoubtedly include self-harm (Smith et al. 2015). Thus, self-harm is not only the visible manifestation of the relationship an individual has with themselves, but is also a way for the individual to "align", to a greater extent, their convictions with the objective reality (since most people do not find the wounds and scars caused by self-harm attractive). In doing so, the individual shows they have a poor self-image, they do not care for themselves to such an extent that they are willing to self-mutilate, and in this way they also self-harm – and not only through the activity itself (by feeling pain from self-harm) but also through its consequences (wounds, scars), which make the individual less attractive to others. This interpretation has been confirmed by the results of some studies which have highlighted the fact that self-harming individuals do not take care of themselves (Kittila 2012), and have a significantly lower level of body protection than healthy individuals (Cerutti et al. 2012),

A negative self-image may also be manifested in other ways within self-harming behaviour – individuals who are convinced that they are unattractive often use other maladaptive forms to solve their problem, such as eating disorders. The correlation between self-harm and eating disorders has been confirmed by several studies (Muehlenkamp et al. 2009; Peebles et al. 2011; Smithuis et al. 2018). In the context of self-harm, these individuals may exhibit forms that lead to a supposed improvement in their appearance, for example, through excessive exercise, a reduction in weight by limiting food intake, sleep or abusing laxatives.

A low level of self-confidence also indirectly reinforces the retention and increase in self-harming behaviour. It is assumed that individuals with low self-confidence and a negative self-image will only seek a minimal amount of social support and help from

---

211 This means that the individual may be well aware of the fact that others are not critical of them (that they are not considered ugly), but they may still be dissatisfied with their appearance.

others, which has a considerable effect on the likelihood of an intervention and thus treatment of this high-risk behaviour. Even if help is offered, in addition to the obstacles normally present with other mental problems, self-harmers tend not to believe that others care for them, that they can be worried about them or even like them. They cannot believe this is why they want to help. If it is professional help, they have hard time believing that anybody would waste their time and energy for their benefit or that they are worth the effort. Therefore, professional help should expect this, and an intervention aimed at improving self-confidence and self-image should be part of the therapy for self-harmers (Hooley & St. Germain 2014).

Negative Perfectionism

The link between higher levels of perfectionism and the presence of self-harm has been proven by many studies (see Gu et al. 2020; Gyori & Balazs 2021; Janssen & Hamza 2022), both in adolescents (Luyckx et al. 2015), as well as adults (Claes et al. 2012) and in both clinical (Claes et al. 2012) and non-clinical samples (Hoff & Muehlenkamp 2009). In the context of self-harm, we mainly speak about "negative perfectionism"[212]. Self-harming individuals are often characterised by their effort to achieve excellence, regardless of the circumstances and consequences (Claes et al. 2012; Gyori & Balazs 2021), which has negative impacts on both their mental well-being and mental health. Oftentimes, self-harming individuals do not lower their standards, even if their goals are unlikely to be obtainable or would require enormous, excessive effort, they might even set goals that are unachievable. In doing so, they fur-

---

[212] Perfectionism itself does not necessarily have to present a risk to the mental well-being of an individual. In addition to the one-dimensional model of perfectionism that describes this characteristic as the uncompromising effort to achieve high standards despite the negative consequences (Shafran et al. 2002), there are also multidimensional models of perfectionism that distinguish healthy (Stumpf & Parker 2000)/adaptive (Rice & Mirzadeh 2000)/functional (Rheaume et al. 2000)/positive (Terry-Short et al. 1995) perfectionism from unhealthy/maladaptive/dysfunctional/negative perfectionism. Research observing the risk/contributing factors of self-harm has mainly focused on negative (or maladaptive/dysfunctional/unhealthy) perfectionism.

ther contribute to their false cognitions – if they do not achieve their goal to a sufficient extent, or not at all, as it was unrealistic, it reinforces their view of their lack of ability. Perfectionists tend to undervalue their performance (although objectively they may be exceptional), they consider it to be unsatisfactory, which once more reinforces their conviction that they are not capable, and thus unworthy of attention, respect, dignity or affection. Studies confirm that perfectionism tends to co-occur with high levels of self-criticism in self-harming individuals (Frost et al. 1990).

The negative impact of dysfunctional (maladaptive) perfectionism is not only exhibited in the self-evaluation and the self-image of the self-harmer; the individual also has unrealistic expectations of the events in their life – they expect things to work perfectly, all of their experiences and events have to be extraordinary... Naturally enough these expectations lead to disappointment and frustration, giving the impression that life just keeps dealing out one blow after another. Perfectionism is not only retained in the repertoire of cognitive schemes of self-harmers because it is associated with other core cognitive schemes whose combined effects act as a multiplier but also because setting overly high goals (even unattainable) is in itself a form of self-harm – the individual deliberately exaggerates their goals, and the inevitable experience of failure is a way to trigger mental distress, discomfort and pain. Janssen and Hamza attempted to identify the factors that are associated with self-harm and perfectionism. Their research concluded that perfectionism increases the risk of the occurrence of self-harm by simultaneously: (a) increasing the desire to self-punish and (b) diminishing the individual's level of self-worth (Janssen & Hamza 2022). Considering that perfectionism is an inappropriate cognitive scheme that contributes to the onset (Gu et al. 2020) or retention of self-harm, the treatment of self-harm requires the individual to be able to understand and identify it as a maladaptive thought pattern and to work on it as such. In this context, there is another specific element (facet) of perfectionism that is often discussed – the "perfectionism cognitions" (Janssen & Hamza 2022), which manifest as automatisms. Here, it appears that it would be useful to practice the technique of improving mindfulness (Per et al. 2022; Gu et al. 2022). This is the ability of an individual to achieve a state of mind, where they can become aware of the present and accept their current thoughts, experiences and feelings and not judge them (Nicastro et al. 2010; Yu & Clark 2015). To be aware of, understand and accept one's own emotions is a key element of therapy dedicated to self-harmers, since deficits in affect regulation are one of the primary factors in the aetiology of this high-risk behaviour.

Rumination

The vicious circle of negative conviction (as well as negative emotionality[213]) includes rumination. It is a specific enduring cognitive mindset of an individual which results in them primarily focusing their attention on negatives (present, past and future), which leads to a considerable degree of emotional discomfort and suffering (Sansone & Sansone, 2012). Rumination has two essential elements – overthinking (paying excessive attention and mental activity to certain types of impulses) and negative emotionality (drawing attention to, thinking about and experiencing impulses accompanied by negative emotions). As a result of the presence of this cognitive mindset, the individual is constantly (it is an enduring characteristic) flooded by memories, worries and impulses that are accompanied by a wide range of negative emotional states – from fear, worry, anxiety, hopelessness, frustration through to panic, or depression. The individual specific focus of attention, mindset and memory focus that is a result of rumination cause the individual to ignore any positive impulses – they have less of a memory of them from the past and minimise their value for the future, or do not even expect them to occur in the future. Thus, negative emotions are constant and dominant. Many studies have pointed out that rumination is closely linked to depressivity (Robinson & Alloy 2003), hopelessness (Lam et al. 2003), poor problem-solving abilities (Watkins & Moulds 2005), anxiety (Nolen-Hoeksema 1991) and suicidality (Morrison & O'Connor 2008), but it is also an element found within self-harming behaviour (Selby et al. 2010; Johnson et al. 2022; Nagy et al. 2022).

---

213 See the following section.

Both self-harming behaviour and rumination are maladaptive mechanisms of affect regulation (Nicolai et al. 2016) – their link can be observed in the pathological cycle of experience and behaviour: rumination draws attention to the negative events in an individual's life, thus increasing the frequency of negative experiences and moods. The individual tries to regulate their negative emotions through self-harming behaviour, which is a maladaptive pattern of behaviour that ultimately leads to the reappearance of negative emotions (feelings of guilt, the return of negative emotions after the pain and the effects of self-harm disappear...). Both mechanisms – rumination and self-harm – are thus unsuccessful attempts to regulate emotion, and ultimately both result in a deterioration of emotional experience (Tait et al. 2014).

Hopelessness

Compared to the other cognitive characteristics of self-harming individuals, hopelessness is arguably the most destructive. While a negative self-image or high levels of perfectionism can, under certain circumstances, be corrected (e.g., through positive experiences or by mindfulness training), hopelessness defeats any effort or tendency for change. When an individual is affected by feelings of hopelessness, they are convinced that making any effort will be in vain and completely useless, that there is no possibility that they can be helped or that things for them can be improved.

Historically, the psychological construct of hopelessness is mainly associated with the studies of A. T. Beck, who, unlike the approach taken by others, who preferred a single dimensional definition of this characteristic (see e.g., Hanna et al. 2011), identified three types (factors) of hopelessness: affective (hope, enthusiasm, faith and happiness), motivational (giving up) and cognitive (negative expectations for the future) (Beck 1974). The importance of this multi-dimensional approach in the study of hopelessness was later confirmed by several other studies (Bouvard et al. 1992; Brodbeck et al. 2014; Boduszek & Dhingra 2016). In the context of self-harm, Pérez Rodriguez et al. observed the differences in the levels of the individual dimensions of hopelessness within a clinical sample of adult self-harmers and non-self-harmers. They found differences between the two groups, especially within motivational and cognitive hopelessness (Pérez Rodríguez et al. 2017). Analyses of the link between self-harm and hopelessness highlight that hopelessness is one of the most important predictors of self-harm (Fox et al. 2015). The presence of hopelessness is also associated with the more serious forms of self-harm, such as suicidal thoughts and attempted suicide (Mazza & Reynolds 1998; Horwitz et al. 2017) and other symptoms of internalisation, such as sadness, weeping, feelings of guilt and loss of pleasure (Case et al. 2020) which only cause further deterioration in the overall mental state. Intervention is also highly problematic in this case – individuals with high levels of hopelessness do not make the effort or expend energy in order to work at therapy, and even worse, they do not seek any professional or untrained help, or they reject it as it will be useless (they are convinced that things cannot get better).

A Low Level of Optimism

Optimism tends to be defined in many different ways – as a personality trait (Carver et al. 2010), as a cognitive bias (Weinstein 1980), a disposition (Scheier & Carver 1985; Burešová et al. 2020) or as an attributional style (Peterson & Seligman (1987), but at its core, it always refers to differences in the extent to which individuals expect future events to be favourable (Carver et al. 2010). Extensive research has been dedicated to the study of optimism in psychology, since it is considered to be a major protective factor for affective disorders, anxiety disorders, alcohol abuse (Öcal et al. 2022), suicide (Chang et al. 2018), suicidal thoughts (Hirsch et al. 2009) and other mental problems. A high level of optimism positively correlates with overall mental health (Scheier & Carver 1985) and well-being (Conversano et al. 2010), while a low level is associated with many mental disorders or makes them worse (Kennes et al. 2021).

Since there is such a close link between self-harm and depressivity, anxiousness, desperation, hopelessness and rumination[214] as characteristics which produce a pessimistic outlook (not only) for the future, but we may also assume that there is a negative

---

214 See previous sections dedicated to mental disorders (5.1) and cognition (5.4).

correlation between optimism and self-harm. This assumption has been confirmed by studies – just as rumination acts as a mediator between negative emotionality and self-harming behaviour, optimism represents an important mediating factor between psychological distress and self-harm (Tanner et al. 2014). If an individual has low levels of optimism, it is possible to observe a positive correlation with distress and self-harm (ibid.). Within the adult population Melson and O'Connor (2019) found lower levels of optimism in those with a history of self-harm when compared to those who have not self-harmed.

5.6 Emotionality

Self-harming individuals are characterised by negative emotional mood (negative affectivity), which intervenes with other areas of the psyche – it is associated with cognitive characteristics (how we process, interpret and retain information), psychomotor rate (a tendency to bradypsychia) and interpersonal interactions (self-isolation, affiliation with specific groups and subcultures). This characteristic has several components – facets – such as depressivity or hostility (see Table 35). Several studies have demon-

Table 35. Levels of negative affectivity and its facets in individuals with non-suicidal self-injury and those without (MANCOVA)

		NSSI		nNSSI		MANCOVA	
		M	SD	M	SD	F	p
Negative affectivity		68.39	20.40	56.66	17.19	11.27	0.001
Facets	Emotional lability	9.47	4.57	6.78	4.12	13.36	<0.001
	Anxiousness	11.86	6.88	8.61	5.49	10.30	0.001
	Depressivity[215]	6.72	4.66	5.82	3.71	7.58	0.006
	Separation insecurity	9.17	4.94	6.98	3.79	8.95	0.003
	Hostility	10.83	6.28	8.13	4.68	9.88	0.002

Notes: NSSI – individuals with non-suicidal self-injury; nNSSI – individuals without non-suicidal self-injury
Source: Smets & Claes (2017, 98)

---

[215] Originally, it was referred to as "restricted affectivity".

strated the presence of negative affectivity in self-harming individuals (Nicolai et al. 2016; Somma et al. 2019) as well as increased levels of its facets (Tang et al. 2013; Martorana 2015; Smets & Claes 2017; Evans & Simms 2019).

Emotional Lability

Self-harming individuals often experience and/or express their reactions to events and experiences with unusual intensity and a negative mindset. These expressions of emotion are often unpredictable, change quickly and are described by the concept of emotional lability [216] (Van Liefferinge et al. 2018). A high level of emotional lability is typical (compared to the period of childhood and adolescence) during adolescence (Larson et al. 2002); but there are individuals who have higher levels when compared to their peers. Emotional lability is a symptom that is associated with many mental disorders and clinical diagnoses (ADHD, Tourette's syndrome, affective disorders... – APA 2013); with regard to self-harm, researchers are mostly concerned with borderline personality disorder, which has a considerable degree of co-morbidity with self-harm (Reichl & Kaess 2021). The problem with lability lies on one hand in the lack of predictability of emotions (especially due to their frequent and rapid changes) and on the other their intensity. An inability to anticipate one's own emotional reactions and their powerful intensity makes it difficult for the individual to regulate them[217]; self-harm is a way to cope with them. Although it is a maladaptive strategy, it allows the individual (through the pain that accompanies self-harm) to quieten unbearable emotions; unlike the emotions, the pain inflicted by self-harm as a substitute

---

216 Another name for this phenomenon is "affective instability".
217 Emotional dysregulation frequently occurs in self-harming individuals (Wolff et al. 2019). It is demonstrated through a lack of awareness, understanding or acceptance of one's own emotions; through an inability to control one's own behaviour when emotionally distressed; by the lack of adaptive strategies for modulating the length and/or intensity of aversive emotional experiences; and by the unwillingness to experience emotional constraints (Gratz & Roemer 2004). The concept of emotional (dys)regulation was described in more detail in section "2.5 Regulatory Concepts".

can be regulated – the individual chooses when, for how long and to what intensity they will inflict it. It is readily availability (our bodies are always readily available for self-harm) and highly effective (the physical pain distracts us from the emotional pain). These are the high-risk characteristics that encourage the onset and retention of this behaviour in the repertoire of maladaptive regulation mechanisms in individuals with a high level of emotional lability.

Many studies have dealt with the relationship between emotional lability and self-harm (You et al. 2012; Peters et al. 2016; Wolff et al. 2019, etc.). For example, You et al. (2012) studied a sample of more than 4,500 adolescents and discovered that emotional lability (together with deteriorated interpersonal relationships and impulsivity) significantly correlates with present and future self-harm. Similar conclusions were also reached by Brickman et al. – emotional lability (as a symptom of borderline personality disorder) closely correlated with self-harm (Brickman 2014). The meta-analysis of scientific studies that researched the mutual correlations of self-harm and emotional lability confirmed these findings – by analysing the results of 48 published articles, the authors discovered that increased levels of emotional dysregulation are linked to an increased risk of the occurrence of self-harm, both in male and female subjects (Wolff et al. 2019). A study by Peters et al. that considered the relationship between emotional lability and self-harm discovered that emotional lability is not only associated with self-harm, but it is also a major risk factor for the onset of self-harm and its continuation in the future (Peters et al. 2016). Thus, the goal of intervention therapy that focuses on the problem of emotional lability has to take several key issues into account. Firstly, it is necessary to deal with the problem of anticipation – self-harming individuals tend to be surprised by their emotional reactions, they are caught unprepared and thus it is vital for them to learn to better perceive their emotions (greater mindfulness) and understand them (the cognitive aspect). If they learn to do so, they will be able to better deal with their emotional state and opt for a more appropriate problem-solving strategy (Wester & Trepal 2017); ideally, the strategy adopted should be able to regulate the intensity of the emotions they experience[218].

---

218 For an overview of the efficiency of the individual approaches to affect regu-

Anxiousness

Anxiousness (unlike temporary anxiety) is a relatively permanent characteristic of an individual, which affects their anticipation of negative experiences and events. The concepts of anxiety (as a current state) and anxiousness (as a relatively stable characteristic) overlap in research studies; most studies that deal with this phenomenon, in the context of self-harm, utilise the term anxiety, even if they observe its repeated presence in study subjects – in such cases, it would be more accurate to work with the term anxiousness. Anxiousness is mostly discussed as a personality trait, whereas the term "anxiety" is mostly used with regard to negative emotionality, even if the emotional state occurs repeatedly and becomes typical of the individual. An anxious individual worries significantly more... which means that the characteristic is closely linked to rumination[219] and is one of the typical traits found in self-harming individuals (Klonsky et al. 2003; Hack & Martin 2018; Lanfredi et al. 2021). Self-harming individuals describe the presence of anxiousness as persistent feelings of tension and uncertain worries about the near or distant future. As a result, they feel a strong need to keep these unpleasant thoughts under control which is one of the most common reasons for them to start to self-harm (Lloyd-Richardson et al. 2007; Hack & Martin 2018). Favazza and Conterio suggest that self-harming behaviour is a maladaptive way of dealing with feelings of growing tension and anxiousness (Favazza & Conterio 1989). In addition to negative emotionality, anxiousness is also one of the facets of neuroticism (Goldstein et al. 2018), which leads us to its link with other problematic characteristics. The relationship between self-harm and the occurrence of anxiety has been confirmed by several studies. Self-harming individuals differ from their non-self-harming peers in their levels of anxiety and at the same time, the levels of anxiety in actively self-harming individuals are higher than in those who are not active (Hack & Martin 2018). Higher levels of anxiousness in self-harming young people in comparison to their non-self-harming peers were also discov-

---

lation, see Wyman et al. 2010; Boehme et al. 2019; Daros et al. 2021.
219 The relationship between these concepts is described in the previous section "5.4 Cognition".

ered by Lanfredi et al. (2021). Perlman et al. (2018) consider anxiousness to be a significant personality correlate of self-harmers. According to other studies (see Klonsky et al. 2003), the presence of anxiety is a considerably stronger predictor for the occurrence of self-harm than depressivity. Anxiousness also turned out to be a significant predictor of suicidal behaviour (Brezo et al. 2008).

Depressivity

Depressivity is one of the most commonly reported correlates of self-harm. It fits into the overall image of the self-harming individual who typically has a distorted self-image, an increased degree of self-criticism, rumination and elevated levels of hopelessness, with all of these characteristics mutually interacting[220].

It should be pointed out that suffering from depressivity does not necessarily have to mean that an affective disorder – depression – is present; usually, there are elevated levels of depressive symptoms, i.e. an increase in the overall degree of depressivity or depressive mood. To examine the tendencies for the occurrence of depressivity in self-harming individuals, an exploratory study (Démuthová & Rojková 2022) was conducted that focused on the detection of depressive symptoms in children and youths in Slovakia, and especially their prevalence in self-harmers. A sample of adolescents (n = 1,117) was assessed through the CDI – Children's Depression Inventory[221] (Kovacs 1998), which identifies the presence of depressive symptoms, in addition, they were also assessed for self-harm (through the SHI, which monitors the prevalence of self-harm). The gross score for depressivity in self-harming individuals (n = 546) was 18.93 (st. dev. = 8.55). This is statistically significantly

---

220 For instance, as already mentioned with regard to mindfulness in section "2.4. Cognition" – mindfulness acts as a mediator between depressivity and self-harm, and at the same time, it is a protective factor from the negative impacts of depressivity on the occurrence of self-harm (Heath et al. 2016). Furthermore, individuals with a higher level of mindfulness experience less frustration, even during adverse life events (Lisá & Valachová 2021).
221 The questionnaire is frequently used in Slovakia and in nearby countries (see: Trebatická 2017; Jelínek et al. 2021), which simplifies the comparison of the obtained data.

higher (sig. of the single sample test = 0.000) than the standard score from the CDI test (mean value = 8.7). Only 13% (n = 71) of self-harming adolescents had a score lower or equal to the average for the general population. 69.3% of self-harming boys and 77.8% of self-harming girls scored values above the 75th percentile. 9.5% of boys and a quarter (24.5%) of girls reached the 97th percentile or higher (Démuthová & Rojková 2022). At the same time, the data analysis revealed that the higher the rate of depressivity exhibited by a self-harmer, the greater the intensity (the number and frequency of forms of self-harm) of self-harm (see Figure 15).

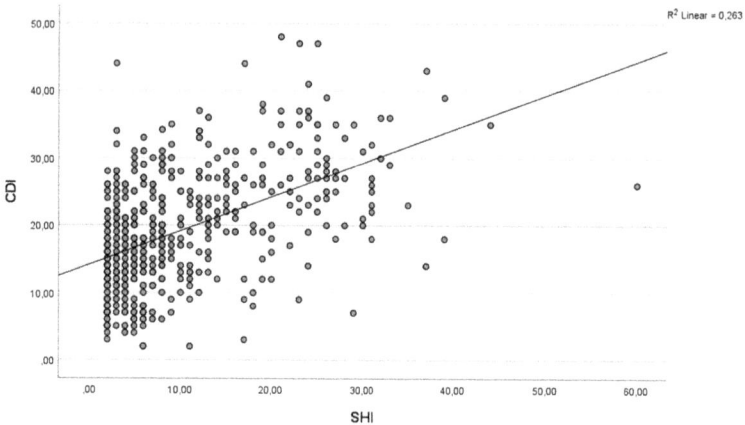

Figure 15. Spearman's non-parametric correlation between levels of depressivity and self-harm

Note: CDI = Children's Depression Inventory; SHI = Self-Harm Inventory
Source: Démuthová & Rojková (2022, 167)

These results generally correspond with the findings of other studies. For example, Giletta et al. 2012, conducted a study on adolescents from three different countries (Italy, the Netherlands and the USA). They found that higher levels of depressive symptoms significantly correlated with self-harm in all three groups. Similar conclusions were reached by studies that dealt with various nationalities and ethnicities (Hamdan et al. 2022). Hence, it appears that the link between depressive symptoms and self-harm is very close indeed. The study by Serra et al. from 2022 is highly topical, they emphasised further specificities of the link between depressivity and self-harm. It was conducted on a sample of adolescents who had been diagnosed with depressivity (according to DSM-5), with the discovery of differences between individuals with self-harm and without self-harm. It turned out that the group of self-harming adolescents had a significantly higher prevalence ($p = 0.0039$) of suicidal thoughts, depressive symptoms ($p = 0.0138$), symptoms of anxiety ($p = 0.0153$) and suffered from a significantly higher degree of emotional dysregulation ($p = 0.0092$) than individuals who have been diagnosed with depression but without self-harm. Therefore, it appears that self-harming is characteristic of the more serious phenotypes of depression in adolescents (Serra et al. 2022).

The mutual links between depressivity and self-harm, along with those they form with other factors are still the subject of research. In addition to studies into correlations or possible differences in the occurrence of depressive symptoms in self-harming and non-self-harming individuals, researchers are also examining potential causal relationships. As stated by Başgöze et al. (2021), in some adolescents, depression occurs first and NSSI only develops later, as a maladaptive strategy for coping with the symptoms; in others, NSSI comes first and is followed by depressive symptoms as a result of the psychological, interpersonal and/or biological consequences of repeated NSSI. There are also individuals in whom self-harm and depressive symptoms appear simultaneously, and they are also at risk of other complications, such as suicidal behaviour. To address this, Wang et al. conducted a meta-analysis of data from 25 studies, in order to identify high-risk factors for self-harm. Major factors in the area of mental disorders included the presence of depressive symptoms and anxiety (Wang et al. 2022).

Separation Insecurity

Another facet of negative emotionality is separation insecurity. It is also one of the characteristic symptoms of borderline personality disorder (APA 2013). It is a consistent fear of rejection and/or separation from someone close, which could be manifested in an excessive degree of dependency and a loss of autonomy (Ferris & Silton 2016). The presence of this characteristic may stem from several aspects of the thought process and emotionality of a self-harming adolescent – low self-confidence, a negative self-image, the conviction that they are not worthy of affection, negativism, rumination and more. All of these contribute to causing the individual to worry that they might be rejected by their significant other. This characteristic can also result from the more distant aetiopathogenesis – individuals with borderline personality disorder as well as individuals that self-harm were often mistreated in childhood, separated from their mother or had an insufficiently strong mother–child bond (Chapman et al. 2022; Serafini et al. 2017). These experiences have a major impact on the broad areas of emotionality and cognition, especially in a social context.

Hostility

Hostility is a broad concept that in addition to affective states characterised by the experience of frequent and intense anger also includes specific behavioural tendencies (exhibited by aggression) and a specific cognitive style (referred to as cynicism) (Thomas et al. 2020). Although self-harm as such draws our attention to internalised rather than externalised expressions of aggression, the connection between hostility and self-harm is not so rare. It can be observed on several levels. Hostility as the cognitive component of aggression (Buss & Warren 2010) is not only related to a lack of trust in others, a vulnerability to stress, poor stress management and frequent concurrent negative emotions but also to anxiety and depression (Felsten & Hill 1999). These characteristics are also frequently considered to be high-risk factors that lead to self-harm (Portzky et al. 2008; Bhui et al. 2007). Another link appears when individuals have issues with the management of difficulties and problem-solving. Individuals with these deficiencies more frequently experience frustration and failure, and what is more, this combination with the frequent occurrence of negative perfectionism, along with an increased degree of self-criticism leads to an individual who very often experiences failure. Generally, the most common reaction to frustration is aggression (Berkowitz 1989), and hostile behaviour is one form. A self-harming individual may express hostility more often, especially as a consequence of their frequent experience of frustration.

Researchers have attempted to unveil some of the possible connections and links. Scocco et al. examined the levels of hostility in the clinical population and discovered that individuals who also self-harmed (on top of their primary diagnoses), score significantly higher on the scale of indirect aggression in the Buss-Durkee Hostility Inventory than non-self-harming individuals (Scocco et al. 2019). The connection between hostility and self-harm is not only related to the clinical population – increased levels of hostility, verbal and indirect, were also reported in self-harming adolescents (compared to their non-self-harming peers) Tang et al. (2013). Hostility is also associated with the risk of continued self-harming behaviour – it was discovered that individuals who continued to self-harm, had significantly higher levels of hopelessness and intropunitive hostility than those who did not repeatedly self-harm (Brittlebank et al. 1990). Dillon et al. (2021) attempted to find an answer to the question of whether hostility predicts self-harm or if hostility is a consequence of self-harm. Using a multi-level modelling methodology, they discovered that hostile and aggressive situations provoke self-harm, not the other way around. Thus, it appears that anger and hostility are predictors or triggers of self-harm; however, these results cannot be generalised, since the authors only worked with a very specific sample of military veterans. It seems that the exact mechanism of the interaction or mutual influence of self-harm and hostility needs further investigation. This is shown by the large number of studies that have confirmed the existence of a mutual relationship (e.g., Jacobson & Gould 2007; Mullins-Sweatt et al. 2013; Tang et al. 2013).

Conclusion

Conclusion

The effort to find the answers to scientific problems often leads to an even greater number of questions. And yet, we should not refrain from the study of these phenomena, quite the opposite. By gradually revealing the specificities of highly complex topics, some of their aspects are clarified, while others – despite their persistent lack of clarity – stand out as an inspiration for further investigation.

In the context of current research into self-harm, the key findings of this monograph cover several facts. Firstly, self-harm includes a wide range of actions that are intended to harm or inflict pain upon oneself. This means that in addition to the general concept of activities that lead to the visible damage of bodily tissues (cuts, bruises, burns...), it is also necessary to study many other indirect forms, which may cause covert physical damage or forms which lead to mental suffering. It is the findings related to the prevalence of "mental" forms of self-harm as well as "indirect physical" forms that suggest that these may be more prevalent forms than the more commonly discussed "direct physical" forms. Although the existence of these types of self-harm as separate groups (factors) is yet to be proven, it is crucial to take them into consideration in the definition of self-harm. Thus, it may be necessary to re-evaluate the criteria for the definition of self-harm beyond that suggested by the fifth revision of the Diagnostic and Statistical Manual of Mental Disorders of the American Psychiatric Association (DSM-5).

Another important finding is that self-harm is a highly prevalent phenomenon that especially occurs during adolescence. It is more common in girls and individuals who use it as a maladaptive coping strategy. The aetiology of self-harm includes several causal and concurrent factors – it appears that the individuals who are most vulnerable to self-harm are those whose experiences have weakened their ability to cope with stress and pressure. This may be the consequence of childhood abuse, the absence of high quality, permanent and safe relationships, life experiences that the individual finds they cannot cope with, or a specific (especially cognitive and emotional) mindset that life is extraordinarily difficult. As a result of these life experiences, the individual fails in the search for and use of adaptive patterns of behaviour and instead opts to use a high-risk maladaptive strategy in the form of self-harm.

Although self-harm is a symptom of some clinical diagnoses (intellectual disorders, borderline personality disorder, eating disorders, etc.), its increase in prevalence is especially apparent in the non-clinical adolescent population. Analyses aimed at the discovery of potential pressures have identified several accented (but still non-pathological) personality traits (depressivity, emotional lability, neuroticism, psychoses, perfectionism, etc.), and it appears that the more striking these personality traits are, the more serious the self-harming behaviour (as to the frequency, intensity and prognosis). There is no truly systemic research in this area – the absence of a clinical diagnosis may not mean the absence of a disorder (due to the difficulty in the identification of mental problems in childhood and adolescence); moreover, when it comes to the deterioration of the mental health of the population (including the mental health of children and adolescents), it is possible that the increased prevalence of these adverse phenomena, including self-harm, stems from the increasing number of mental disorders and problems. The contribution of these factors to the prevalence of self-harm could be identified by a longitudinal study that observes the further developments, course and disappearance of self-harm in the ontogenesis, or possibly the onset and development of consequent mental disorders.

Last but not least, this leads us to the extensive topic of psychological interventions aimed at self-harming behaviour. This behaviour is the result of the simultaneous impact (and sometimes also malfunction) of a whole complex of mental mechanisms. Even though this monograph had no ambitions to deal with this area, when describing cognitivist, psycho-dynamic, interpersonal or biological concepts, possible questions and incentives naturally arise for corrective actions, which could potentially help to prevent the onset of self-harm, or to reduce or remove it from the repertoire of maladaptive forms of reaction to pressure.

There are still many topics and questions open for discussion in research into self-harm. This monograph, along with other future works in this area, will hopefully make it possible for the most precious in our society – our youth, who embody our future, to be able to live high-quality, valuable lives, and to create space for the healthy development of not only individuals but also the whole of society, not only for today but also for the generations who follow.

References

Acosta, M., Pirani, S., Garcia, A., Wainwright, K., & Osman, A. (2020). Evaluation of the psychometric properties of the Multidimensional Revenge Attitudes Inventory-21. *Psychological assessment, 32*(12), 1172–1183. https://doi.org/10.1037/pas0000951

Adler, P. A., & Adler, P. (2011). *The tender cut: Inside the hidden world of self-injury.* New York University Press.

Afshar, H., Roohafza, H., Sadeghi, M., Saadaty, A., Salehi, M., Motamedi, M., Matinpour, M., Isfahani, H. N., & Asadollahi, G. (2011). Positive and negative perfectionism and their relationship with anxiety and depression in Iranian school students. *Journal of research in medical sciences : the official journal of Isfahan University of Medical Sciences, 16*(1), 79–86.

Agos, K. C. M., Batino D. T. D., & Marasigan, P. R. (2021). Personality Traits and Non-Suicidal Self-Injury among Young Adolescents. *International Review of Social Sciences Research, 1*(4), 24–46. https://doi.org/10.53378/352084

Aizenman, M., & Jensen, M. A. C. (2007). Speaking Through the Body: The Incidence of Self-Injury, Piercing, and Tattooing Among College Students. *Journal of College Counseling, 10*(1), 27–43. https://doi.org/10.1002/J.2161-1882.2007.TB00004.X

Albores-Gallo, L., Méndez-Santos, J. L., Xóchitl-García Luna, A., Delgadillo-González, Y., Chávez-Flores, C. I., & Martínez, O. L. (2014). Nonsuicidal self-injury in a community sample of older children and adolescents of Mexico City. *Actas espanolas de psiquiatria, 42*(4), 159–168.

Alharbi, R., Varese, F., Husain, N., & Taylor, P. J. (2020). Posttraumatic stress symptomology and non-suicidal self-injury: The role of intrusion and arousal symptoms. *Journal of affective disorders, 276*, 920–926. https://doi.org/10.1016/j.jad.2020.07.084

Allen, C. (1995). Helping with deliberate self-harm: Some practical guidelines. *Journal of Mental Health, 4* (3), 243–250. https://doi.org/10.1080/09638239550037523

Allen, J. D., Fox, K. R., Schatten, H. T., & Hooley, J. M. (2019). Frequency of nonsuicidal self-injury is associated with impulsive decision-making during criticism. *Psychiatry research, 271*, 68. https://doi.org/10.1016/j.psychres.2018.11.022

Allen, K. J., & Hooley, J. M. (2015). Inhibitory control in people who self-injure: evidence for impairment and enhancement. *Psychiatry research, 225*(3), 631–637. https://doi.org/10.1016/j.psychres.2014.11.033

Allroggen, M., Kleinrahm, R., Rau, T. A., Weninger, L., Ludolph, A. G., & Plener, P. L. (2014). Nonsuicidal self-injury and its relation to personality traits in medical students. *The Journal of nervous and mental disease, 202*(4), 300–304.

Alm, S., Brolin Låftman, S., & Bohman, H. (2019). Poor Family Relationships in Adolescence and the Risk of Premature Death: Findings from the Stockholm Birth Cohort Study. *International journal of environmental research and public health, 16*(10), 1690. https://doi.org/10.3390/ijerph16101690

Alonso-Stuyck P. (2019). Which Parenting Style Encourages Healthy Lifestyles in Teenage Children? Proposal for a Model of Integrative Parenting Styles. *International journal of environmental research and public health, 16*(11), 2057. https://doi.org/10.3390/ijerph16112057

American Psychiatric Association. (1994). Diagnostic and statistical manual of mental disorders, 4th ed.(DSM-IV). *American Journal of Psychiatry 1995, 152* (8), 1228-1228. https://doi.org/10.1176/appi.books.9780890425596

Ammerman, B. A., Jacobucci, R., Kleiman, E. M., Uyeji, L. L., & McCloskey, M. S. (2018). The Relationship Between Nonsuicidal Self-Injury Age of Onset and Severity of Self-Harm. *Suicide & life-threatening behavior, 48*(1), 31–37. https://doi.org/10.1111/sltb.12330

Andover M. S. (2012). A Cognitive-Behavioral Approach to Case Formulations for Nonsuicidal Self-Injury. *Journal of cognitive psychotherapy, 26*(4), 318–330. https://doi.org/10.1891/0889-8391.26.4.318

Andover M. S. (2014). Non-suicidal self-injury disorder in a community sample of adults. *Psychiatry research, 219*(2), 305–310. https://doi.org/10.1016/j.psychres.2014.06.001

Andover, M. S., & Morris, B. W. (2014). Expanding and clarifying the role of emotion regulation in nonsuicidal self-injury. *The Canadian Journal of Psychiatry, 59*(11), 569–575. https://doi.org/10.1177/070674371405901102

Andover, M. S., Pepper, C. M., Ryabchenko, K. A., Orrico, E. G., & Gibb, B. E. (2005). Self-mutilation and symptoms of depression, anxiety, and borderline personality disorder. *Suicide & life-threatening behavior, 35*(5), 581–591. https://doi.org/10.1521/suli.2005.35.5.581

Andrews, J. L., Foulkes, L., & Blakemore, S. J. (2020). Peer Influence in Adolescence: Public-Health Implications for COVID-19. *Trends in cognitive sciences, 24*(8), 585–587. https://doi.org/10.1016/j.tics.2020.05.001

APA (2013). *Diagnostic and Statistical Manual of Mental Disorders.* Fifth Edition. American Psychiatric Association.

Arendt, F., Scherr, S., & Romer, D. (2019). Effects of exposure to self-harm on social media: Evidence from a two-wave panel study among young adults. *New Media & Society, 21*(11-12), 2422–2442. https://doi.org/10.1177/1461444819850106

Armiento, J., Hamza, C. A., Stewart, S. L., & Leschied, A. (2016). Direct and indirect forms of childhood maltreatment and nonsuicidal self-injury among clinically-referred children and youth. *Journal of affective disorders, 200*, 212–217. https://doi.org/10.1016/j.jad.2016.04.041

Arnett, J. J. (2014). *Emerging adulthood: The winding road from the late teens through the twenties.* Oxford University Press.

Arnett, J. J. (2018). *Adolescence and Emerging Adulthood: A Cultural Approach.* 6th Edition. Pearson.

Asch, S. S. (1971). Wrist Scratching as a Symptom of Anhedonia: a Predepressive State. *Psychoanalytic Quarterly 40*(4), 603–613.

Assavedo, B. L., & Anestis, M. D. (2016). The relationship between non-suicidal self-injury and both perceived burdensomeness and thwarted belongingness. *Journal of Psychopathology and Behavioral Assessment, 38*(2), 251-257. https://doi.org/10.1007/s10862-015-9508-8

Bae, Y., Seong, Y., Kim, S. H., & Kim, S. (2020). Clinical Characteristics of Non-Suicidal Self-Injury and Suicide Attempts among Psychiatric Patients in Korea: A Retrospective Chart Review. *Psychiatry investigation, 17*(4), 320-330. https://doi.org/10.30773/pi.2019.0269

Baer, M. M., Tull, M. T., Forbes, C. N., Richmond, J. R., & Gratz, K. L. (2020). Methods Matter: Nonsuicidal Self-Injury in the Form of Cutting is Uniquely Associated with Suicide Attempt Severity in Patients with Substance Use Disorders. *Suicide & life-threatening behavior, 50*(2), 397-407. https://doi.org/10.1111/sltb.12596

Baetens, I., Claes, L., Hasking, P. et al. The Relationship Between Parental Expressed Emotions and Non-suicidal Self-injury: The Mediating Roles of Self-criticism and Depression. *J Child Fam Stud 24*, 491-498 (2015). https://doi.org/10.1007/s10826-013-9861-8

Bai, Y. M., Liu, C. Y., & Lin, C. C. (1997). Risk factors for parasuicide among psychiatric inpatients. *Psychiatric services, 48*(9), 1201-1203. https://doi.org/10.1176/ps.48.9.1201

Bailey, D., Wright, N., & Kemp, L. (2017). Self-harm in young people: a challenge for general practice. *British Journal of General Practice 2017; 67* (665): 542-543. https://doi.org/10.3399/bjgp17X693545

Balázs, J., Győri, D., Horváth, L. O., Mészáros, G., & Szentiványi, D. (2018). Attention-deficit hyperactivity disorder and nonsuicidal self-injury in a clinical sample of adolescents: the role of comorbidities and gender. *BMC psychiatry, 18*(1), 34. https://doi.org/10.1186/s12888-018-1620-3

Balzer, B. W., Duke, S. A., Hawke, C. I., & Steinbeck, K. S. (2015). The effects of estradiol on mood and behavior in human female adolescents: a systematic review. *European journal of pediatrics, 174*(3), 289-298. https://doi.org/10.1007/s00431-014-2475-3

Bandura, A. (1977). Self-efficacy: Toward a unifying theory of behavioral change. *Psychological Review, 84*(2), 191-215. https://doi.org/10.1037/0033-295X.84.2.191

Bandura, A. (1986). The explanatory and predictive scope of self-efficacy theory. *Journal of Social and Clinical Psychology, 4*(3), 359-373. https://doi.org/10.1521/jscp.1986.4.3.359

Bandura, A. (1997). *Self-efficacy: The exercise of control.* W H Freeman/Times Books/ Henry Holt & Co.

Baralla, F., Ventura, M., Negay, N., Di Napoli, A., Petrelli, A., Mirisola, C., & Sarchiapone, M. (2021). Clinical Correlates of Deliberate Self-Harm Among Migrant Trauma-Affected Subgroups. *Frontiers in psychiatry, 12*, 529361. https://doi.org/10.3389/fpsyt.2021.529361

Barrocas, A. L., Hankin, B. L., Young, J. F., & Abela, J. R. (2012). Rates of non-suicidal self-injury in youth: age, sex, and behavioral methods in a community sample. *Pediatrics, 130*(1), 39–45. https://doi.org/10.1542/peds.2011-2094

Barry, T. J., Hallford, D. J., Hitchcock, C., Takano, K., & Raes, F. (2021). The current state of memory Specificity Training (MeST) for emotional disorders. *Current opinion in psychology, 41,* 28–33. https://doi.org/10.1016/j.copsyc.2021.02.002

Başgöze, Z., Wiglesworth, A., Carosella, K. A., Klimes-Dougan, B., & Cullen, K. R. (2021). Depression, Non-Suicidal Self-Injury, and Suicidality in Adolescents: Common and Distinct Precursors, Correlates, and Outcomes. *Journal of psychiatry and brain science, 6*(5), e210018. https://doi.org/10.20900/jpbs.20210018

Batey, H., May, J., & Andrade, J. (2010). Negative intrusive thoughts and dissociation as risk factors for self-harm. *Suicide & life-threatening behavior, 40*(1), 35–49. https://doi.org/10.1521/suli.2010.40.1.35

Bauman, Z. (2000). *Liquid modernity*. Polity Press, Cambridge.

Beck A. T. (1988). *Beck Hopelessness Scale*. The Psychological Corporation.

Beck A. T. (2008). The evolution of the cognitive model of depression and its neurobiological correlates. *The American journal of psychiatry, 165*(8), 969–977. https://doi.org/10.1176/appi.ajp.2008.08050721

Beck, A. T., Brown, G., & Steer, R. A. (1989). Prediction of eventual suicide in psychiatric inpatients by clinical ratings of hopelessness. *Journal of consulting and clinical psychology, 57*(2), 309–310. https://doi.org/10.1037//0022-006x.57.2.309

Beck, A. T., Brown, G., Berchick, R. J., Stewart, B. L., & Steer, R. A. (1990). Relationship between hopelessness and ultimate suicide: a replication with psychiatric outpatients. *The American journal of psychiatry, 147*(2), 190–195. https://doi.org/10.1176/ajp.147.2.190

Beck, A. T., Weissman, A., Lester, D., & Trexler, L. (1974). The measurement of pessimism: the hopelessness scale. *Journal of consulting and clinical psychology, 42*(6), 861–865. https://doi.org/10.1037/h0037562

Benzel, S. (2019). Selbstverletzende Handlungen in der Adoleszenz. [Self-injurious acts in adolescence]. In S. Benzel (ed.): Die Bedeutung des Körpers bei Selbstverletzungen junger Frauen. Adoleszenzforschung (Zur Theorie und Empirie der Jugend aus transdisziplinärer Perspektive). [The role of the body in self-harm in young women. *Adolescence research [On the theory and empiricism of youth from a transdisciplinary perspective]*. Springer. https://doi.org/10.1007/978-3-658-27947-9_2

Berardelli, I., Sarubbi, S., Rogante, E., Hawkins, M., Cocco, G., Erbuto, D., Lester, D., & Pompili, M. (2019). The Role of Demoralization and Hopelessness in Suicide Risk in Schizophrenia: A Review of the Literature. *Medicina 55*(5), 200. https://doi.org/10.3390/medicina55050200

Berkowitz L. (1989). Frustration-aggression hypothesis: examination and reformulation. *Psychological bulletin, 106*(1), 59–73. https://doi.org/10.1037/0033-2909.106.1.59

Bhui, K., McKenzie, K., & Rasul, F. (2007). Rates, risk factors & methods of self harm among minority ethnic groups in the UK: a systematic review. *BMC Public Health, 7*, 336. https://doi.org/10.1186/1471-2458-7-336

Bieling, P. J., Israeli, A. L., & Antony, M. M. (2004). Is perfectionism good, bad, or both? Examining models of the perfectionism construct. *Personality and Individual Differences, 36*(6), 1373–1385. https://doi.org/10.1016/S0191-8869(03)00235-6

Black, E. B., Garratt, M., Beccaria, G., Mildred, H., & Kwan, M. (2019). Body image as a predictor of nonsuicidal self-injury in women: A longitudinal study. *Comprehensive psychiatry, 88*, 83–89. https://doi.org/10.1016/j.comppsych.2018.11.010

Black, M., Erulkar, J., Kerfoot, M., Meadow, R. & Baderman, H. (1982) The management of parasuicide in young people under sixteen. *Bulletin of the Royal College of Psychiatrists, 6*, (10). 182–185. https://doi.org/10.1192/S0140078900007069

Blakemore, S.-J. (2018). *Avoiding Social Risk in Adolescence. Journal of Material Culture, 27*(2), 408–427. https://doi.org/10.1177/1359183520954462

Blasco-Fontecilla, H., Fernández-Fernández, R., Colino, L., Fajardo, L., Perteguer-Barrio, R., & de Leon, J. (2016). The Addictive Model of Self-Harming (Non-suicidal and Suicidal) Behavior. *Frontiers in psychiatry, 7*, 8. https://doi.org/10.3389/fpsyt.2016.00008

Boduszek, D., & Dhingra, K. (2016). Construct validity of the Beck Hopelessness Scale (BHS) among university students: A multitrait-multimethod approach. *Psychological assessment, 28*(10), 1325–1330. https://doi.org/10.1037/pas0000245

Boduszek, D., Debowska, A., Ochen, E. A., Fray, C., Nanfuka, E. K., Powell-Booth, K., Turyomurugyendo, F., Nelson, K., Harvey, R., Willmott, D., & Mason, S. J. (2021). Prevalence and correlates of non-suicidal self-injury, suicidal ideation, and suicide attempt among children and adolescents: Findings from Uganda and Jamaica. *Journal of affective disorders, 283*, 172–178. https://doi.org/10.1016/j.jad.2021.01.063

Boehme, S., Biehl, S. C., & Mühlberger, A. (2019). Effects of Differential Strategies of Emotion Regulation. *Brain sciences, 9*(9), 225. https://doi.org/10.3390/brainsci9090225

Bolognini, M., Plancherel, B., Laget, J., Stéphan, P., & Halfon, O. (2003). Adolescents' self-mutilation–Relationship with dependent behaviour. *Swiss Journal of Psychology / Schweizerische Zeitschrift für Psychologie / Revue Suisse de Psychologie, 62*(4), 241–249. https://doi.org/10.1024/1421-0185.62.4.241

Boričević Maršanić, V., Aukst Margetić, B., Ožanić Bulić, S., Đuretić, I., Kniewald, H., Jukić, T., & Paradžik, L. (2015). Non-suicidal self-injury among psychiatric outpatient adolescent offspring of Croatian posttraumatic stress disorder male war veterans: Prevalence and psychosocial correlates. *The International journal of social psychiatry, 61*(3), 265–274. https://doi.org/10.1177/0020764014541248

Borschmann, R., & Kinner, S. A. (2019). Responding to the rising prevalence of self-harm. *The lancet. Psychiatry, 6*(7), 548–549. https://doi.org/10.1016/S2215-0366(19)30210-X

Bosmia, A. N., Tubbs, R. S., Griessenauer, C. J., & Haddad, V., Jr (2015). Ritualistic envenomation by bullet ants among the Sateré-Mawé Indians in the Brazilian Amazon. *Wilderness & environmental medicine, 26*(2), 271–273. https://doi.org/10.1016/j.wem.2014.09.003

Bošiaková, L. (2013). Príčiny automutilácií psychiatrických pacientov vo väzenských podmienkach. [Causes of self-mutilation of psychiatric patients in prison condition]. *Psychiatrie pro praxi, 14*(2), 66–68.

Bouvard, M., Charles, S., Guérin, J., Aimard, G., & Cottraux, J. (1992). Etude de l'échelle de désespoir de Beck (hopelessness scale). Validation et analyse factorielle [Study of Beck's hopelessness scale. Validation and factor analysis]. *L'Encephale, 18*(3), 237–240.

Boyd, A. S., & Dewan, A. (2015). Dermatitis artefacta in an adolescent female. *Journal of cutaneous pathology, 42*(9), 660–661. https://doi.org/10.1111/cup.12499

Brager-Larsen, A., Zeiner, P., Klungsøyr, O., & Mehlum, L. (2022). Is age of self-harm onset associated with increased frequency of non-suicidal self-injury and suicide attempts in adolescent outpatients?. *BMC psychiatry, 22*(1), 58. https://doi.org/10.1186/s12888-022-03712-w

Brausch, A. M., & Gutierrez, P. M. (2010). Differences in non-suicidal self-injury and suicide attempts in adolescents. *Journal of youth and adolescence, 39*(3), 233–242. https://doi.org/10.1007/s10964-009-9482-0

Brausch, A. M., & Woods, S. E. (2019). Emotion Regulation Deficits and Nonsuicidal Self-Injury Prospectively Predict Suicide Ideation in Adolescents. *Suicide & life-threatening behavior, 49*(3), 868–880. https://doi.org/10.1111/sltb.12478

Brausch, A. M., Muehlenkamp, J. J., Fergerson, A. K., Laves, E. H., Whitfield, M. B., & Clapham, R. B. (2020). Examining Nonsuicidal Self-Injury Features as Motivational Moderators in the Relationship Between Hopelessness and Suicide Ideation. *Archives of suicide research : official journal of the International Academy for Suicide Research*, 1–14. https://doi.org/10.1080/13811118.2020.1853638

Brausch, A. M., Nichols, P. M., Laves, E. H., & Clapham, R. B. (2021). Body Investment as a Protective Factor in the Relationship Between Acquired Capability for Suicide and Suicide Attempts. *Behavior therapy, 52*(5), 1114–1122. https://doi.org/10.1016/j.beth.2021.02.008

Bresin, K., & Schoenleber, M. (2015). Gender differences in the prevalence of nonsuicidal self-injury: A meta-analysis. *Clinical psychology review, 38*, 55–64. https://doi.org/10.1016/j.cpr.2015.02.009

Brezo, J., Barker, E. D., Paris, J., Hébert, M., Vitaro, F., Tremblay, R. E., & Turecki, G. (2008). Childhood trajectories of anxiousness and disruptiveness as predictors of suicide attempts. *Archives of pediatrics & adolescent medicine, 162*(11), 1015-1021. https://doi.org/10.1001/archpedi.162.11.1015

Brickman, L. J., Ammerman, B. A., Look, A. E., Berman, M. E., & McCloskey, M. S. (2014). The relationship between non-suicidal self-injury and borderline personality disorder symptoms in a college sample. *Borderline personality disorder and emotion dysregulation, 1*, 14. https://doi.org/10.1186/2051-6673-1-14

Briere, J., & Gil, E. (1998). Self-mutilation in clinical and general population samples: prevalence, correlates, and functions. *The American journal of orthopsychiatry, 68*(4), 609-620. https://doi.org/10.1037/h0080369

Brittlebank, A. D., Cole, A., Hassanyeh, F., Kenny, M., Simpson, D., & Scott, J. (1990). Hostility, hopelessness and deliberate self-harm: a prospective follow-up study. *Acta psychiatrica Scandinavica, 81*(3), 280-283. https://doi.org/10.1111/j.1600-0447.1990.tb06497.x

Brodbeck, J., Goodyer, I. M., Abbott, R. A., Dunn, V. J., St Clair, M. C., Owens, M., Jones, P. B., & Croudace, T. J. (2014). General distress, hopelessness-suicidal ideation and worrying in adolescence: concurrent and predictive validity of a symptom-level bifactor model for clinical diagnoses. *Journal of affective disorders*, 152-154, 299-305. https://doi.org/10.1016/j.jad.2013.09.029

Brooksbank, D. (1985). Suicide and Parasuicide in Childhood and Early Adolescence. *British Journal of Psychiatry, 146*(5), 459-463. https://doi.ogr/10.1192/bjp.146.5.459

Brown, J. T., Volk, F., & Gearhart, G. L. (2018). A psychometric analysis of the Ottawa self-injury inventory-f. *Journal of American college health : J of ACH, 66*(1), 23-31. https://doi.org/10.1080/07448481.2017.1366496

Brown, M. Z., Comtois, K. A., & Linehan, M. M. (2002). Reasons for suicide attempts and nonsuicidal self-injury in women with borderline personality disorder. *Journal of abnormal psychology, 111*(1), 198-202. https://doi.org/10.1037//0021-843x.111.1.198

Brunner, R., Kaess, M., Parzer, P., Fischer, G., Carli, V., Hoven, C. W., Wasserman, C., Sarchiapone, M., Resch, F., Apter, A., Balazs, J., Barzilay, S., Bobes, J., Corcoran, P., Cosmanm, D., Haring, C., Iosuec, M., Kahn, J. P., Keeley, H., Meszaros, G., ... Wasserman, D. (2014). Life-time prevalence and psychosocial correlates of adolescent direct self-injurious behavior: a comparative study of findings in 11 European countries. *Journal of child psychology and psychiatry, and allied disciplines, 55*(4), 337-348. https://doi.org/10.1111/jcpp.12166

Buelens, T., Luyckx, K., Verschueren, M., Schoevaerts, K., Dierckx, E., Depestele, L., & Claes, L. (2020). Temperament and Character Traits of Female Eating Disorder Patients with(out) Non-Suicidal Self-Injury. *Journal of clinical medicine, 9*(4), 1207. https://doi.org/10.3390/jcm9041207

Burešová, I. (2016). Self-Harm Classification System Development: Theoretical Study. *Review of Social Sciences, 1*(4), 13-20. https://doi.org/10.18533/rss.v1i4.21

Burešová, I., Jelinek, M., Dosedlová, J., & Klimusová, H. (2020). Predictors of Mental Health in Adolescence: The Role of Personality, Dispositional Optimism, and Social Support. *SAGE Open, 10*(2). https://doi.org/10.1177/2158244020917963

Burke, T. A., Hamilton, J. L., Abramson, L. Y., & Alloy, L. B. (2015). Non-suicidal self-injury prospectively predicts interpersonal stressful life events and depressive symptoms among adolescent girls. *Psychiatry research, 228*(3), 416–424. https://doi.org/10.1016/j.psychres.2015.06.021

Burke, T. A., Jacobucci, R., Ammerman, B. A., Piccirillo, M., McCloskey, M. S., Heimberg, R. G., & Alloy, L. B. (2018). Identifying the relative importance of non-suicidal self-injury features in classifying suicidal ideation, plans, and behavior using exploratory data mining. *Psychiatry research, 262*, 175–183. https://doi.org/10.1016/j.psychres.2018.01.045

Buss, A. H., & Warren, W. L. (2010). *The aggression questionnaire manual.* Western Psychological Services.

Cadigan, J. M., Duckworth, J. C., Parker, M. E., & Lee, C. M. (2019). Influence of developmental social role transitions on young adult substance use. *Current opinion in psychology, 30*, 87–91. https://doi.org/10.1016/j.copsyc.2019.03.006

Calvete, E., Orue, I., Aizpuru, L., & Brotherton, H. (2015). Prevalence and functions of non-suicidal self-injury in Spanish adolescents. *Psicothema, 27*(3), 223–228. https://doi.org/10.7334/psicothema2014.262

Carli, V., Jovanović, N., Podlesek, A., Roy, A., Rihmer, Z., Maggi, S., Marusic, D., Cesaro, C., Marusic, A., & Sarchiapone, M. (2010). The role of impulsivity in self-mutilators, suicide ideators and suicide attempters - a study of 1265 male incarcerated individuals. *Journal of affective disorders, 123*(1-3), 116–122. https://doi.org/10.1016/j.jad.2010.02.119

Carr, M. J., Ashcroft, D. M., Kontopantelis, E., Awenat, Y., Cooper, J., Chew-Graham, C., Kapur, N., & Webb, R. T. (2016). The epidemiology of self-harm in a UK-wide primary care patient cohort, 2001-2013. *BMC psychiatry, 16*, 53. https://doi.org/10.1186/s12888-016-0753-5

Carvalho, C. B., Nunes, C., Castilho, P., da Motta, C., Caldeira, S., & Pinto-Gouveia, J. (2015). Mapping non suicidal self-injury in adolescence: Development and confirmatory factor analysis of the Impulse, Self-harm and Suicide Ideation Questionnaire for Adolescents (ISSIQ-A). *Psychiatry research, 227*(2-3), 238–245. https://doi.org/10.1016/j.psychres.2015.01.031

Carver, C. S., Scheier, M. F., & Segerstrom, S. C. (2010). Optimism. *Clinical psychology review, 30*(7), 879–889. https://doi.org/10.1016/j.cpr.2010.01.006

Case, J., Burke, T. A., Siegel, D. M., Piccirillo, M. L., Alloy, L. B., & Olino, T. M. (2020). Functions of Non-Suicidal Self-Injury in Late Adolescence: A Latent Class Analysis. *Archives of suicide research : official journal of the International Academy for Suicide Research, 24*(sup2), S165–S186. https://doi.org/10.1080/13811118.2019.1586607

Case, J., Mattoni, M., & Olino, T. M. (2021). Examining the Neurobiology of Non-Suicidal Self-Injury in Children and Adolescents: The Role of Reward Responsivity. *Journal of clinical medicine, 10*(16), 3561. https://doi.org/10.3390/jcm10163561

Caspi, A., McClay, J., Moffitt, T. E., Mill, J., Martin, J., Craig, I. W., Taylor, A., & Poulton, R. (2002). Role of genotype in the cycle of violence in maltreated children. *Science, 297*(5582), 851-854. https://www.jstor.org/stable/3832002

Cassels, M., Neufeld, S., van Harmelen, A. L., Goodyer, I., & Wilkinson, P. (2020). Prospective Pathways From Impulsivity to Non-Suicidal Self-Injury Among Youth. Archives of suicide research : official journal of the International Academy for Suicide Research, 1-14. https://doi.org/10.1080/13811118.2020.1811180

CDC - Centers for Disease Control and Prevention (2021). U.S. Department of Health & Human Services.https://phinvads.cdc.gov/vads/SearchVocab.actionhttps://phinvads.cdc.gov/vads/ViewCodeSystemConcept.action?oid=2.16.840.1.113883.6.96&code=402737007

Cerutti, R., Presaghi, F., Manca, M., & Gratz, K. L. (2012). Deliberate self-harm behavior among Italian young adults: correlations with clinical and nonclinical dimensions of personality. *The American journal of orthopsychiatry, 82*(3), 298-308. https://doi.org/10.1111/j.1939-0025.2012.01169.x

Chamberlain, S. R., Redden, S. A., & Grant, J. E. (2017). Associations between self-harm and distinct types of impulsivity. Psychiatry research, 250, 10-16. https://doi.org/10.1016/j.psychres.2017.01.050

Chand SP, Kuckel DP, Huecker MR. (2021). Cognitive Behavior Therapy. StatPearls Publishing. https://www.ncbi.nlm.nih.gov/books/NBK470241/

Chang, E. C., Chang, O. D., Martos, T., Sallay, V., Li, X., Lucas, A. G., & Lee, J. (2018). Does optimism weaken the negative effects of being lonely on suicide risk? Death studies, 42(1), 63-68. https://doi.org/10.1080/07481187.2017.1332115

Chapman, A. L., Gratz, K. L., & Brown, M. Z. (2006). Solving the puzzle of deliberate self-harm: the experiential avoidance model. Behaviour research and therapy, 44(3), 371-394. https://doi.org/10.1016/j.brat.2005.03.005

Chapman, J., Jamil, R. T., & Fleisher, C. (2022). Borderline Personality Disorder. StatPearls Publishing.

Chen, C. Y., Lin, S. H., Li, P., Huang, W. L., & Lin, Y. H. (2015). The role of the harm avoidance personality in depression and anxiety during the medical internship. Medicine, 94(2). https://doi.org/10.1097/MD.0000000000000389

Chibanda, D., Sebit, M. B., & Acuda, S. W. (2002). Prevalence of major depression in deliberate self-harm individuals in Harare, Zimbabwe. East African medical journal, 79(5), 263-266. https://doi.org/10.4314/eamj.v79i5.8866

Cho, J., & Choi, Y. (2020). Patterns of wrist cutting: A retrospective analysis of 115 suicide attempts. Archives of plastic surgery, 47(3), 250-255. https://doi.org/10.5999/aps.2020.00059

Christie, D., & Viner, R. (2005). Adolescent development. BMJ (Clinical research ed.), 330(7486), 301-304. https://doi.org/10.1136/bmj.330.7486.301

Chu, C., Rogers, M. L., & Joiner, T. E. (2016). Cross-sectional and temporal association between non-suicidal self-injury and suicidal ideation in young adults: The explanatory roles of thwarted belongingness and perceived burdensomeness. Psychiatry research, 246, 573-580. https://doi.org/10.1016/j.psychres.2016.07.061

Cipriano, A., Cella, S., & Cotrufo, P. (2017). Nonsuicidal Self-injury: A Systematic Review. *Frontiers in psychology, 8,* 1946. https://doi.org/10.3389/fpsyg.2017.01946

Claes, L., Soenens, B., Vansteenkiste, M., & Vandereycken, W. (2012). The scars of the inner critic: perfectionism and nonsuicidal self-injury in eating disorders. *European eating disorders review : the journal of the Eating Disorders Association, 20*(3), 196-202. https://doi.org/10.1002/erv.1158

Claes, L., Turner, B., Dierckx, E., Luyckx, K., Verschueren, M., & Schoevaerts, K. (2018). Different Clinical Presentations in Eating Disorder Patients with Non-Suicidal Self-Injury Based on the Co-Occurrence of Borderline Personality Disorder. *Psychologica Belgica, 58*(1), 243-255. https://doi.org/10.5334/pb.420

Claes, L., Vandereycken, W., & Vertommen, H. (2001). Self-injurious behaviors in eating-disordered patients. *Eating behaviors, 2*(3), 263-272. https://doi.org/10.1016/s1471-0153(01)00033-2

Claes, L., Vandereycken, W., & Vertommen, H. (2007). Self-injury in female versus male psychiatric patients: a comparison of characteristics, psychopathology and aggression regulation. *Personality and Individual Differences, 42*(4), 611-621. https://doi.org/10.1016/j.paid.2006.07.021

Clausen, L., Rosenvinge, J. H., Friborg, O., & Rokkedal, K. (2011). Validating the Eating Disorder Inventory-3 (EDI-3): A Comparison Between 561 Female Eating Disorders Patients and 878 Females from the General Population. *Journal of psychopathology and behavioral assessment, 33*(1), 101-110. https://doi.org/10.1007/s10862-010-9207-4

Clements, C., Jones, S., Morriss, R., Peters, S., Cooper, J., While, D., & Kapur, N. (2015). Self-harm in bipolar disorder: findings from a prospective clinical database. *Journal of affective disorders, 173,* 113-119. https://doi.org/10.1016/j.jad.2014.10.012

Cloninger C. R. (1987). A systematic method for clinical description and classification of personality variants. A proposal. *Archives of general psychiatry, 44*(6), 573-588. https://doi.org/10.1001/archpsyc.1987.01800180093014

Cloninger, C. R., Svrakic, D. M., & Przybeck, T. R. (1993). A psychobiological model of temperament and character. *Archives of general psychiatry, 50*(12), 975-990. https://doi.org/10.1001/archpsyc.1993.01820240059008

Committee on Improving the Health, Safety, and Well-Being of Young Adults; Board on Children, Youth, and Families; Institute of Medicine; National Research Council; Bonnie RJ, Stroud C, Breiner H, (eds.) (2015). *Investing in the Health and Well-Being of Young Adults.* National Academies Press https://www.ncbi.nlm.nih.gov/books/NBK284782/

Conversano, C., Rotondo, A., Lensi, E., Della Vista, O., Arpone, F., & Reda, M. A. (2010). Optimism and its impact on mental and physical well-being. *Clinical practice and epidemiology in mental health : CP & EMH, 6, 25–29. https://doi.org/10.2174/1745017901006010025

Costa, R., Peixoto, A., Lucas, C., Falcão, D. N., Farias, J., Viana, L., Pereira, M., Sandes, M., Lopes, T. B., Mousinho, K. C., & Trindade-Filho, E. M. (2021). Profile of non-suicidal self-injury in adolescents: interface with impulsiveness and loneliness. *Jornal de pediatria, 97*(2), 184–190. https://doi.org/10.1016/j.jped.2020.01.006

Cox, B. J., Borger, S. C., Asmundson, G. J. G., & Taylor, S. (2000). Dimensions of hypochondriasis and the five-factor model of personality. *Personality and Individual Differences, 29*(1), 99–108. https://doi.org/10.1016/S0191-8869(99)00180-4

Craig A. D. (2002). How do you feel? Interoception: the sense of the physiological condition of the body. *Nature reviews. Neuroscience, 3*(8), 655–666. https://doi.org/10.1038/nrn894

Craigie, T. A., Brooks-Gunn, J., & Waldfogel, J. (2012). Family Structure, Family Stability, and Outcomes of Five-Year-Old Children. *Families, relationships and societies : in international journal of research and debate, 1*(1), 43–61. https://doi.org/10.1332/204674312X633153

Cservenka, A., Herting, M. M., Seghete, K. L., Hudson, K. A., & Nagel, B. J. (2013). High and low sensation seeking adolescents show distinct patterns of brain activity during reward processing. *NeuroImage, 66*, 184–193. https://doi.org/10.1016/j.neuroimage.2012.11.003

Dahlgren, M. K., Hooley, J. M., Best, S. G., Sagar, K. A., Gonenc, A., & Gruber, S. A. (2018). Prefrontal cortex activation during cognitive interference in non-suicidal self-injury. *Psychiatry research. Neuroimaging, 277*, 28–38. https://doi.org/10.1016/j.pscychresns.2018.04.006

Daldin, H. J. (1988). A contribution to the understanding of self-mutilating behaviour in adolescence. *Journal of Child Psychotherapy, 14*(1), 61–66. https://doi.org/10.1080/00754178808254819

D'Alessandro, M., & Lester, D. (2000). Self-destructiveness and manic-depressive tendencies. *Psychological reports, 87*(2), 466. https://doi.org/10.2466/pr0.2000.87.2.466

Daros, A. R., Haefner, S. A., Asadi, S., Kazi, S., Rodak, T., & Quilty, L. C. (2021). A meta-analysis of emotional regulation outcomes in psychological interventions for youth with depression and anxiety. *Nature human behaviour, 5*(10), 1443–1457. https://doi.org/10.1038/s41562-021-01191-9

Daukantaitė, D., Lundh, L. G., Wångby-Lundh, M., Claréus, B., Bjärehed, J., Zhou, Y., & Liljedahl, S. I. (2021). What happens to young adults who have engaged in self-injurious behavior as adolescents? A 10-year follow-up. *European child & adolescent psychiatry, 30*(3), 475–492. https://doi.org/10.1007/s00787-020-01533-4

Dawkins, J. C., Hasking, P. A., Boyes, M. E., Greene, D., & Passchier, C. (2019). Applying a cognitive-emotional model to nonsuicidal self-injury. *Stress and health : journal of the International Society for the Investigation of Stress, 35*(1), 39–48. https://doi.org/10.1002/smi.2837

De Leo, D., & Heller, T. S. (2004). Who are the kids who self-harm? An Australian self-report school survey. *The Medical journal of Australia, 181*(3), 140–144. https://doi.org/10.5694/j.1326-5377.2004.tb06204.x

De Smet, L., Van Houdenhove, B., & Fabry, G. (1997). Escalation of automutilation of the hand. *Acta orthopaedica belgica, 63*(3), 212–214.

Démuth, A., & Démuthová, S. (2019). Forms of deliberate self-harm and their prevalence in adolescence. In: *International Conference on Research in Psychology* (23-38). Diamond Scientific Publication. https://www.doi.org/10.33422/icrpconf.2019.03.140

Démuthová S., & Démuth, A. (2019a). The prevalence and most frequent forms of self-harm in adolescents. In: *International Conference on Research in Psychology* (39-51). Diamond Scientific Publication. https://www.doi.org/10.33422/icrpconf.2019.03.139

Démuthová, S., & Démuth, A. (2019b). The specifics of self-harmers who attempt suicide. In: *Proceedings of The 2nd International Conference on Advanced Research in Social Sciences* (1–7). Diamond Scientific Publication.

Démuthová, S., & Démuth, A. (2019c). The specificities of the motivation for self-harm in adolescents. In: *ASNet International Multidisciplinary Academic Conference (AIMAC 2019)* (130–138), Selangor.

Démuthová, S., & Démuth, A. (2020). Self-harm in adolescence as maladaptive coping. *Brain : broad research in artificial intelligence and neuroscience, 11*(2), 37-47, https://doi.org/10.18662/brain/11.2Sup1/92

Démuthová, S., & Doktorová, D. (2019). Interpohlavné rozdiely v prevalencii jednotlivých foriem sebapoškodzovania u adolescentov. [Gender differences in the prevalence of individual forms of self-harm in adolescents]. In A. Baranovská (ed.), *Kondášove dni 2018. [Kondas´ Days 2018]* (19–32). Univerzita sv. Cyrila a Metoda.

Démuthová, S., & Doktorová, D. (2021). Symptoms of eating disorders in young women with and without self-harming behaviour. *AD ALTA : Journal of interdisciplinary research, 11*(1), 65–77.

Démuthová, S., & Rojková, Z. (2019). Špecifiká osobnosti sebapoškodzujúcich sa adolescentov s výskytom suicidálnych pokusov [The special personal characteristics of self-harming adolescents with the history of suicidal attempt]. In S. Démuthová, & A. Baranovská (eds.), *Kondášove dni 2019. [Kondas´ Days 2019]* (18–25). Univerzita sv. Cyrila a Metoda.

Démuthová, S., & Rojková, Z. (2022). Depressive Symptoms among Self-Harming Adolescents.In: *Lumen Proceedings,* (164-174). Lumen publishing house. https://doi.org/10.18662/wlc2021

Démuthova, S., & Spasovski, O. (2020). The analysis of drop-out in the potential diagnostic systems for self-harm in the adolescent population. AD ALTA : *Journal of Interdisciplinary Research, 10*(2), 51–55.

Démuthová, S., & Václaviková, I. (2019). Rozdiely v motivácii k sebapoškodzovaniu u adolescentov so suicidálnymi pokusmi a bez nich. [The differences in the motivation for self-harm in adolescents who have attempted suicide and those who have not]. In S. Démuthová, & A. Baranovská (eds.), *Kondášove dni 2019. [Kondas´ Days 2019]* (26-34). Univerzita sv. Cyrila a Metoda.

Démuthová, S., Vavrová, M., & Sirotová, M. (2020). Prítomnosť depresívnych symptómov u sebapoškodzujúcich sa adolescentov v jednotlivých typoch sebapoškodzovania [The presence of depressive symptoms in self-harming adolescents within individual types of self-harm]. In: A. Baranovská, & D. Kochanová (eds.): Kondášove dni 2020 : zborník vedeckých recenzovaných príspevkov z konferencie. [Kondas´days 2020 : proceedings of scientific peer-reviewed papers from the conference], 7–17, Katedra psychológie FF UCM.

Dennis, M. S., Wakefield, P., Molloy, C., Andrews, H., & Friedman, T. (2007). A study of self-harm in older people: Mental disorder, social factors and motives. *Aging & Mental Health, 11*(5), 520–525. https://doi.org/10.1080/13607860601086611

Dickstein, D. P., Puzia, M. E., Cushman, G. K., Weissman, A. B., Wegbreit, E., Kim, K. L., Nock, M. K., & Spirito, A. (2015). Self-injurious implicit attitudes among adolescent suicide attempters versus those engaged in nonsuicidal self-injury. *Journal of child psychology and psychiatry, and allied disciplines, 56*(10), 1127–1136. https://doi.org/10.1111/jcpp.12385

Dillon, K. H., Glenn, J. J., Dennis, P. A., LoSavio, S. T., Cassiello-Robbins, C., Gromatsky, M. A., Beckham, J. C., Calhoun, P. S., & Kimbrel, N. A. (2021). Anger Precedes and Predicts Nonsuicidal Self-Injury in Veterans: Findings from an Ecological Momentary Assessment Study. *Journal of psychiatric research, 135*, 47. https://doi.org/10.1016/j.jpsychires.2021.01.011

Dixon-Gordon, K. L., Tull, M. T., & Gratz, K. L. (2014). Self-injurious behaviors in posttraumatic stress disorder: an examination of potential moderators. *Journal of affective disorders, 166*, 359–367. https://doi.org/10.1016/j.jad.2014.05.033

Drzał-Fiałkiewcz, E., Makarewicz, A., Walczak, M., Walczak, A., Futyma-Jędrzejewska, M., Kozak, G., Frończuk, P., & Karakuła-Juchnowicz, H. (2017). Self-harm - an overview of the tools used to assess non-suicidal self-harming behaviors. *Curr Probl Psychiatry, 18*(4): 342–359.

Du, N., Ouyang, Y., Xiao, Y., & Li, Y. (2021). Psychosocial Factors Associated With Increased Adolescent Non-suicidal Self-Injury During the COVID-19 Pandemic. *Frontiers in psychiatry, 12*, 743526. https://doi.org/10.3389/fpsyt.2021.743526

Duell, N., Steinberg, L., Icenogle, G., Chein, J., Chaudhary, N., Di Giunta, L., Dodge, K. A., Fanti, K. A., Lansford, J. E., Oburu, P., Pastorelli, C., Skinner, A. T., Sorbring, E., Tapanya, S., Uribe Tirado, L. M., Alampay, L. P., Al-Hassan, S. M., Takash, H., Bacchini, D., & Chang, L. (2018). Age Patterns in Risk Taking Across the World. *Journal of youth and adolescence, 47*(5), 1052–1072. https://doi.org/10.1007/s10964-017-0752-y

Eddleston M. (2000). Patterns and problems of deliberate self-poisoning in the developing world. *QJM : monthly journal of the Association of Physicians, 93*(11), 715–731. https://doi.org/10.1093/qjmed/93.11.715

Eddleston, M., Karunaratne, A., Weerakoon, M., Kumarasinghe, S., Rajapakshe, M., Sheriff, M. H., Buckley, N. A., & Gunnell, D. (2006). Choice of poison for intentional self-poisoning in rural Sri Lanka. *Clinical toxicology (Philadelphia, Pa.), 44*(3), 283–286. https://doi.org/10.1080/15563650600584444

Ennis, J., Barnes, R. A., Kennedy, S., & Trachtenberg, D. D. (1989). Depression in self-harm patients. *The British journal of psychiatry : the journal of mental science, 154*, 41–47. https://doi.org/10.1192/bjp.154.1.41

Erikson, E. H. (1972). *Childhood and society (Repr. ed. ed.)*. Harmondsworth, Middlesex: Penguin Books.

Ersen, B., Kahveci, R., Saki, M. C., Tunali, O., & Aksu, I. (2017). Analysis of 41 suicide attempts by wrist cutting: a retrospective analysis. *European journal of trauma and emergency surgery : official publication of the European Trauma Society, 43*(1), 129–135. https://doi.org/10.1007/s00068-015-0599-4

Esaki, Y., Obayashi, K., Saeki, K., Fujita, K., Iwata, N., & Kitajima, T. (2020). Higher prevalence of intentional self-harm in bipolar disorder with evening chronotype: A finding from the APPLE cohort study. *Journal of affective disorders, 277*, 727–732. https://doi.org/10.1016/j.jad.2020.08.068

ESPAD. (2019). European School Survey Project on Alcohol and Other Drugs. http://www.espad.org/

Esposito-Smythers, C., Goldstein, T., Birmaher, B., Goldstein, B., Hunt, J., Ryan, N., Axelson, D., Strober, M., Gill, M. K., Hanley, A., & Keller, M. (2010). Clinical and psychosocial correlates of non-suicidal self-injury within a sample of children and adolescents with bipolar disorder. *Journal of affective disorders, 125*(1-3), 89–97. https://doi.org/10.1016/j.jad.2009.12.029

Evans, C. M., & Simms, L. J. (2019). The latent structure of self-harm. *Journal of abnormal psychology, 128*(1), 12–24. https://doi.org/10.1037/abn0000398

Evans, K., Tyrer, P., Catalan, J., Schmidt, U., Davidson, K., Dent, J., Tata, P., Thornton, S., Barber, J., & Thompson, S. (1999). Manual-assisted cognitive-behaviour therapy (MACT): a randomized controlled trial of a brief intervention with bibliotherapy in the treatment of recurrent deliberate self-harm. *Psychological medicine, 29*(1), 19–25. https://doi.org/10.1017/s003329179800765x

Favazza, A. R. (1998). The coming of age of self-mutilation. *Journal of Nervous and MentalDisease, 186*(5), 259–268.

Favazza, A. R. (2009). A cultural understanding of nonsuicidal self-injury. In: M. K. Nock (ed.). Understanding nonsuicidal self-injury: *Origins, assessment, and treatment, 19–35*, American Psychological Association.

Favazza, A. R., & Conterio, K. (1989). Female habitual self-mutilators. *Acta psychiatrica Scandinavica, 79*(3), 283–289. https://doi.org/10.1111/j.1600-0447.1989.tb10259.x

Faye P. (1995). Addictive characteristics of the behavior of self-mutilation. *Journal of psychosocial nursing and mental health services, 33*(6), 36–39. https://doi.org/10.3928/0279-3695-19950601-08

Felsten, G., & Hill, V. (1999). Aggression Questionnaire hostility scale predicts anger in response to mistreatment. *Behaviour research and therapy, 37*(1), 87–97. https://doi.org/10.1016/s0005-7967(98)00104-1

Fergusson, D. M., Woodward, L. J., & Horwood, L. J. (2000). Risk factors and life processes associated with the onset of suicidal behaviour during adolescence and early adulthood. *Psychological medicine, 30*(1), 23–39. https://doi.org/10.1017/s003329179900135x

Ferková, Š. (2015). Úloha školského psychológa pri riešení problému sebapoškodzovania dospievajúcich. [The role of a school psychologist in solving the problem of self-harm in adolescents]. *Školní psycholog, 16*(1), 82-90.

Ferrara, M., Terrinoni, A., & Williams, R. (2012). Non-suicidal self-injury (NSSI) in adolescent inpatients: assessing personality features and attitude toward death. *Child and adolescent psychiatry and mental health*, 6 (12). https://doi.org/10.1186/1753-2000-6-12

Ferreira de Castro, E., Cunha, M. A., Pimenta, F., & Costa, I. (1998). Parasuicide and mental disorders. *Acta psychiatrica Scandinavica, 97*(1), 25–31. https://doi.org/10.1111/j.1600-0447.1998.tb09958.x

Ferreira Gonçalves, S., Martins, C., Rosendo, A. P., Machado, B. C., & Silva, E. (2012). Self-injurious behavior in Portuguese adolescents. *Psicothema, 24*(4), 536–541.

Ferris, A., & Silton, N. R. (2016). Separation Insecurity. In: Zeigler-Hill, V., Shackelford, T. (eds.) *Encyclopedia of Personality and Individual Differences*. Springer, Cham. https://doi.org/10.1007/978-3-319-28099-8_1111-1

Figueroa, M. D. (1988). A dynamic taxonomy of self-destructive behaviour. *Psychotherapy, 25*(2),280–287.

Fikke, L. T., Melinder, A., & Landrø, N. I. (2013). The effects of acute tryptophan depletion on impulsivity and mood in adolescents engaging in nonsuicidal self-injury. *Human psychopharmacology, 28*(1), 61–71. https://doi.org/10.1002/hup.2283

Finkelstein, Y., Macdonald, E. M., Hollands, S., Sivilotti, M. L., Hutson, J. R., Mamdani, M. M., Koren, G., Juurlink, D. N., & Canadian Drug Safety and Effectiveness Research Network (CDSERN) (2015). Risk of Suicide Following Deliberate Self-poisoning. *JAMA psychiatry, 72*(6), 570–575. https://doi.org/10.1001/jamapsychiatry.2014.3188

Finore, E. D., Andreoli, E., Alfani, S., Palermi, G., Pedicelli, C., & Paradisi, M. (2007). Dermatitis artefacta in a child. *Pediatric dermatology, 24*(5), E51–E56. https://doi.org/10.1111/j.1525-1470.2007.00441.x

Fischer, G., Ameis, N., Parzer, P., Plener, P. L., Groschwitz, R., Vonderlin, E., Kölch, M., Brunner, R., & Kaess, M. (2014). The German version of the self-injurious thoughts and behaviors interview (SITBI-G): a tool to assess nonsuicidal self-injury and suicidal behavior disorder. *BMC psychiatry, 14*, 265. https://doi.org/10.1186/s12888-014-0265-0

Fliege, H., Kocalevent, R. D., Walter, O. B., Beck, S., Gratz, K. L., Gutierrez, P. M., & Klapp, B. F. (2006). Three assessment tools for deliberate self-harm and suicide behavior: evaluation and psychopathological correlates. *Journal of psychosomatic research, 61*(1), 113–121. https://doi.org/10.1016/j.jpsychores.2005.10.006

Fodstad, J. C., Kirsch, A., Faidley, M., & Bauer, N. (2018). Demonstration of Parent Training to Address Early Self-Injury in Young Children with Intellectual and Developmental Delays. *Journal of autism and developmental disorders, 48*(11), 3846–3857. https://doi.org/10.1007/s10803-018-3651-5

Fomby, P., & Osborne, C. (2017). Family instability, multipartner fertility, and behavior in middle childhood. *Journal of Marriage and the Family, 79*(1), 75 - 93, https://doi.org/10.1111/jomf.12349

Forrester, R. L., Slater, H., Jomar, K., Mitzman, S., & Taylor, P. J. (2017). Self-esteem and non-suicidal self-injury in adulthood: A systematic review. *Journal of affective disorders, 221,* 172–183. https://doi.org/10.1016/j.jad.2017.06.027

Fox, K. R., Franklin, J. C., Ribeiro, J. D., Kleiman, E. M., Bentley, K. H., & Nock, M. K. (2015). Meta-analysis of risk factors for nonsuicidal self-injury. *Clinical psychology review, 42,* 156–167. https://doi.org/10.1016/j.cpr.2015.09.002

Fox, K. R., Harris, J. A., Wang, S. B., Millner, A. J., Deming, C. A., & Nock, M. K. (2020). Self-Injurious Thoughts and Behaviors Interview—Revised: Development, reliability, and validity. *Psychological Assessment, 32*(7), 677–689. https://doi.org/10.1037/pas0000819

Franklin, A. (2012). A lonely society?: Loneliness and liquid modernity in Australia. *Australian Journal of Social Issues, 47,* 11-28 .https://doi.org/10.1002/j.1839-4655.2012.tb00232.x

Freud S (1917) Mourning and melancholia. *The Standard Edition of the Complete Psychological Works of Sigmund Freud, 12,* 243–58. Hogarth Press.

Freud, S. (2005). *Civilization and Its Discontents.* Norton.

Froreich, F. V., Vartanian, L. R., Grisham, J. R., & Touyz, S. W. (2016). Dimensions of control and their relation to disordered eating behaviours and obsessive-compulsive symptoms. *Journal of eating disorders, 4,* 14. https://doi.org/10.1186/s40337-016-0104-4

Frost, R. O., Marten, P., Lahart, C., & Rosenblate, R. (1990). The dimensions of perfectionism. *Cognitive Therapy and Research, 14*(5), 449–468. https://doi.org/10.1007/BF01172967

Fuhrmann, D., Knoll, L. J., & Blakemore, S. J. (2015). Adolescence as a Sensitive Period of Brain Development. *Trends in cognitive sciences, 19*(10), 558–566. https://doi.org/10.1016/j.tics.2015.07.008

Gao, Y., Xiong, Y., Liu, X., & Wang, H. (2021). The Effects of childhood maltreatment on non-suicidal self-injury in male adolescents: the moderating roles of the Monoamine Oxidase A (MAOA) gene and the Catechol-O-Methyltransferase (COMT) gene. *International journal of environmental research and public health, 18*(5), 2598. https://doi.org/10.3390/ijerph18052598

García-Nieto, R., Carballo, J. J., Díaz de Neira Hernando, M., de León-Martinez, V., & Baca-García, E. (2015). Clinical Correlates of Non-Suicidal Self-

Injury (NSSI) in an Outpatient Sample of Adolescents. *Archives of suicide research : official journal of the International Academy for Suicide Research, 19*(2), 218–230. https://doi.org/10.1080/13811118.2014.957447

Garisch, J. A., & Wilson, M. S. (2015). Prevalence, correlates, and prospective predictors of non-suicidal self-injury among New Zealand adolescents: cross-sectional and longitudinal survey data. *Child and adolescent psychiatry and mental health, 9*, 28. https://doi.org/10.1186/s13034-015-0055-6

Gartland, N., Rosmalen, J., & O'Connor, D. B. (2022). Effects of childhood adversity and cortisol levels on suicidal ideation and behaviour: Results from a general population study. *Psychoneuroendocrinology, 138*, 105664. https://doi.org/10.1016/j.psyneuen.2022.105664

Gattu, S., Rashid, R. M., & Khachemoune, A. (2009). Self-induced skin lesions: a review of dermatitis artefacta. *Cutis, 84*(5), 247–251.

Gaudreau, P., & Thompson, A. (2010). Testing a 2×2 model of dispositional perfectionism. *Personality and Individual Differences, 48*(5), 532–537. https://doi.org/10.1016/j.paid.2009.11.031

Germain, S.A., & Hooley, J.M. (2012). Direct and indirect forms of non-suicidal self-injury: Evidence for a distinction. *Psychiatry Research, 197*, 78-84. https://doi.org/10.1016/j.psychres.2011.12.050

Giletta, M., Scholte, R. H., Engels, R. C., Ciairano, S., & Prinstein, M. J. (2012). Adolescent non-suicidal self-injury: a cross-national study of community samples from Italy, the Netherlands and the United States. *Psychiatry research, 197*(1-2), 66–72. https://doi.org/10.1016/j.psychres.2012.02.009

Gillies, D., Christou, M. A., Dixon, A. C., Featherston, O. J., Rapti, I., Garcia-Anguita, A., Villasis-Keever, M., Reebye, P., Christou, E., Al Kabir, N., & Christou, P. A. (2018). Prevalence and Characteristics of Self-Harm in Adolescents: Meta-Analyses of Community-Based Studies 1990-2015. *Journal of the American Academy of Child and Adolescent Psychiatry, 57*(10), 733–741. https://doi.org/10.1016/j.jaac.2018.06.018

Glenn, C. R., & Klonsky, E. D. (2013). Nonsuicidal self-injury disorder: an empirical investigation in adolescent psychiatric patients. *Journal of clinical child and adolescent psychology : the official journal for the Society of Clinical Child and Adolescent Psychology, American Psychological Association, Division 53, 42*(4), 496–507. https://doi.org/10.1080/15374416.2013.794699

Glenn, C. R., Kleiman, E. M., Cha, C. B., Nock, M. K., & Prinstein, M. J. (2016). Implicit cognition about self-injury predicts actual self-injurious behavior: results from a longitudinal study of adolescents. *Journal of child psychology and psychiatry, and allied disciplines, 57*(7), 805–813. https://doi.org/10.1111/jcpp.12500

Glenn, J. J., Werntz, A. J., Slama, S. J., Steinman, S. A., Teachman, B. A., & Nock, M. K. (2017). Suicide and self-injury-related implicit cognition: A large-scale examination and replication. *Journal of abnormal psychology, 126*(2), 199–211. https://doi.org/10.1037/abn0000230

Godina, E., & Zadorozhnaya, L. (2016). Self-perception of Physical Appearance in Adolescents: Gender, Age and Ethnic Aspects. *Collegium antropologicum, 40*(2), 73-81.

Goldberg, J. S., & Carlson, M. J. (2014). Parents' Relationship Quality and Children's Behavior in Stable Married and Cohabiting Families. *Journal of marriage and the family, 76*(4), 762-777. https://doi.org/10.1111/jomf.12120

Goldstein, B. L., Kotov, R., Perlman, G., Watson, D., & Klein, D. N. (2018). Trait and facet-level predictors of first-onset depressive and anxiety disorders in a community sample of adolescent girls. *Psychological medicine, 48*(8), 1282-1290. https://doi.org/10.1017/S0033291717002719

Gómez-Expósito, A., Wolz, I., Fagundo, A. B., Granero, R., Steward, T., Jiménez-Murcia, S., Agüera, Z., & Fernández-Aranda, F. (2016). Correlates of Nonsuicidal Self-Injury and Suicide Attempts in Bulimic Spectrum Disorders. *Frontiers in psychology, 7,* 1244. https://doi.org/10.3389/fpsyg.2016.01244

Gordon D. E. (1990). Formal operational thinking: the role of cognitive-developmental processes in adolescent decision-making about pregnancy and contraception. *The American journal of orthopsychiatry, 60*(3), 346-356. https://doi.org/10.1037/h0079156

Gottfried, J. (2019). České normativní skóry Beckovy škály depresivity: metaanalýza. *Testfórum, 7*(12), 30-46. https://doi.org/10.5817/TF2019-12-12246

Graff, H., & Mallin, R. (1967). The syndrome of the wrist cutter. *The American journal of psychiatry, 124*(1), 36-42. https://doi.org/10.1176/ajp.124.1.36

Grandclerc, S., De Labrouhe, D., Spodenkiewicz, M., Lachal, J., & Moro, M. R. (2016). Relations between Nonsuicidal Self-Injury and Suicidal Behavior in Adolescence: A Systematic Review. *PloS one, 11*(4), e0153760. https://doi.org/10.1371/journal.pone.0153760

Gratz, K. L. (2001). Measurement of deliberate self-harm: preliminary data on the deliberate self-harm inventory. *J Psychopathol Behav Assess* 23(4):253-263. https://doi.org/10.1023/A:1012779403943

Gratz, K. L., & Roemer, L. (2004). Multidimensional assessment of emotion regulation and dysregulation: Development, factor structure, and initial validation of the difficulties in emotion regulation scale. *Journal of Psychopathology and Behavioral Assessment, 26*(1), 41-54. https://doi.org/10.1023/B:JOBA.0000007455.08539.94

Gratz, K. L., & Tull, M. T. (2012). Exploring the relationship between posttraumatic stress disorder and deliberate self-harm: the moderating roles of borderline and avoidant personality disorders. *Psychiatry research, 199*(1), 19-23. https://doi.org/10.1016/j.psychres.2012.03.025

Gratz, K. L., Dixon-Gordon, K. L., Chapman, A. L., & Tull, M. T. (2015). Diagnosis and Characterization of DSM-5 Nonsuicidal Self-Injury Disorder Using the Clinician-Administered Nonsuicidal Self-Injury Disorder Index. *Assessment, 22*(5), 527-539. https://doi.org/10.1177/1073191114565878

Gratz, K. L., Chapman, A. L., Dixon-Gordon, K. L., & Tull, M. T. (2016). Exploring the association of deliberate self-harm with emotional relief using a novel Implicit Association Test. *Personality disorders, 7*(1), 91–102. https://doi.org/10.1037/per0000138

Gray, N. S., Knowles, J., George, D., Harvey, A., Powell, R., Zadeh, M. V., Wansing, C., & Snowden, R. J. (2021). Explicit and Implicit Hopelessness and Self-injury. *Suicide & life-threatening behavior, 51*(3), 606–615. https://doi.org/10.1111/sltb.12743

Green, A. H. (1978.) Self-destructive behaviour in battered children. *The American Journal of Psychiatry, 135*, 579–582.

Greenberger, E. (1984). Defining psychosocial maturity in adolescence. *Advances in Child Behavioral Analysis & Therapy, 3*, 1–37.

Greene, D., Boyes, M., & Hasking, P. (2020). The associations between alexithymia and both non-suicidal self-injury and risky drinking: A systematic review and meta-analysis. *Journal of affective disorders, 260*, 140–166. https://doi.org/10.1016/j.jad.2019.08.088

Greene, D., Hasking, P., & Boyes, M. (2021). A comparison of the associations between alexithymia and both non-suicidal self-injury and risky drinking: The roles of explicit outcome expectancies and refusal self-efficacy. *Stress and health : journal of the International Society for the Investigation of Stress, 37*(2), 272–284. https://doi.org/10.1002/smi.2991

Greif, E. B., & Ulman, K. J. (1982). The psychological impact of menarche on early adolescent females: a review of the literature. *Child development, 53*(6), 1413–1430.

Greydanus, D. E., & Apple, R. W. (2011). The relationship between deliberate self-harm behavior, body dissatisfaction, and suicide in adolescents: current concepts. *Journal of multidisciplinary healthcare, 4*, 183–189. https://doi.org/10.2147/JMDH.S11569

Griffin, E., McMahon, E., McNicholas, F. , Corcoran, P., Perry, I. J., & Arensman, E. (2018). Increasing rates of self-harm among children, adolescents and young adults: a 10-year national registry study 2007-2016. *Social Psychiatry and Psychiatric Epidemiology, 53*, 663–671. https://doi.org/10.1007/s00127-018-1522-1

Groschwitz, R. C., Kaess, M., Fischer, G., Ameis, N., Schulze, U. M., Brunner, R., Koelch, M., & Plener, P. L. (2015). The association of non-suicidal self-injury and suicidal behavior according to DSM-5 in adolescent psychiatric inpatients. *Psychiatry research, 228*(3), 454–461. https://doi.org/10.1016/j.psychres.2015.06.019

Gross, J. J. (1998). The emerging field of emotion regulation: An integrative review. *Review of General Psychology, 2*(3), 271–299. https://doi.org/10.1037/1089-2680.2.3.271

Grunebaum, H. U., & Klerman, G. L. (1967). Wrist slashing. *The American journal of psychiatry, 124*(4), 527–534. https://doi.org/10.1176/ajp.124.4.52

Gu, H., Hu, C., & Wang, L. (2022). Maladaptive perfectionism and adolescent NSSI: A moderated mediation model of psychological distress and mindfulness. *Journal of clinical psychology, 78*(6), 1137-1150. https://doi.org/10.1002/jclp.23304

Gu, J. H., & Jeong, S. H. (2012). Self-wrist cutting injury: a traumatologic and psychological analysis. *Plastic and reconstructive surgery, 129*(4), 763e-764e. https://doi.org/10.1097/PRS.0b013e318245e8c5

Guénolé, F., Spiers, S., Gicquel, L., Delvenne, V., Robin, M., Corcos, M., Pham-Scottez, A., & Speranza, M. (2021). Interpersonal Relatedness and Non-suicidal Self-Injurious Behaviors in Female Adolescents With Borderline Personality Disorder. *Frontiers in psychiatry, 12*, 731629. https://doi.org/10.3389/fpsyt.2021.731629

Guérin-Marion, C., Martin, J., Deneault, A. A., Lafontaine, M. F., & Bureau, J. F. (2018). The functions and addictive features of non-suicidal self-injury: A confirmatory factor analysis of the Ottawa self-injury inventory in a university sample. *Psychiatry research, 264*, 316-321. https://doi.org/10.1016/j.psychres.2018.04.019

Gulbas, L. E., Hausmann-Stabile, C., De Luca, S. M., Tyler, T. R., & Zayas, L. H. (2015). An exploratory study of nonsuicidal self-injury and suicidal behaviors in adolescent Latinas. *The American journal of orthopsychiatry, 85*(4), 302-314. https://doi.org/10.1037/ort0000073

Güney, E., Alnıak, İ., & Erkıran, M. (2020). Predicting factors for non-suicidal self-injury in patients with schizophrenia spectrum disorders and the role of substance use. *Asian journal of psychiatry, 52*, 102068. https://doi.org/10.1016/j.ajp.2020.102068

Gupta, R., Narnoli, S., Das, N., Sarkar, S., & Balhara, Y. (2019). Patterns and predictors of self-harm in patients with substance-use disorder. *Indian journal of psychiatry, 61*(5), 431-438. https://doi.org/10.4103/psychiatry.IndianJPsychiatry_578_18

Gutierrez, P. M., Osman, A., Barrios, F. X., & Kopper, B. A. (2001). Development and initial validation of the Self-harm Behavior Questionnaire. *Journal of personality assessment, 77*(3), 475-490. https://doi.org/10.1207/S15327752JPA7703_08

Guyer, A. E., Silk, J. S., & Nelson, E. E. (2016). The neurobiology of the emotional adolescent: From the inside out. *Neuroscience and biobehavioral reviews, 70*, 74-85. https://doi.org/10.1016/j.neubiorev.2016.07.037

Gyori, D., & Balazs, J. (2021). Nonsuicidal Self-Injury and Perfectionism: A Systematic Review. *Frontiers in psychiatry, 12*, 691147. https://doi.org/10.3389/fpsyt.2021.691147

Hack, J., & Martin, G. (2018). Expressed Emotion, Shame, and Non-Suicidal Self-Injury. *International journal of environmental research and public health, 15*(5), 890. https://doi.org/10.3390/ijerph15050890

Halama, P., Kohút, M., Soto, C. J., & John, O. P. (2020). Slovak Adaptation of the Big Five Inventory (BFI-2): Psychometric Properties and Initial Validation. *Studia Psychologica, 62*(1), 74-87. https://doi.org/10.31577/sp.2020.01.792

Hallensleben, N., Spangenberg, L., Kapusta, N. D., Forkmann, T., & Glaesmer, H. (2016). The German version of the Interpersonal Needs Questionnaire (INQ)--Dimensionality, psychometric properties and population-based norms. *Journal of affective disorders, 195*, 191–198. https://doi.org/10.1016/j.jad.2016.01.045

Hamdan, S., Apter, A., & Levi-Belz, Y. (2022). Non-suicidal Self-Injury Among Adolescents From Diverse Ethnocultural Groups in Israel: The Association With Sleep Problems and Internet Addiction. *Frontiers in psychiatry, 13*. https://doi.org/10.3389/fpsyt.2022.899956

Hamza, C. A., Stewart, S. L., & Willoughby, T. (2012). Examining the link between nonsuicidal self-injury and suicidal behavior: a review of the literature and an integrated model. *Clinical psychology review, 32*(6), 482–495. https://doi.org/10.1016/j.cpr.2012.05.003

Hamza, C. A., Willoughby, T., & Heffer, T. (2015). Impulsivity and nonsuicidal self-injury: A review and meta-analysis. *Clinical psychology review, 38*, 13–24. https://doi.org/10.1016/j.cpr.2015.02.010

Hankin, B. L., Barrocas, A. L., Young, J. F., Haberstick, B., & Smolen, A. (2015). 5-HTTLPR × interpersonal stress interaction and nonsuicidal self-injury in general community sample of youth. *Psychiatry research, 225*(3), 609–612. https://doi.org/10.1016/j.psychres.2014.11.037

Hanna, D., White, R., Lyons, K., McParland, M. J., Shannon, C., & Mulholland, C. (2011). The structure of the Beck Hopelessness Scale: A confirmatory factor analysis in UK students. *Personality and Individual Differences, 51*(1), 17–22. https://doi.org/10.1016/j.paid.2011.03.001

Harman, G., Kliamovich, D., Morales, A. M., Gilbert, S., Barch, D. M., Mooney, M. A., Feldstein Ewing, S. W., Fair, D. A., & Nagel, B. J. (2021). Prediction of suicidal ideation and attempt in 9 and 10 year-old children using transdiagnostic risk features. *PloS one, 16*(5), e0252114. https://doi.org/10.1371/journal.pone.0252114

Harris, C. N., & Rai, K. (1976). The self-inflicted wrist slash. *The Journal of trauma, 16*(9), 743–745. https://doi.org/10.1097/00005373-197609000-00011

Harris, I. M., Beese, S., & Moore, D. (2019). Predicting future self-harm or suicide in adolescents: a systematic review of risk assessment scales/tools. *BMJ open, 9*(9), e029311. https://doi.org/10.1136/bmjopen-2019-029311

Hasking, P. A., Di Simplicio, M., McEvoy, P. M., & Rees, C. S. (2018). Emotional cascade theory and non-suicidal self-injury: the importance of imagery and positive affect. *Cognition & emotion, 32*(5), 941–952. https://doi.org/10.1080/02699931.2017.1368456

Hasking, P., & Rose, A. (2016). A Preliminary Application of Social Cognitive Theory to Nonsuicidal Self-Injury. *Journal of youth and adolescence, 45*(8), 1560–1574. https://doi.org/10.1007/s10964-016-0449-7

Hasking, P., Whitlock, J., Voon, D., & Rose, A. (2017). A cognitive-emotional model of NSSI: using emotion regulation and cognitive processes to explain why people self-injure. *Cognition & emotion, 31*(8), 1543–1556. https://doi.org/10.1080/02699931.2016.1241219

Hauber, K., Boon, A., & Vermeiren, R. (2019). Non-suicidal Self-Injury in Clinical Practice. *Frontiers in psychology, 10*, 502. https://doi.org/10.3389/fpsyg.2019.00502

Haw, C., Hawton, K., Houston, K., & Townsend, E. (2001). Psychiatric and personality disorders in deliberate self-harm patients. *The British journal of psychiatry : the journal of mental science, 178*(1), 48-54. https://doi.org/10.1192/bjp.178.1.48

Haw, C., Hawton, K., Sutton, L., Sinclair, J., & Deeks, J. (2005). Schizophrenia and deliberate self-harm: a systematic review of risk factors. *Suicide & life-threatening behavior, 35*(1), 50-62. https://doi.org/10.1521/suli.35.1.50.59260

Hawton, K., Saunders, K. E., & O'Connor, R. C. (2012). Self-harm and suicide in adolescents. *The Lancet 379*(9834), 2373-2382. https://doi.org/10.1016/S0140-6736(12)60322-5

Hawton, K., Saunders, K., Topiwala, A., & Haw, C. (2013). Psychiatric disorders in patients presenting to hospital following self-harm: a systematic review. *Journal of affective disorders, 151*(3), 821-830. https://doi.org/10.1016/j.jad.2013.08.02

Heath, N. L., Carsley, D., De Riggi, M. E., Mills, D., & Mettler, J. (2016). The Relationship Between Mindfulness, Depressive Symptoms, and Non-Suicidal Self-Injury Amongst Adolescents. *Archives of suicide research : official journal of the International Academy for Suicide Research, 20*(4), 635-649. https://doi.org/10.1080/13811118.2016.1162243

Hefti, S., In-Albon, T., Schmeck, K., & Schmid, M. (2013). Temperaments-und Charaktereigenschaften und selbstverletzendes Verhalten bei Jugendlichen. *Nervenheilkunde, 32*(01/02), 45-53.

Heilbron, N., Franklin, J. C., Guerry, J. D., & Prinstein, M. J. (2014). Social and ecological approaches to understanding suicidal behaviors and nonsuicidal self-injury. In: M. K. Nock (ed.), *The Oxford Handbook of Suicide and Self-Injury* (308-320). Oxford University Press. https://doi.org/10.1016/j.jad.2016.01.045

Henderson, A. S., Hartigan, J., Davidson, J., Lance, G. N., Duncan-Jones, P., Koller, K. M., Ritchie, K., McAuley, H., Williams, C. L., & Slaghuis, W. (1977). A typology of parasuicide. *British journal of psychiatry, 131* (6), 631-641. https://doi.org/10.1192/bjp.131.6.631

Henderson, S., & Lance, G. N. (1979). Types of attempted suicide (parasuicide). *Acta psychiatrica Scandinavica, 59*(1), 31-39. https://doi.org/10.1111/j.1600-0447.1979.tb06944.x

Henneberger, A.K., Mushonga, D.R. & Preston, A.M.(2021) Peer Influence and Adolescent Substance Use: A Systematic Review of Dynamic Social Network Research. *Adolescent Res Rev 6*, 57-73). https://doi.org/10.1007/s40894-019-00130-0

Henry, N., Parthiban, S., & Farroha, A. (2021). The effect of COVID-19 lockdown on the incidence of deliberate self-harm injuries presenting to the emergency room. *International journal of psychiatry in medicine, 56*(4), 266-277. https://doi.org/10.1177/0091217420982100

Himelein-Wachowiak, M., Giorgi, S., Kwarteng, A., Schriefer, D., Smitterberg, C., Yadeta, K., Bragard, E., Devoto, A., Ungar, L., & Curtis, B. (2022). Getting "clean" from nonsuicidal self-injury: Experiences of addiction on the subreddit r/selfharm. *Journal of behavioral addictions, 11*(1), 128–139. https://doi.org/10.1556/2006.2022.00005

Hirsch, J. K., Wolford, K., Lalonde, S. M., Brunk, L., & Parker-Morris, A. (2009). Optimistic explanatory style as a moderator of the association between negative life events and suicide ideation. *Crisis, 30*(1), 48–53. https://doi.org/10.1027/0227-5910.30.1.48

Hirsch, S. R., Walsh, C., & Draper, R. (1983). The concept and efficacy of the treatment of parasuicide. *British journal of clinical pharmacology, 15*(2), 189S–194S. https://doi.org/10.1111/j.1365-2125.1983.tb05865.x

Hodas, N. O., & Lerman, K. (2014). The simple rules of social contagion. *Scientific reports, 4*, 4343. https://doi.org/10.1038/srep04343

Hoff, E. R., & Muehlenkamp, J. J. (2009). Nonsuicidal self-injury in college students: The role of perfectionism and rumination. *Suicide and Life-Threatening Behavior, 39*(6), 576–587. https://doi.org/10.1521/suli.2009.39.6.576

Hooley, J. M., & St. Germain, S. A. (2014). Nonsuicidal self-injury, pain, and self-criticism: Does changing self-worth change pain endurance in people who engage in self-injury? *Clinical Psychological Science, 2*(3), 297–305. https://doi.org/10.1177/2167702613509372

Hooley, J. M., Fox, K. R., & Boccagno, C. (2020). Nonsuicidal Self-Injury: Diagnostic Challenges And Current Perspectives. *Neuropsychiatric disease and treatment, 16*, 101–112. https://doi.org/10.2147/NDT.S198806

Horrocks, J., Price, S., House, A., & Owens, D. (2003). Self-injury attendances in the accident and emergency department: Clinical database study. *The British journal of psychiatry : the journal of mental science, 183*, 34–39. https://doi.org/10.1192/bjp.183.1.34

Horváth, L. O., Győri, D., Komáromy, D., Mészáros, G., Szentiványi, D., & Balázs, J. (2020). Nonsuicidal Self-Injury and Suicide: The Role of Life Events in Clinical and Non-Clinical Populations of Adolescents. *Frontiers in psychiatry, 11*, 370. https://doi.org/10.3389/fpsyt.2020.00370

Horwitz, A. G., Berona, J., Czyz, E. K., Yeguez, C. E., & King, C. A. (2017). Positive and Negative Expectations of Hopelessness as Longitudinal Predictors of Depression, Suicidal Ideation, and Suicidal Behavior in High-Risk Adolescents. *Suicide & life-threatening behavior, 47*(2), 168–176. https://doi.org/10.1111/sltb.12273

Houben, M., Claes, L., Vansteelandt, K., Berens, A., Sleuwaegen, E., & Kuppens, P. (2017). The emotion regulation function of nonsuicidal self-injury: A momentary assessment study in inpatients with borderline personality disorder features. *Journal of abnormal psychology, 126*(1), 89–95. https://doi.org/10.1037/abn0000229

Hu, Y.-Q., & Gan, Y.-Q. (2008). Development and psychometric validity of the Resilience Scale for Chinese Adolescents. *Acta Psychologica Sinica, 40*(8), 902–912. https://doi.org/10.3724/SP.J.1041.2008.00902

Huband, N., & Tantam, D. (2004). Repeated self-wounding: women's recollection of pathways to cutting and of the value of different interventions. *Psychology and psychotherapy, 77* (4), 413–428. https://doi.org/10.1348/1476083042555370

ICD-10 (2016). International Statistical Classification of Diseases and Related Health Problems. World Health Organization. https://www.who.int/classifications/icd/icdonlineversions/en/

In-Albon, T., Bürli, M., Ruf, C., & Schmid, M. (2013). Non-suicidal self-injury and emotion regulation: a review on facial emotion recognition and facial mimicry. *Child and adolescent psychiatry and mental health, 7*(1), 5. https://doi.org/10.1186/1753-2000-7-5

In-Albon, T., Ruf, C., & Schmid, M. (2013). Proposed Diagnostic Criteria for the DSM-5 of Nonsuicidal Self-Injury in Female Adolescents: Diagnostic and Clinical Correlates. *Psychiatry journal,* 159208. https://doi.org/10.1155/2013/159208

In-Albon, T., Tschan, T., Schwarz, D., & Schmid, M. (2015). Emotionsregulation bei Jugendlichen mit Nichtsuizidalen Selbstverletzungen [Emotion Regulation in Adolescents with Nonsuicidal Self-Injury]. *Praxis der Kinderpsychologie und Kinderpsychiatrie, 64*(5), 386–403. https://doi.org/10.13109/prkk.2015.64.5.386

ISAS measure (n.d.). Inventory of statements about self-injury (ISAS) – Section I.Behaviors. https://www2.psych.ubc.ca/~klonsky/publications/ISASmeasure.pdf

Iskric, A., Ceniti, A. K., Bergmans, Y., McInerney, S., & Rizvi, S. J. (2020). Alexithymia and self-harm: A review of nonsuicidal self-injury, suicidal ideation, and suicide attempts. *Psychiatry research, 288,* 112920. https://doi.org/10.1016/j.psychres.2020.11292

Islam, M. A., Steiger, H., Jimenez-Murcia, S., Israel, M., Granero, R., Agüera, Z., Castro, R., Sánchez, I., Riesco, N., Menchón, J. M., & Fernández-Aranda, F. (2015). Non-suicidal Self-injury in Different Eating Disorder Types: Relevance of Personality Traits and Gender. *European eating disorders review : the journal of the Eating Disorders Association, 23*(6), 553–560. https://doi.org/10.1002/erv.2374

Iwata, B. A., Pace, G. M., Kissel, R. C., Nau, P. A., & Farber, J. M. (1990). The Self-Injury Trauma (SIT) Scale: a method for quantifying surface tissue damage caused by self-injurious behavior. *Journal of applied behavior analysis, 23*(1), 99–110. https://doi.org/10.1901/jaba.1990.23-99

Izadi-Mazidi, M., Yaghubi, H., Mohammadkhani, P., & Hassanabadi, H. (2019). Assessing the Functions of Non-Suicidal Self-Injury: Factor Analysis of Functional Assessment of Self-Mutilation among Adolescents. *Iranian journal of psychiatry, 14*(3), 184–191.

Izáková, Ľ., Novotný, V., & André, I. (2006). Klinické aspekty suicidality. [Clinical aspects of suicidality]. *Česká a slovenská psychiatrie, 102*(3), 137-141.

Jacobson, C. M., & Batejan, K. (2014). Comprehensive Theoretical Models of Nonsuicidal Self-Injury. In M. K. Nock (ed.), *The Oxford Handbook of Suicide and Self-Injury* (308–320). Oxford University Press.

Jacobson, C. M., & Gould, M. (2007). The epidemiology and phenomenology of non-suicidal self-injurious behavior among adolescents: a critical review of the literature. *Archives of suicide research : official journal of the International Academy for Suicide Research, 11*(2), 129–147. https://doi.org/10.1080/13811110701247602

Jacobson, C. M., Muehlenkamp, J. J., Miller, A. L., & Turner, J. B. (2008). Psychiatric impairment among adolescents engaging in different types of deliberate self-harm. *Journal of clinical child and adolescent psychology 37*(2), 363–375. https://doi.org/10.1080/15374410801955771

Janssen, W. F., & Hamza, C. A. (2022). What Do We Still Need to Know? Pressing Issues and Promising Directions in Research on Perfectionism and Nonsuicidal Self-injury. *Frontiers in psychology, 13*, 873410. https://doi.org/10.3389/fpsyg.2022.873410

Jarahi, L., Dadgarmoghaddam, M., Naderi, A., & Ghalibaf, A. M. (2021). Self-harm prevalence and associated factors among street children in Mashhad, North East of Iran. *Archives of public health = Archives belges de sante publique, 79*(1), 139. https://doi.org/10.1186/s13690-021-00660-x

Jaworska, N., & MacQueen, G. (2015). Adolescence as a unique developmental period. *Journal of psychiatry & neuroscience : JPN, 40*(5), 291–293. https://doi.org/10.1503/jpn.150268

Jelínek, M., Květon, P., Burešová, I., & Klimusová, H. (2021). Measuring depression in adolescence: Evaluation of a hierarchical factor model of the Children's Depression Inventory and measurement invariance across boys and girls. *PloS one, 16*(4), e0249943. https://doi.org/10.1371/journal.pone.0249943

Jeong, J. Y., & Kim, D. H. (2021). Gender Differences in the Prevalence of and Factors Related to Non-Suicidal Self-Injury among Middle and High School Students in South Korea. *International journal of environmental research and public health, 18*(11), 5965. https://doi.org/10.3390/ijerph18115965

Jiang, W., Hu, G., Zhang, J., Chen, K., Fan, D., & Feng, Z. (2020). Distinct effects of over-general autobiographical memory on suicidal ideation among depressed and healthy people. *BMC psychiatry, 20*(1), 501. https://doi.org/10.1186/s12888-020-02877-6

Jiao, X. Y., Xu, C. Z., Chen, Y., Peng, Q. L., Ran, H. L., Che, Y. S., Fang, D., Peng, J. W., Chen, L., Wang, S. F., & Xiao, Y. Y. (2022). Personality traits and self-harm behaviors among Chinese children and adolescents: The mediating effect of psychological resilience. *World journal of psychiatry, 12*(3), 494–504. https://doi.org/10.5498/wjp.v12.i3.494

Johnson, S. L., Robison, M., Anvar, S., Swerdlow, B. A., & Timpano, K. R. (2022). Emotion-related impulsivity and rumination: Unique and conjoint effects on suicidal ideation, suicide attempts, and nonsuicidal self-injury across two samples. *Suicide & life-threatening behavior, 52*(4), 642–654. https://doi.org/10.1111/sltb.12849

Joiner, T. E., Van Orden, K. A., Witte, T. K., Selby, E. A., Ribeiro, J. D., Lewis, R., & Rudd, M. D. (2009). Main predictions of the interpersonal-psychological theory of suicidal behavior: empirical tests in two samples of young adults. *Journal of abnormal psychology, 118*(3), 634–646. https://doi.org/10.1037/a0016500

Jollant, F., Lawrence, N. L., Olié, E., Guillaume, S., & Courtet, P. (2011). The suicidal mind and brain: a review of neuropsychological and neuroimaging studies. *The world journal of biological psychiatry : the official journal of the World Federation of Societies of Biological Psychiatry, 12*(5), 319–339. https://doi.org/10.3109/15622975.2011.556200

Jourdy, R., & Petot, J.-M. (2017). Relationships between personality traits and depression in the light of the "Big Five" and their different facets. *L'Évolution Psychiatrique, 82*(4), e27–e37. https://doi.org/10.1016/j.evopsy.2017.08.002

Joyce, P. R., McKenzie, J. M., Mulder, R. T., Luty, S. E., Sullivan, P. F., Miller, A. L., & Kennedy, M. A. (2006). Genetic, developmental and personality correlates of self-mutilation in depressed patients. *The Australian and New Zealand journal of psychiatry, 40*(3), 225–229. https://doi.org/10.1080/j.1440-1614.2006.01778.x

Jung, K. Y., Kim, T., Hwang, S. Y., Lee, T. R., Yoon, H., Shin, T. G., Sim, M. S., Cha, W. C., & Jeon, H. J. (2018). Deliberate Self-harm among Young People Begins to Increase at the Very Early Age: a Nationwide Study. *Journal of Korean medical science, 33*(30), e191. https://doi.org/10.3346/jkms.2018.33.e191

Kądziela-Olech, H., Zak, G., Kalinowska, B., Wągrocka, A., Perestret, G., & Bielawski, M. (2015). The prevalence of Non-suicidal Self-Injury (NSSI) among high school students in relation to age and sex. *Psychiatria polska, 49*(4), 765–778. https://doi.org/10.12740/psychiatriapolska.pl/online-first/3

Kaess, M., Parzer, P., Mattern, M., Plener, P. L., Bifulco, A., Resch, F., & Brunner, R. (2013). Adverse childhood experiences and their impact on frequency, severity, and the individual function of nonsuicidal self-injury in youth. *Psychiatry research, 206*(2-3), 265–272. https://doi.org/10.1016/j.psychres.2012.10.012

Kahn, N. F., & Graham, R. (2019). Promoting Positive Adolescent Health Behaviors and Outcomes: Thriving in the 21st Century. Washington (DC): National Academies Press (US); 2019. Available from: https://www.ncbi.nlm.nih.gov/books/NBK554988/

Kalivas, P. W., & Nakamura, M. (1999). Neural systems for behavioral activation and reward. *Current opinion in neurobiology, 9*(2), 223–227. https://doi.org/10.1016/s0959-4388(99)80031-2

Kalivodová, V. (2021). *Sebapoškodzovanie: vymedzenie, prevalencia a typológia sebapoškodzujúcich sa adolescentov* [Dizertačná práca].Univerzita sv. Cyrila a Metoda v Trnave.

Kapur, N., Cooper, J., O'Connor, R. C., & Hawton, K. (2013). Non-suicidal self-injury v. attempted suicide: new diagnosis or false dichotomy?. *The British journal of psychiatry : the journal of mental science, 202*(5), 326–328. https://doi.org/10.1192/bjp.bp.112.116111

Katz, S. E., & Levendusky, P. G. (1990). Cognitive-behavioral approaches to treating borderline and self-mutilating patients. *Bulletin of the Menninger Clinic, 54*(3), 398–408.

Kennes, A., Peeters, S., Janssens, M., Reijnders, J., Simons, M., Lataster, J., & Jacobs, N. (2021). Optimism and Mental Health in Adolescence: a Prospective Validation Study of the Dutch Life-Orientation Test-Revised (LOT-R-A) for Adolescents. *Psychologica Belgica, 61*(1), 104–115. https://doi.org/10.5334/pb.799

Kern, R. S., Kuehnel, T. G., Teuber, J., & Hayden, J. L. (1997). Multimodal cognitive-behavior therapy for borderline personality disorder with self-injurious behavior. *Psychiatric services, 48*(9), 1131–1133. https://doi.org/10.1176/ps.48.9.1131

Kessel, N., & McCulloch, W. (1966). Repeated acts of self-poisoning and self-injury. *Proceedings of the Royal Society of Medicine, 59*(2), 89–92.

Khalsa, S. S., & Lapidus, R. C. (2016). Can Interoception Improve the Pragmatic Search for Biomarkers in Psychiatry?. *Frontiers in psychiatry, 7*, 121. https://doi.org/10.3389/fpsyt.2016.00121

Kiekens, G., Hasking, P., Claes, L., Mortier, P., Auerbach, R. P., Boyes, M., Cuijpers, P., Demyttenaere, K., Green, J. G., Kessler, R. C., Nock, M. K., & Bruffaerts, R. (2018). The DSM-5 nonsuicidal self-injury disorder among incoming college students: Prevalence and associations with 12-month mental disorders and suicidal thoughts and behaviors. *Depression and anxiety, 35*(7), 629–637. https://doi.org/10.1002/da.22754

Kienhorst, C., De Wilde, E., Van Den Bout, J., Diekstra, R., & Wolters, W. (1990). Characteristics of Suicide Attempters in a Population-Based Sample of Dutch Adolescents. *British Journal of Psychiatry, 156*(2), 243-248. https://doi.org/10.1192/bjp.156.2.243

Kim, J. H., Yoo, H., & Eun, S. (2021). A pilot study of 17 wrist-cutting suicide injuries in single institution: perspectives from a hand surgeon. *BMC emergency medicine, 21*(1), 40. https://doi.org/10.1186/s12873-021-00432-4

Kim, S. J., Lee, S. J., Yune, S. K., Sung, Y. H., Bae, S. C., Chung, A., Kim, J., & Lyoo, I. K. (2006). The relationship between the biogenetic temperament and character and psychopathology in adolescents. *Psychopathology, 39*(2), 80–86. https://doi.org/10.1159/000090597

Kittila, A.K., (2012). *Emotion and Nonsuicidal Self-injury* [Doctoral Dissertation]. Griffith University. https://www120.secure.griffith.edu.au/rch/file/5097ec1f-f668-04a8-7f5b-3bdaee02a1d9/1/Kittila_2013_02Thesis.pdf

Kleindienst, N., Bohus, M., Ludäscher, P., Limberger, M. F., Kuenkele, K., Ebner-Priemer, U. W., Chapman, A. L., Reicherzer, M., Stieglitz, R. D., & Schmahl, C. (2008). Motives for nonsuicidal self-injury among women with borderline personality disorder. *The Journal of nervous and mental disease, 196*(3), 230–236. https://doi.org/10.1097/NMD.0b013e3181663026

Klemera, E., Brooks, F. M., Chester, K. L., Magnusson, J., & Spencer, N. (2017). Self-harm in adolescence: protective health assets in the family, school and community. *International journal of public health, 62*(6), 631–638. https://doi.org/10.1007/s00038-016-0900-2

Klimes-Dougan, B., Begnel, E., Almy, B., Thai, M., Schreiner, M. W., & Cullen, K. R. (2019). Hypothalamic-pituitary-adrenal axis dysregulation in depressed adolescents with non-suicidal self-injury. *Psychoneuroendocrinology, 102*, 216–224. https://doi.org/10.1016/j.psyneuen.2018.11.004

Klonsky E. D. (2007). The functions of deliberate self-injury: a review of the evidence. *Clinical psychology review, 27*(2), 226–239. https://doi.org/10.1016/j.cpr.2006.08.002

Klonsky E. D. (2009). The functions of self-injury in young adults who cut themselves: clarifying the evidence for affect-regulation. *Psychiatry research, 166*(2-3), 260–268. https://doi.org/10.1016/j.psychres.2008.02.008

Klonsky, E. D., & Glenn, C. R. (2009). Assessing the functions of non-suicidal self-injury: Psychometric properties of the Inventory of Statements About Self-injury (ISAS). *Journal of psychopathology and behavioral assessment, 31*(3), 215–219. https://doi.org/10.1007/s10862-008-9107-z

Klonsky, E. D., & Moyer, A. (2008). Childhood sexual abuse and non-suicidal self-injury: meta-analysis. *The British journal of psychiatry : the journal of mental science, 192*(3), 166–170. https://doi.org/10.1192/bjp.bp.106.030650

Klonsky, E. D., & Olino, T. M. (2008). Identifying clinically distinct subgroups of self-injurers among young adults: A latent class analysis. *Journal of Consulting and Clinical Psychology, 76*(1), 22–27. https://doi.org/10.1037/0022-006X.76.1.22

Klonsky, E. D., Kotov, R., Bakst, S., Rabinowitz, J., & Bromet, E. J. (2012). Hopelessness as a predictor of attempted suicide among first admission patients with psychosis: a 10-year cohort study. *Suicide & life-threatening behavior, 42*(1), 1–10. https://doi.org/10.1111/j.1943-278X.2011.00066.x

Klonsky, E. D., Oltmanns, T. F., & Turkheimer, E. (2003). Deliberate self-harm in a nonclinical population: prevalence and psychological correlates. *The American journal of psychiatry, 160*(8), 1501–1508. https://doi.org/10.1176/appi.ajp.160.8.1501

Klonsky, E. D., Victor, S. E., & Saffer, B. Y. (2014). Nonsuicidal self-injury: what we know, and what we need to know. *Canadian journal of psychiatry. Revue canadienne de psychiatrie, 59*(11), 565–568. https://doi.org/10.1177/070674371405901101

Knipe, D., Metcalfe, C., Hawton, K., Pearson, M., Dawson, A., Jayamanne, S., Konradsen, F., Eddleston, M., & Gunnell, D. (2019). Risk of suicide and repeat self-harm after hospital attendance for non-fatal self-harm in Sri Lanka: a cohort study. *The Lancet, 6*(8), 659–666. https://doi.org/10.1016/S2215-0366(19)30214-7

Knorr, A. C., Tull, M. T., Anestis, M. D., Dixon-Gordon, K. L., Bennett, M. F., & Gratz, K. L. (2016). The Interactive Effect of Major Depression and Non-suicidal Self-Injury on Current Suicide Risk and Lifetime Suicide Attempts. *Archives of suicide research : official journal of the International Academy for Suicide Research, 20*(4), 539–552. https://doi.org/10.1080/13811118.2016.1158679

Kokkevi, A., Rotsika, V., Arapaki, A., & Richardson, C. (2012). Adolescents' self-reported suicide attempts, self-harm thoughts and their correlates across 17 European countries. *Journal of child psychology and psychiatry, and allied disciplines, 53*(4), 381–389. https://doi.org/10.1111/j.1469-7610.2011.02457.x

Koposov, R., Stickley, A., & Ruchkin, V. (2021). Non-Suicidal Self-Injury Among Incarcerated Adolescents: Prevalence, Personality, and Psychiatric Comorbidity. *Frontiers in psychiatry, 12*, 652004. https://doi.org/10.3389/fpsyt.2021.652004

Kose, S. (2003). A Psychobiological Model of Temperament and Character: TCI. *Yeni Symposium: psikiyatri, nöroloji ve davranış bilimleri dergisi, 41*(2), 86–97.

Kostić, J., Žikić, O., Stankovic, M., & Nikolić, G. (2019). Nonsuicidal self-injury among adolescents in south-east Serbia. *International journal of pediatrics & adolescent medicine, 6*(4), 131–134. https://doi.org/10.1016/j.ijpam.2019.06.002

Kovacs, M. (1998). CDI. Sebaposudzovacia škála depresivity pre deti. [Children´s Depressivity Inventory]. Bratislava: Psychodiagnostika, a.s.

Kubiak, A. (2012). *Dylematy związane z badaniem bezpośrednich zachowań autodestruktywnych w Nowoczesne metody badawcze w psychologii.* Paluchowski W. et spp. Poznań, 49-65.

Kumar, G., Pepe, D., & Steer, R. A. (2004). Adolescent psychiatric inpatients' self-reported reasons for cutting themselves. *The Journal of nervous and mental disease, 192*(12), 830–836. https://doi.org/10.1097/01.nmd.0000146737.18053.d2

Kurtz, P. F., Chin, M. D., Huete, J. M., & Cataldo, M. F. (2012). Identification of Emerging Self-Injurious Behavior in Young Children: A Preliminary Study. *Journal of mental health research in intellectual disabilities, 5*(3-4), 260–285. https://doi.org/10.1080/19315864.2011.600809

Lai, S., Su, C., Song, S., Yan, M., Tang, C., Zhang, Q., Yin, F., & Liu, Q. (2021). Depression and Deliberate Self-Harm Among Rural Adolescents of Sichuan Province in Western China: A 2-Year Longitudinal Study. *Frontiers in psychiatry, 12*, 605785. https://doi.org/10.3389/fpsyt.2021.605785

Lam, D., Schuck, N., Smith, N., Farmer, A., & Checkley, S. (2003). Response style, interpersonal difficulties and social functioning in major depressive disorder. *Journal of affective disorders, 75*(3), 279–283. https://doi.org/10.1016/s0165-0327(02)00058-7

Lan, T., Jia, X., Lin, D., & Liu, X. (2019). Stressful Life Events, Depression, and Non-Suicidal Self-Injury Among Chinese Left-Behind Children: Moderating Effects of Self-Esteem. *Frontiers in psychiatry, 10*, 244. https://doi.org/10.3389/fpsyt.2019.00244

Lanfredi, M., Macis, A., Ferrari, C., Meloni, S., Pedrini, L., Ridolfi, M. E., Zonca, V., Cattane, N., Cattaneo, A., & Rossi, R. (2021). Maladaptive behaviours in adolescence and their associations with personality traits, emotion dysregulation and other clinical features in a sample of Italian students: a cross-sectional study. *Borderline personality disorder and emotion dysregulation, 8*(1), 14. https://doi.org/10.1186/s40479-021-00154-w

Lang, J., & Yao, Y. (2018). Prevalence of nonsuicidal self-injury in chinese middle school and high school students: A meta-analysis. *Medicine, 97*(42), e12916. https://doi.org/10.1097/MD.0000000000012916

Larson, R. W., Moneta, G., Richards, M. H., & Wilson, S. (2002). Continuity, stability, and change in daily emotional experience across adolescence. *Child development*, *73*(4), 1151–1165. https://doi.org/10.1111/1467-8624.00464

Laskyte, A., & Zemaitiene, N. (2009). Lietuvos paaugliu samoningo saves zalojimo paplitimas ir būdai [The types of deliberate self-harm and its prevalence among Lithuanian teenagers]. *Medicina 45*(2), 132–139.

Latimer, S., Covic, T., Cumming, S.R. et al. Psychometric analysis of the Self-Harm Inventory using Rasch modelling. *BMC Psychiatry 9*, (53).https://doi.org/10.1186/1471-244X-9-53

Lauw, M., How, C. H., & Loh, C. (2015). PILL Series. Deliberate self-harm in adolescents. *Singapore medical journal*, *56*(6), 306–309. https://doi.org/10.11622/smedj.2015087

Laye-Gindhu, A., & Schonert-Reichl, K. A. (2005). Nonsuicidal Self-Harm Among Community Adolescents: Understanding the "Whats" and "Whys" of Self-Harm. *Journal of Youth and Adolescence*, *34*(5), 447–457. https://doi.org/10.1007/S10964-005-7262-Z

Laye-Gindhu, A., Schonert-Reichl, K.A. (2005). Nonsuicidal Self-Harm Among Community Adolescents: Understanding the "Whats" and "Whys" of Self-Harm. *J Youth Adolescence 34*, 447–457.https://doi.org/10.1007/s10964-005-7262-z

LeBlanc, R. (1993). Educational management of self-injurious behavior. *Acta paedopsychiatrica*, *56*(2), 91–98.

Lee, E. M., Klement, K. R., Ambler, J. K., Loewald, T., Comber, E. M., Hanson, S. A., Pruitt, B., & Sagarin, B. J. (2016). Altered States of Consciousness during an Extreme Ritual. *PloS one*, *11*(5), e0153126. https://doi.org/10.1371/journal.pone.0153126

Leiva Pereira, J. E., & Concha Landeros, A. M. (2019). Autolesiones no suicidas y su relación con el estilo de apego en una muestra no clínica de adolescentes chilenos. [Non-suicidal self-harm and their relationship with attachment style in a non-clinical sample of chilean adolescents]. *Salud & Sociedad*, *10*(1), 84-99. https://doi.org/10.22199/S07187475.2019.0001.00006

Lena, S. M., & Bijoor, S. (1990). Wrist cutting: a dare game among adolescents. *CMAJ : Canadian Medical Association journal = journal de l'Association medicale canadienne*, *142*(2), 131–132.

Lepistö, S., Astedt-Kurki, P., Joronen, K., Luukkaala, T., & Paavilainen, E. (2010). Adolescents' experiences of coping with domestic violence. *Journal of advanced nursing*, *66*(6), 1232–1245. https://doi.org/10.1111/j.1365-2648.2010.05289.x

Lerner, R. M., & Ohannessian, C. M. (2014). *Risks and Problem Behaviors in Adolescence*. Taylor & Francis.

Lewis, S. P., & Heath, N. L. (2013). Nonsuicidal self-injury. *CMAJ : Canadian Medical Association journal = journal de l'Association medicale canadienne*, *185*(6), 505. https://doi.org/10.1503/cmaj.120969

Lewis, S. P., Heath, N. L., Michal, N. J., & Duggan, J. M. (2012). Non-suicidal self-injury, youth, and the Internet: What mental health professionals need to know. *Child and adolescent psychiatry and mental health, 6*(1), 13. https://doi.org/10.1186/1753-2000-6-13

Liang, S. G., Yan, J., Zhu, C. Z., Situ, M. J., Du, N., Fu, X. Y., & Huang, Y. (2014). Sichuan da xue xue bao. Yi xue ban [Personality traits of Chinese adolescents with non-suicidal self injury and suicide attempt]. *Medical science edition, 45*(6), 970–973.

Lifshitz, M., & Gavrilov, V. (2002). Deliberate self-poisoning in adolescents. *The Israel Medical Association journal : IMAJ, 4*(4), 252–254

Lim, K. S., Wong, C. H., McIntyre, R. S., Wang, J., Zhang, Z., Tran, B. X., Tan, W., Ho, C. S., & Ho, R. C. (2019). Global Lifetime and 12-Month Prevalence of Suicidal Behavior, Deliberate Self-Harm and Non-Suicidal Self-Injury in Children and Adolescents between 1989 and 2018: A Meta-Analysis. *International journal of environmental research and public health, 16*(22), 4581. https://doi.org/10.3390/ijerph16224581

Limburg, K., Watson, H. J., Hagger, M. S., & Egan, S. J. (2017). The Relationship Between Perfectionism and Psychopathology: A Meta-Analysis. *Journal of clinical psychology, 73*(10), 1301–1326. https://doi.org/10.1002/jclp.22435

Linehan, M. M., Comtois, K. A., Brown, M. Z., Heard, H. L., & Wagner, A. (2006). Suicide Attempt Self-Injury Interview (SASII): development, reliability, and validity of a scale to assess suicide attempts and intentional self-injury. *Psychological assessment, 18*(3), 303–312. https://doi.org/10.1037/1040-3590.18.3.303

Linhartová, P., Širůček, J., Bartecek, R., Theiner, P., Jeřábková, B., Rudišinová, D., & Kasparek, T. (2017). České verze sebeposuzovacích modelů impulzivity Barrattovy škály a škály UPPS-P a jejich psychometrické charakteristiky [Czech versions of impulsIvity self-report scales the Barratt Scale and the UPPS-P Scale and their psychometric properties]. *Česká a Slovenská Psychiatrie, 113*(4), 149–157.

Lisá, E. & Valachová, M. (2021). Dispositional mindfulness as a mediator between basic psychological needs and dark triad traits. *Personality and Individual Differences, 181*, 111057. https://doi.org/10.1016/j.paid.2021.111057

Liu, R. T., Cheek, S. M., & Nestor, B. A. (2016). Non-suicidal self-injury and life stress: A systematic meta-analysis and theoretical elaboration. *Clinical psychology review, 47*, 1–14. https://doi.org/10.1016/j.cpr.2016.05.005

Llamocca, E. N., Fristad, M. A., Bridge, J. A., Brock, G., Steelesmith, D. L., Axelson, D. A., & Fontanella, C. A. (2022). Correlates of deliberate self-harm among youth with bipolar disorder. *Journal of affective disorders, 302*, 376–384. https://doi.org/10.1016/j.jad.2022.01.085

Lloyd, E. E. (1997). *Self-Mutilation in a Community Sample of Adolescents.* [LSU Historical Dissertations and Theses. 6546.] https://digitalcommons.lsu.edu/gradschool_disstheses/6546

Lloyd-Richardson, E. E., Perrine, N., Dierker, L., & Kelley, M. L. (2007). Characteristics and functions of non-suicidal self-injury in a community sample of adolescents. *Psychological medicine, 37*(8), 1183–1192. https://doi.org/10.1017/S003329170700027X

Low, G., Jones, D., MacLeod, A., Power, M., & Duggan, C. (2000). Childhood trauma, dissociation and self-harming behaviour: a pilot study. *The British journal of medical psychology, 73* (2), 269–278. https://doi.org/10.1348/000711200160363

Lüdtke, J., Weizenegger, B., Rauber, R., Contin, B., In-Albon, T., & Schmid, M. (2017). The influence of personality traits and emotional and behavioral problems on repetitive nonsuicidal self-injury in a school sample. *Comprehensive psychiatry, 74,* 214–223. https://doi.org/10.1016/j.comppsych.2017.02.005

Lundh, L. G., Wångby-Lundh, M., Paaske, M., Ingesson, S., & Bjärehed, J. (2011). Depressive symptoms and deliberate self-harm in a community sample of adolescents: a prospective study. *Depression research and treatment, 2011,* 935871. https://doi.org/10.1155/2011/935871

Luthar, S. S. (ed.). (2003). *Resilience and vulnerability: Adaptation in the context of childhood adversities.* Cambridge University Press. https://doi.org/10.1017/CBO9780511615788

Luyckx, K., Gandhi, A., Bijttebier, P., & Claes, L. (2015). Non-suicidal self-injury in female adolescents and psychiatric patients: A replication and extension of the role of identity formation. *Personality and Individual Differences, 77,* 91–96. https://doi.org/10.1016/j.paid.2014.12.057

Lynam, D. R., Miller, J. D., Miller, D. J., Bornovalova, M. A., & Lejuez, C. W. (2011). Testing the relations between impulsivity-related traits, suicidality, and nonsuicidal self-injury: a test of the incremental validity of the UPPS model. *Personality disorders, 2*(2), 151–160. https://doi.org/10.1037/a0019978

Lyon, K. A., Juhasz, G., Brown, L., & Elliott, R. (2020). Big Five personality facets explaining variance in anxiety and depressive symptoms in a community sample. *Journal of affective disorders, 274,* 515–521. https://doi.org/10.1016/j.jad.2020.05.047

Maciejewski, D. F., Renteria, M. E., Abdellaoui, A., Medland, S. E., Few, L. R., Gordon, S. D., Madden, P. A., Montgomery, G., Trull, T. J., Heath, A. C., Statham, D. J., Martin, N. G., Zietsch, B. P., & Verweij, K. J. (2017). The Association of Genetic Predisposition to Depressive Symptoms with Non-suicidal and Suicidal Self-Injuries. *Behavior genetics, 47*(1), 3–10. https://doi.org/10.1007/s10519-016-9809-z

MacLaren, V. V., & Best, L. A. (2010). Nonsuicidal self-injury, potentially addictive behaviors, and the five factor model in undergraduates. *Personality and Individual Differences, 49*(5), 521–525. https://doi.org/10.1016/j.paid.2010.05.019

MacLeod, C. M. (2005). The Stroop Task in Cognitive Research. In A. Wenzel & D. C. Rubin (eds.), *Cognitive methods and their application to clinical research* (17–40). American Psychological Association. https://doi.org/10.1037/10870-002

Maddox, B. B., Trubanova, A., & White, S. W. (2017). Untended wounds: Non-suicidal self-injury in adults with autism spectrum disorder. *Autism : the international journal of research and practice, 21*(4), 412–422. https://doi.org/10.1177/1362361316644731

Madge, N., Hewitt, A., Hawton, K., de Wilde, E. J., Corcoran, P., Fekete, S., van Heeringen, K., De Leo, D., & Ystgaard, M. (2008). Deliberate self-harm within an international community sample of young people: comparative findings from the Child & Adolescent Self-harm in Europe (CASE) Study. *Journal of child psychology and psychiatry, and allied disciplines, 49*(6), 667–677. https://doi.org/10.1111/j.1469-7610.2008.01879.x

Mareš, P., Rabušic, L., & Soukup, P. (2015). *Analýza sociálněvědných dat (nejen) v psychologii. [Analysis of social science data (not only) in psychology].* Muni Press.

Marchant, A., Hawton, K., Burns, L., Stewart, A., & John, A. (2021). Impact of Web-Based Sharing and Viewing of Self-Harm-Related Videos and Photographs on Young People: Systematic Review. *Journal of medical Internet research, 23*(3), e18048. https://doi.org/10.2196/18048

Martens, K., Barry, T. J., Takano, K., & Raes, F. (2019). The transportability of Memory Specificity Training (MeST): Adapting an intervention derived from experimental psychology to routine clinical practices. *BMC Psychology, 7,* Article 5. https://doi.org/10.1186/s40359-019-0279-y

Martin, J., Cloutier, P. F., Levesque, C., Bureau, J. F., Lafontaine, M. F., & Nixon, M. K. (2013). Psychometric properties of the functions and addictive features scales of the Ottawa Self-Injury Inventory: a preliminary investigation using a university sample. *Psychological assessment, 25*(3), 1013–1018. https://doi.org/10.1037/a0032575

Martorana G. (2015). Characteristics and associated factors of non-suicidal self-injury among Italian young people: a survey through a thematic website. *Journal of behavioral addictions, 4*(2), 93–100. https://doi.org/10.1556/2006.4.2015.001

Masi, G., Milone, A., Montesanto, A. R., Valente, E., & Pisano, S. (2018). Non suicidal self-injury in referred adolescents with mood disorders and its association with cyclothymic-hypersensitive temperament. *Journal of affective disorders, 227,* 477–482. https://doi.org/10.1016/j.jad.2017.11.049

Maslowsky, J., Owotomo, O., Huntley, E. D., & Keating, D. (2019). Adolescent Risk Behavior: Differentiating Reasoned And Reactive Risk-taking. *Journal of youth and adolescence, 48*(2), 243–255. https://doi.org/10.1007/s10964-018-0978-3

Matera, E., Margari, M., Serra, M., Petruzzelli, M.G., Gabellone, A., Piarulli, F.M., Pugliese, A., Tassiello, A.R., Croce, F., Matera, E., Margari, M., Serra, M., Petruzzelli, M. G., Gabellone, A., Piarulli, F. M., Pugliese, A., Tassiello, A. R., Croce, F., Renna, C., & Margari, A. (2021). Non-Suicidal Self-Injury: An Observational Study in a Sample of Adolescents and Young Adults. *Brain sciences, 11*(8), 974. https://doi.org/10.3390/brainsci11080974

Matsumoto, T., Yamaguchi, A., Chiba, Y., Asami, T., Iseki, E., & Hirayasu, Y. (2004). Patterns of self-cutting: a preliminary study on differences in clinical implications between wrist- and arm-cutting using a Japanese juvenile detention center sample. *Psychiatry and clinical neurosciences, 58*(4), 377–382. https://doi.org/10.1111/j.1440-1819.2004.01271.x

Mazza, J. J., & Reynolds, W. M. (1998). A longitudinal investigation of depression, hopelessness, social support, and major and minor life events and their relation to suicidal ideation in adolescents. *Suicide & life-threatening behavior, 28*(4), 358–374. https://doi.org/10.1111/j.1943-278X.1998.tb00972.x

McAdams, D. P. (2001). The psychology of life stories. *Review of General Psychology, 5*(2), 100–122. https://doi.org/10.1037/1089-2680.5.2.100

McGaughey, J., Long, A., & Harrisson, S. (1995). Suicide and parasuicide: a selected review of the literature. *Journal of psychiatric and mental health nursing, 2*(4), 199–206. https://doi.org/10.1111/j.1365-2850.1995.tb00058.x

McHugh, C. M., Chun Lee, R. S., Hermens, D. F., Corderoy, A., Large, M., & Hickie, I. B. (2019). Impulsivity in the self-harm and suicidal behavior of young people: A systematic review and meta-analysis. *Journal of psychiatric research, 116*, 51–60. https://doi.org/10.1016/j.jpsychires.2019.05.012

McManus, S., Gunnell, D., Cooper, C., Bebbington, P. E., Howard, L. M., Brugha, T., Jenkins, R., Hassiotis, A., Weich, S., & Appleby, L. (2019). Prevalence of non-suicidal self-harm and service contact in England, 2000-14: repeated cross-sectional surveys of the general population. *The lancet. Psychiatry, 6*(7), 573–581. https://doi.org/10.1016/S2215-0366(19)30188-9

McManus, S., Hassiotis, A., Jenkins, R., Dennis, M., Aznar, C., & Appleby, L. (2016*). Chapter 12: suicidal thoughts, suicide attempts and self-harm*. In S. McManus, P. Bebbington, R. Jenkins, & T. Brugha (eds). Mental Health and Wellbeing in England: Adult Psychiatric Morbidity Survey 2014. NHS Digital.

Meeus, W., Iedema, J., Maassen, G., & Engels, R. (2005). Separation-individuation revisited: on the interplay of parent-adolescent relations, identity and emotional adjustment in adolescence. *Journal of adolescence, 28*(1), 89–106. https://doi.org/10.1016/j.adolescence.2004.07.003

Melendez, J. C., Mayordomo, T., Sancho, P., & Tomás, J. M. (2012). Coping strategies: gender differences and development throughout life span. *The Spanish journal of psychology, 15*(3), 1089–1098. https://doi.org/10.5209/rev_sjop.2012.v15.n3.39399

Melson, A. J., & O'Connor, R. C. (2019). Differentiating adults who think about self-harm from those who engage in self-harm: the role of volitional alcohol factors. *BMC psychiatry, 19*(1), 319. https://doi.org/10.1186/s12888-019-2292-3

Menninger, K. (1938). *Man against Himself*. Harcourt Brace World.

Merrill, J., Milner, G., Owens, J., & Vale, A. (1992). Alcohol and attempted suicide. *British journal of addiction, 87*(1), 83–89. https://doi.org/10.1111/j.1360-0443.1992.tb01903.x

Mészáros, G., Győri, D., Horváth, L. O., Szentiványi, D., & Balázs, J. (2020). Nonsuicidal Self-Injury: Its Associations With Pathological Internet Use and Psychopathology Among Adolescents. *Frontiers in psychiatry, 11*, 814. https://doi.org/10.3389/fpsyt.2020.00814

Millard C. (2013). Making the cut: The production of 'self-harm' in post-1945 Anglo-Saxon psychiatry. *History of the human sciences, 26*(2), 126–150. https://doi.org/10.1177/0952695112473619

Mitchell, M. R., & Potenza, M. N. (2014). Addictions and Personality Traits: Impulsivity and Related Constructs. *Current behavioral neuroscience reports, 1*(1), 1–12. https://doi.org/10.1007/s40473-013-0001-y

Mitchell, M. R., & Potenza, M. N. (2014). Recent Insights into the Neurobiology of Impulsivity. *Current addiction reports, 1*(4), 309–319. https://doi.org/10.1007/s40429-014-0037-4

Moffatt C. (2000). Self-inflicted wounding. 2: Identification, assessment and management. *British journal of community nursing, 5*(1), 34–40. https://doi.org/10.12968/bjcn.2000.5.1.7433

Mohandas, P., Ravenscroft, J. C., & Bewley, A. (2018). Dermatitis artefacta in childhood and adolescence: a spectrum of disease. *G Ital Dermatol Venereol, 153*(4), 525–534. https://doi.org/10.23736/S0392-0488.18.06019-4

Moir, A., & Moir, B. (1998). *Why Men Don't Iron: The Real Science of Gender Studies*. Harper Collins.

Molaie, A. M., Chiu, C. Y., Habib, Z., Galynker, I., Briggs, J., Rosenfield, P. J., Calati, R., & Yaseen, Z. S. (2019). Emotional Pain Mediates the Link Between Preoccupied Attachment and Non-suicidal Self-Injury in High Suicide Risk Psychiatric Inpatients. *Frontiers in psychology, 10*, 289. https://doi.org/10.3389/fpsyg.2019.00289

Moran, P., Coffey, C., Romaniuk, H., Olsson, C., Borschmann, R., Carlin, J. B., & Patton, G. C. (2012). The natural history of self-harm from adolescence to young adulthood: a population-based cohort study. *Lancet, 379*(9812), 236–243. https://doi.org/10.1016/S0140-6736(11)61141-0

Moreira, P. A., Cloninger, C. R., Dinis, L., Sá, L., Oliveira, J. T., Dias, A., & Oliveira, J. (2015). Personality and well-being in adolescents. *Frontiers in psychology, 5*, 1494. https://doi.org/10.3389/fpsyg.2014.01494

Morey, Y., Mellon, D., Dailami, N., Verne, J., & Tapp, A. (2017). Adolescent self-harm in the community: an update on prevalence using a self-report survey of adolescents aged 13-18 in England. *Journal of public health, 39*(1), 58–64. https://doi.org/10.1093/pubmed/fdw010

Morgan, C., Webb, R. T., Carr, M. J., Kontopantelis, E., Green, J., Chew-Graham, C. A., Kapur, N., & Ashcroft, D. M. (2017). Incidence, clinical management, and mortality risk following self harm among children and adolescents: cohort study in primary care. *BMJ (Clinical research ed.), 359*, j4351. https://doi.org/10.1136/bmj.j4351

Morrison, R., & O'Connor, R. C. (2008). A systematic review of the relationship between rumination and suicidality. *Suicide & life-threatening behavior*, 38(5), 523–538. https://doi.org/10.1521/suli.2008.38.5.523

Muehlenkamp, J. J., & Brausch, A. M. (2012). Body image as a mediator of non-suicidal self-injury in adolescents. *Journal of adolescence*, 35(1), 1–9. https://doi.org/10.1016/j.adolescence.2011.06.010

Muehlenkamp, J. J., & Gutierrez, P. M. (2007). Risk for suicide attempts among adolescents who engage in non-suicidal self-injury. *Archives of suicide research : official journal of the International Academy for Suicide Research*, 11(1), 69–82. https://doi.org/10.1080/13811110600992902

Muehlenkamp, J. J., Claes, L., Havertape, L., & Plener, P. L. (2012). International prevalence of adolescent non-suicidal self-injury and deliberate self-harm. *Child and adolescent psychiatry and mental health*, 6, 10. https://doi.org/10.1186/1753-2000-6-10

Muehlenkamp, J. J., Cowles, M. L., & Gutierrez, P. M. (2010). Validity of the Self-Harm Behavior Questionnaire with diverse adolescents. *Journal of Psychopathology and Behavioral Assessment*, 32(2), 236–245. https://doi.org/10.1007/s10862-009-9131-7

Muehlenkamp, J. J., Engel, S. G., Wadeson, A., Crosby, R. D., Wonderlich, S. A., Simonich, H., & Mitchell, J. E. (2009). Emotional states preceding and following acts of non-suicidal self-injury in bulimia nervosa patients. *Behaviour research and therapy*, 47(1), 83–87. https://doi.org/10.1016/j.brat.2008.10.011

Muehlenkamp, J. J., Hilt, L. M., Ehlinger, P. P., & McMillan, T. (2015). Non-suicidal self-injury in sexual minority college students: a test of theoretical integration. *Child and adolescent psychiatry and mental health*, 9, 16. https://doi.org/10.1186/s13034-015-0050-y

Muehlenkamp, J. J., Xhunga, N., & Brausch, A. M. (2019). Self-injury Age of Onset: A Risk Factor for NSSI Severity and Suicidal Behavior. *Archives of suicide research : official journal of the International Academy for Suicide Research*, 23(4), 551–563. https://doi.org/10.1080/13811118.2018.1486252

Mueller, S. C., Cromheeke, S., Siugzdaite, R., & Nicolas Boehler, C. (2017). Evidence for the triadic model of adolescent brain development: Cognitive load and task-relevance of emotion differentially affect adolescents and adults. *Developmental cognitive neuroscience*, 26, 91–100. https://doi.org/10.1016/j.dcn.2017.06.004

Müller, A., Claes, L., Smits, D., Brähler, E., & de Zwaan, M. (2016). Prevalence and Correlates of Self-Harm in the German General Population. *PloS one*, 11(6), e0157928. https://doi.org/10.1371/journal.pone.0157928

Müller, A., Claes, L., Smits, D., Schag, K., & de Zwaan, M. (2018). Lifetime Self-Harm Behaviors Are Not More Prevalent in Bariatric Surgery Candidates than in Community Controls with Obesity. *Obesity facts*, 11(2), 109–115. https://doi.org/10.1159/000486484

Mullick, M. S., Karim, M. E., & Khanam, M. (1994). Depression in deliberate self harm patients. *Bangladesh Medical Research Council bulletin*, 20(3), 123–128.

Mullins-Sweatt, S. N., Lengel, G. J., & Grant, D. M. (2013). Non-suicidal self-injury: the contribution of general personality functioning. *Personality and mental health, 7*(1), 56–68. https://doi.org/10.1002/pmh.1211

Muyibi, A. S., Ajayi, I., Irabor, A. E., & Ladipo, M. (2010). Relationship between adolescents' family function with socio-demographic characteristics and behaviour risk factors in a primary care facility. *African Journal of Primary Health Care & Family Medicine, 2*(1), 177. https://doi.org/10.4102/phcfm.v2i1.177

Nagy, L. M., Shanahan, M. L., & Baer, R. A. (2021). An experimental investigation of the effects of self-criticism and self-compassion on implicit associations with non-suicidal self-injury. *Behaviour research and therapy, 139*, 103819. https://doi.org/10.1016/j.brat.2021.103819

Nagy, L. M., Shanahan, M. L., & Seaford, S. P. (2022). Nonsuicidal self-injury and rumination: A meta-analysis. Journal of clinical psychology, 10.1002/jclp.23394. Advance online publication. https://doi.org/10.1002/jclp.23394

National Academies of Sciences, Engineering, and Medicine; Health and Medicine Division; Division of Behavioral and Social Sciences and Education; Board on Children, Youth, and Families; Committee on the Neurobiological and Socio-behavioral Science of Adolescent Development and Its Applications; Backes EP, Bonnie RJ, (eds.)(2019) *The Promise of Adolescence: Realizing Opportunity for All Youth.* National Academies Press. https://www.ncbi.nlm.nih.gov/books/NBK545476/

National Collaborating Centre for Mental Health.(2012). Self-Harm: Longer-Term Management. *British Psychological Society, 133* (4) https://www.ncbi.nlm.nih.gov/books/NBK126796/

Nelson, A., & Muehlenkamp, J. J. (2012). Body attitudes and objectification in non-suicidal self-injury: comparing males and females. *Archives of suicide research : official journal of the International Academy for Suicide Research,, 16*(1), 1–12. https://doi.org/10.1080/13811118.2012.640578

Nester, M. S., Boi, C., Brand, B. L., & Schielke, H. J. (2022). The reasons dissociative disorder patients self-injure. *European journal of psychotraumatology, 13*(1), 2026738. https://doi.org/10.1080/20008198.2022.2026738

Nicastro, R., Jermann, F., Bondolfi, G., & McQuillan, A. (2010). Assessment of mindfulness with the French version of the Kentucky Inventory of Mindfulness Skills in community and borderline personality disorder samples. *Assessment, 17*(2), 197–205. https://doi.org/10.1177/1073191110363551

Nicolai, K. A., Wielgus, M. D., & Mezulis, A. (2016). Identifying Risk for Self-Harm: Rumination and Negative Affectivity in the Prospective Prediction of Nonsuicidal Self-Injury. *Suicide & life-threatening behavior, 46*(2), 223–233. https://doi.org/10.1111/sltb.12186

Nicolai, K. A., Wielgus, M. D., & Mezulis, A. (2016). Identifying Risk for Self-Harm: Rumination and Negative Affectivity in the Prospective Prediction of Nonsuicidal Self-Injury. *Suicide & life-threatening behavior, 46*(2), 223–233. https://doi.org/10.1111/sltb.12186

Nitkowski, D., & Petermann, F. (2011). Selbstverletzendes Verhalten und komorbide psychische Störungen: ein Überblick [Non-suicidal self-injury and comorbid mental disorders: a review]. *Fortschritte der Neurologie-Psychiatrie, 79*(1), 9–20. https://doi.org/10.1055/s-0029-1245772

Nixon, M. K., &Cloutier, P.(2005). Ottawa self-injury inventory. http://www.insync-group.ca/publications/OSI-2015-English-v3.1.pdf

Nixon, M. K., Cloutier, P. F., & Aggarwal, S. (2002). Affect regulation and addictive aspects of repetitive self-injury in hospitalized adolescents. *Journal of the American Academy of Child and Adolescent Psychiatry, 41*(11), 1333–1341. https://doi.org/10.1097/00004583-200211000-00015

Nixon, M. K., Cloutier, P., & Jansson, S. M. (2008). Nonsuicidal self-harm in youth: a population-based survey. *CMAJ : Canadian Medical Association journal = journal de l'Association medicale canadienne, 178*(3), 306–312. https://doi.org/10.1503/cmaj.061693

Nixon, M. K., Levesque, C., Preyde, M., Vanderkooy, J., & Cloutier, P. F. (2015). The Ottawa Self-Injury Inventory: Evaluation of an assessment measure of nonsuicidal self-injury in an inpatient sample of adolescents. *Child and adolescent psychiatry and mental health, 9*, 26. https://doi.org/10.1186/s13034-015-0056-5

Nock, M. K. (2009). Why do People Hurt Themselves? New Insights Into the Nature and Functions of Self-Injury. *Current directions in psychological science, 18*(2), 78–83. https://doi.org/10.1111/j.1467-8721.2009.01613.x

Nock, M. K., & Cha, Ch. (2009). Psychological models of nonsuicidal self-injury. In: M. K. Nock (ed.). *Understanding nonsuicidal self-injury: Origins, assessment, and treatment*, 65–77, American Psychological Association.

Nock, M. K., & Prinstein, M. J. (2004). A functional approach to the assessment of self-mutilative behavior. *Journal of consulting and clinical psychology, 72*(5), 885–890. https://doi.org/10.1037/0022-006X.72.5.885

Nock, M. K., & Prinstein, M. J. (2005). Contextual features and behavioral functions of self-mutilation among adolescents. *Journal of abnormal psychology, 114*(1), 140–146. https://doi.org/10.1037/0021-843X.114.1.140

Nock, M. K., Holmberg, E. B., Photos, V. I., & Michel, B. D. (2007). Self-Injurious Thoughts and Behaviors Interview: development, reliability, and validity in an adolescent sample. *Psychological assessment, 19*(3), 309–317. https://doi.org/10.1037/1040-3590.19.3.309

Nock, M. K., Joiner, T. E., Gordon, K. H., Lloyd-Richardson, E., and Prinstein, M. J. (2006). Nonsuicidal self-injury among adolescents: diagnostic correlates and relation to suicide attempts. *Psychiatry Res. 144*, 65–72. https://doi.org/10.1016/j.psychres.2006.05.010

Nolen-Hoeksema S. (1991). Responses to depression and their effects on the duration of depressive episodes. *Journal of abnormal psychology, 100*(4), 569–582. https://doi.org/10.1037//0021-843x.100.4.569

Nosek, B. A., Bar-Anan, Y., Sriram, N., Axt, J., & Greenwald, A. G. (2014). Understanding and using the brief Implicit Association Test: recommended scoring procedures. *PloS one, 9*(12), e110938. https://doi.org/10.1371/journal.pone.0110938

Noshpitz J. D. (1994). Self-destructiveness in adolescence. *American journal of psychotherapy, 48*(3), 330–346. https://doi.org/10.1176/appi.psychotherapy.1994.48.3.330

Öcal, E. E., Demirtaş, Z., Atalay, B. I., Önsüz, M. F., Işıklı, B., Metintaş, S., & Yenilmez, Ç. (2022). Relationship between Mental Disorders and Optimism in a Community-Based Sample of Adults. *Behavioral sciences,12*(2), 52. https://doi.org/10.3390/bs12020052

O'Connor, R. C., Wetherall, K., Cleare, S., Eschle, S., Drummond, J., Ferguson, E., O'Connor, D. B., & O'Carroll, R. E. (2018). Suicide attempts and non-suicidal self-harm: national prevalence study of young adults. *BJPsych open, 4*(3), 142–148. https://doi.org/10.1192/bjo.2018.14

Offer D, Barglow P (1960). Adolescent and young adult self-mutilation in a general psychiatric hospital. *Arch Gen Psychiatry. 1960;3*(2):194–204. https://doi:10.1001/archpsyc.1960.01710020078010

Ohmann, S., Schuch, B., Konig, M., Blaas, S., Fliri, C., & Popow, C. (2008). Self-injurious behavior in adolescent girls. Association with psychopathology and neuropsychological functions. *Psychopathology, 41*(4), 226–235. https://doi.org/10.1159/000125556

Orbach, I., Bar-Joseph, H., & Dror, N. (1990). Styles of problem solving in suicidal individuals. *Suicide and Life-Threatening Behavior, 20*(1), 56–64.

Ose, S. O., Tveit, T., & Mehlum, L. (2021). Non-suicidal self-injury (NSSI) in adult psychiatric outpatients - A nationwide study. *Journal of psychiatric research, 133*, 1–9. https://doi.org/10.1016/j.jpsychires.2020.11.031

Osuch, E. A., Noll, J. G., & Putnam, F. W. (1999). The motivations for self-injury in psychiatric inpatients. *Psychiatry, 62*(4), 334–346. https://doi.org/10.1080/00332747.1999.11024881

Osuch, E., Ford, K., Wrath, A., Bartha, R., & Neufeld, R. (2014). Functional MRI of pain application in youth who engaged in repetitive non-suicidal self-injury vs. psychiatric controls. *Psychiatry research, 223*(2), 104–112. https://doi.org/10.1016/j.pscychresns.2014.05.003

Ougrin, D., Tranah, T., Leigh, E., Taylor, L., & Asarnow, J. R. (2012). Practitioner review: Self-harm in adolescents. *Journal of child psychology and psychiatry, and allied disciplines, 53*(4), 337–350. https://doi.org/10.1111/j.1469-7610.2012.02525.x

Oumaya, M., Friedman, S., Pham, A., Abou Abdallah, T., Guelfi, J. D., & Rouillon, F. (2008). Personnalité borderline, automutilations et suicide : revue de la littérature [Borderline personality disorder, self-mutilation and suicide: literature review]. *L'Encephale, 34*(5), 452–458.

Paivio, S. C., & McCulloch, C. R. (2004). Alexithymia as a mediator between childhood trauma and self-injurious behaviors. *Child abuse & neglect, 28*(3), 339–354. https://doi.org/10.1016/j.chiabu.2003.11.01

Palese, E. (2013). Zygmunt Bauman. Individual and society in the liquid modernity. *Springer Plus, 2* (1), 191. https://doi.org/10.1186/2193-1801-2-191

Parker, G., Malhi, G., Mitchell, P., Kotze, B., Wilhelm, K., & Parker, K. (2005). Self-harming in depressed patients: pattern analysis. *The Australian and New Zealand journal of psychiatry, 39*(10), 899–906. https://doi.org/10.1080/j.1440-1614.2005.01662

Patel, T. A., Mann, A., Blakey, S. M., Aunon, F. M., Calhoun, P. S., Beckham, J. C., & Kimbrel, N. A. (2021). Diagnostic Correlates of Nonsuicidal Self-Injury Disorder among Veterans with Psychiatric Disorders. *Psychiatry research, 296*, 113672. https://doi.org/10.1016/j.psychres.2020.113672

Pattwell, S. S., Duhoux, S., Hartley, C. A., Johnson, D. C., Jing, D., Elliott, M. D., Ruberry, E. J., Powers, A., Mehta, N., Yang, R. R., Soliman, F., Glatt, C. E., Casey, B. J., Ninan, I., & Lee, F. S. (2012). Altered fear learning across development in both mouse and human. *Proceedings of the National Academy of Sciences of the United States of America, 109*(40), 16318–16323. https://doi.org/10.1073/pnas.1206834109

Paul, E., Tsypes, A., Eidlitz, L., Ernhout, C., & Whitlock, J. (2015). Frequency and functions of non-suicidal self-injury: associations with suicidal thoughts and behaviors. *Psychiatry research, 225*(3), 276–282. https://doi.org/10.1016/j.psychres.2014.12.026

Peebles, R., Wilson, J. L., & Lock, J. D. (2011). Self-injury in adolescents with eating disorders: correlates and provider bias. *The Journal of adolescent health : official publication of the Society for Adolescent Medicine, 48*(3), 310–313. https://doi.org/10.1016/j.jadohealth.2010.06.017

Peng, B., Li, J., Liu, H., Fang, H., Zhao, W., Chen, G., Xiu, M., & Zhang, Y. (2022). Childhood Maltreatment, Low Serum Cortisol Levels, and Non-Suicidal Self-Injury in Young Adults With Major Depressive Disorders. *Frontiers in Pediatrics, 10*. https://doi.org/10.3389/fped.2022.822046

Per, M., Simundic, A., Argento, A., Khoury, B., & Heath, N. (2022). Examining the Relationship Between Mindfulness, Self-Compassion, and Emotion Regulation in Self-Injury. *Archives of suicide research : official journal of the International Academy for Suicide Research, 26*(3), 1286–1301. https://doi.org/10.1080/13811118.2021.1885534

Pérez Rodríguez, S., Marco Salvador, J. H., & Garcia-Alandete, J. (2017). The role of hopelessness and meaning in life in a clinical sample with non-suicidal self-injury and suicide attempts. *Psicothema, 29*(3), 323–328. https://doi.org/10.7334/psicothema2016.284

Perlman, G., Gromatsky, M., Salis, K. L., Klein, D. N., & Kotov, R. (2018). Personality Correlates of Self-Injury in Adolescent Girls: Disentangling the Effects of Lifetime Psychopathology. *Journal of abnormal child psychology, 46*(8), 1677–1685. https://doi.org/10.1007/s10802-018-0403-0

Petermann, F., & Nitkowski, D. (2015). *Selbstverletzendes Verhalten. Erscheinungsformen, Ursachen und Interventionsmöglichkeiten (3., überarb. Aufl.).* Hogrefe.

Peters, E. M., Baetz, M., Marwaha, S., Balbuena, L., & Bowen, R. (2016). Affective instability and impulsivity predict nonsuicidal self-injury in the general population: a longitudinal analysis. *Borderline personality disorder and emotion dysregulation, 3,* 17. https://doi.org/10.1186/s40479-016-0051-3

Peterson, C., & Seligman, M. E. (1987). Explanatory style and illness. *Journal of personality, 55*(2), 237–265. https://doi.org/10.1111/j.1467-6494.1987.tb00436.x

Peterson, C., Xu, L., Leemis, R. W., & Stone, D. M. (2019). Repeat Self-Inflicted Injury Among U.S. Youth in a Large Medical Claims Database. *American journal of preventive medicine, 56*(3), 411–419. https://doi.org/10.1016/j.amepre.2018.09.009

Peterson, J., Freedenthal, S., Sheldon, C., & Andersen, R. (2008). Nonsuicidal Self injury in Adolescents. *Psychiatry, 5*(11), 20–26.

Petersson, S., Clinton, D., Brudin, L., Perseius, K. I., & Norring, C. (2018). Perfectionism in Eating Disorders: Are Long-Term Outcomes Influenced by Extent and Changeability in Initial Perfectionism? *Journal for person-oriented research, 4*(1), 1–14. https://doi.org/10.17505/jpor.2018.01

Plener, P. L., Brunner, R., Fegert, J. M., Groschwitz, R. C., In-Albon, T., Kaess, M., Kapusta, N. D., Resch, F., & Becker, K. (2016). Treating nonsuicidal self-injury (NSSI) in adolescents: consensus based German guidelines. *Child and adolescent psychiatry and mental health, 10,* 46. https://doi.org/10.1186/s13034-016-0134-3

Plener, P. L., Fischer, C. J., In-Albon, T., Rollett, B., Nixon, M. K., Groschwitz, R. C., & Schmid, M. (2013). Adolescent non-suicidal self-injury (NSSI) in German-speaking countries: comparing prevalence rates from three community samples. *Social psychiatry and psychiatric epidemiology, 48*(9), 1439–1445. https://doi.org/10.1007/s00127-012-0645-z

Plener, P. L., Libal, G., Keller, F., Fegert, J. M., & Muehlenkamp, J. J. (2009). An international comparison of adolescent non-suicidal self-injury (NSSI) and suicide attempts: Germany and the USA. *Psychological medicine, 39*(9), 1549–1558. https://doi.org/10.1017/S0033291708005114

Pollock, L. R., & Williams, J. M. G. (2001). Effective problem solving in suicide attempters depends on specific autobiographical recall. *Suicide and Life-Threatening Behavior, 31*(4), 386–396. https://doi.org/10.1521/suli.31.4.386.22041

PORDATA. (2020). *The Database of Contemporary Portugal.* https://www.pordata.pt/en/Europe/Number+of+divorces+per+100+marriages-1566

Portzky, G., De Wilde, E. J., & van Heeringen, K. (2008). Deliberate self-harm in young people: differences in prevalence and risk factors between the Netherlands and Belgium. *European child & adolescent psychiatry, 17*(3), 179–186. https://doi.org/10.1007/s00787-007-0652-x

Posner, K., Brodsky, B., Yershova, K., Buchanan, J., & Mann, J. (2014). The classification of self-injurious behaviors. In M. K. Nock (ed.), *The Oxford Handbook of Suicide and Self-Injury* (7–22). Oxford University Press.

Prinstein, M. J., Guerry, J. D., Browne, C. B. , & Rancourt, D. (2009). Interpersonal models of nonsuicidal self-injury. In: M. K. Nock (ed.). *Understanding nonsuicidal self-injury: Origins, assessment, and treatment*, 79-98, American Psychological Association.

Quarshie, E. N., Shuweihdi, F., Waterman, M., & House, A. (2021). Self-harm among in-school and street-connected adolescents in Ghana: a cross-sectional survey in the Greater Accra region. *BMJ open, 11*(1), e041609. https://doi.org/10.1136/bmjopen-2020-041609

Quarshie, E. N., Waterman, M. G., & House, A. O. (2020). Self-harm with suicidal and non-suicidal intent in young people in sub-Saharan Africa: a systematic review. *BMC psychiatry, 20*(1), 234. https://doi.org/10.1186/s12888-020-02587-z

Raemen, L., Luyckx, K., Müller, A., Buelens, T., Verschueren, M., & Claes, L. (2020). Non-Suicidal Self-Injury and Pathological Buying in Community Adults and Patients with Eating Disorders: Associations with Reactive and Regulative Temperament. *Psychologica Belgica, 60*(1), 396–410. https://doi.org/10.5334/pb.1027

Ragmanauskaite, L., Kim, J., Zhang, Q., Luk, K. M., Getahun, D., Silverberg, M. J., Goodman, M., & Yeung, H. (2020). Self-reported tattoo prevalence and motivations in transgender adults: a cross-sectional survey. *Dermatology online journal, 26*(12), 13030/qt841261s4.

Ran, H., Fang, D., Che, Y., Donald, A. R., Peng, J., Chen, L., Wang, S., & Xiao, Y. (2022). Resilience mediates the association between impulsivity and self-harm in Chinese adolescents. *Journal of affective disorders, 300*, 34-40. https://doi.org/10.1016/j.jad.2021.12.077

Raudales, A. M., Weiss, N. H., Goncharenko, S., Forkus, S. R., & Contractor, A. A. (2020). Posttraumatic stress disorder and deliberate self-harm among military veterans: Indirect effects through negative and positive emotion dysregulation. *Psychological trauma : theory, research, practice and policy, 12*(7), 707–715. https://doi.org/10.1037/tra0000962

Reichl, C., & Kaess, M. (2021). Self-harm in the context of borderline personality disorder. *Current opinion in psychology, 37*, 139–144. https://doi.org/10.1016/j.copsyc.2020.12.007

Reichl, C., Heyer, A., Brunner, R., Parzer, P., Völker, J. M., Resch, F., & Kaess, M. (2016). Hypothalamic-pituitary-adrenal axis, childhood adversity and adolescent nonsuicidal self-injury. *Psychoneuroendocrinology, 74*, 203–211. https://doi.org/10.1016/j.psyneuen.2016.09.011

Reis, M. D., Barbosa, A., Matildes, J., Freitas, J. P., & Rodrigo, F. G. (1997). Dermatite artefacta [Dermatitis artefacta]. *Acta medica portuguesa, 10*(12), 951–954.

Rettew, D. C., & McKee, L. (2005). Temperament and its role in developmental psychopathology. *Harvard review of psychiatry, 13*(1), 14–27. https://doi.org/10.1080/10673220590923146

Rettew, D. C., Doyle, A. C., Kwan, M., Stanger, C., & Hudziak, J. J. (2006). Exploring the boundary between temperament and generalized anxiety disorder: a receiver operating characteristic analysis. *Journal of anxiety disorders, 20*(7), 931–945. https://doi.org/10.1016/j.janxdis.2006.02.002

Rhéaume, J., Freeston, M. H., Ladouceur, R., Bouchard, C., Gallant, L., Talbot, F., & Vallières, A. (2000). Functional and dysfunctional perfectionists: Are they different on compulsive-like behaviors? *Behaviour Research and Therapy, 38*(2), 119–128. https://doi.org/10.1016/S0005-7967(98)00203-4

Rice, K. G., & Mirzadeh, S. A. (2000). Perfectionism, attachment, and adjustment. *Journal of Counseling Psychology, 47*(2), 238–250. https://doi.org/10.1037/0022-0167.47.2.238

Riegel, K. (2015). Osobnostní inventář pro DSM-5: PID-5. [The Personality Inventory for DSM-5 :PID-5]. Hogrefe.

Riegel, K. D. (2018). *Česká verze Osobnostního inventáře pro DSM-5 (PID-5): Teoretická východiska, psychometrické vlastnosti a implikace pro klinickou praxi* [Dizertační práca].Univerzita Karlova. https://dspace.cuni.cz/handle/20.500.11956/102382

Richmond, S., Hasking, P., & Meaney, R. (2017). Psychological Distress and Non-Suicidal Self-Injury: The Mediating Roles of Rumination, Cognitive Reappraisal, and Expressive Suppression. *Archives of suicide research : official journal of the International Academy for Suicide Research, 21*(1), 62–72. https://doi.org/10.1080/13811118.2015.1008160

Roberts, B. W., Jackson, J. J., Fayard, J. V., Edmonds, G., & Meints, J. (2009). Conscientiousness. In: M. R. Leary, & R. H. Hoyle, (eds.) *Handbook of individual differences in social behavior.(369-381)* The Guilford Press.

Robillard, C. L., Chapman, A. L., & Turner, B. J. (2022). Learning from experience: Within- and between-person associations of the consequences, frequency, and versatility of nonsuicidal self-injury. *Suicide and Life-Threatening Behavior, 52*(5), 836– 847. https://doi.org/10.1111/sltb.12867

Robinson, M. S., & Alloy, L. B. (2003). Negative Cognitive Styles and Stress-Reactive Rumination Interact to Predict Depression: A Prospective Study. *Cognitive Therapy and Research, 27*(3), 275–292. https://doi.org/10.1023/A:1023914416469

Romans, S. E., Martin, J. L., Anderson, J. C., Herbison, G. P., & Mullen, P. E. (1995). Sexual abuse in childhood and deliberate self-harm. *The American Journal of Psychiatry, 152*(9), 1336–1342. https://doi.org/10.1176/ajp.152.9.1336

Romer, D., Reyna, V. F., & Satterthwaite, T. D. (2017). Beyond stereotypes of adolescent risk taking: Placing the adolescent brain in developmental context. *Developmental Cognitive Neuroscience, 27*, 19–34. https://doi.org/10.1016/j.dcn.2017.07.007

Rosenthal, R. J., Rinzler, C., Wallsh, R., & Klausner, E. (1972). Wrist-cutting syndrome: the meaning of a gesture. *The American journal of psychiatry, 128*(11), 1363–1368. https://doi.org/10.1176/ajp.128.11.1363

Rozsívalová, E., Trefilová, A, & Paclt, I. (2010). Sebepoškozování u dospívajících. [A Self-harm with Adolescents]. *Česká a Slovenská Psychiatrie, 106*(4), 239–244.

Řičan, P. (1989). *Cesta životem.* [The life journey]. Panorama.

Saha, A., Seth, J., Gorai, S., & Bindal, A. (2015). Dermatitis Artefacta: A Review of Five Cases: A Diagnostic and Therapeutic Challenge. *Indian journal of dermatology, 60*(6), 613–615. https://doi.org/10.4103/0019-5154.169139

Sachsse, U., Von der Heyde, S., & Huether, G. (2002). Stress regulation and self-mutilation. *The American journal of psychiatry, 159*(4), 672. https://doi.org/10.1176/appi.ajp.159.4.672

Sansone, R. A., & Sansone, L. A. (2010). Measuring self-harm behavior with the self-harm inventory. *Psychiatry, 7*(4), 16-20.

Sansone, R. A., & Sansone, L. A. (2012). Rumination: relationships with physical health. *Innovations in clinical neuroscience, 9*(2), 29–34.

Sansone, R. A., Wiederman, M. W., & Sansone, L. A. (1998). The Self-Harm Inventory (SHI): development of a scale for identifying self-destructive behaviors and borderline personality disorder. *Journal of clinical psychology, 54*(7), 973–983. https://doi.org/10.1002/(sici)1097-4679(199811)54:7<973::aid-jclp11>3.0.co;2-h

Sawyer, S. M., Azzopardi, P. S., Wickremarathne, D., & Patton, G. C. (2018). The age of adolescence. *The Lancet Child & Adolescent Health, 2*(3), 223–228. https://doi.org/10.1016/S2352-4642(18)30022-1

Saxe, G. N., Chawla, N., & Van der Kolk, B. (2002). Self-destructive behavior in patients with dissociative disorders. *Suicide & life-threatening behavior, 32*(3), 313–320. https://doi.org/10.1521/suli.32.3.313.22174

Scocco, P., Macis, A., Ferrari, C., Bava, M., Bianconi, G., Bulgari, V., Candini, V., Carrà, G., Cavalera, C., Clerici, M., Conte, G., Cricelli, M., Ferla, M. T., Iozzino, L., Stefana, A., & Girolamo, G. D. (2019). Self-harm behaviour and externally-directed aggression in psychiatric outpatients: a multicentre, prospective study (viormed-2 study). *Scientific Reports, 9.* https://doi.org/10.1038/s41598-019-53993-7

Sedgwick, R., Epstein, S., Dutta, R., & Ougrin, D. (2019). Social media, internet use and suicide attempts in adolescents. *Current opinion in psychiatry, 32*(6), 534–541. https://doi.org/10.1097/YCO.0000000000000547

Selby, E. A., & Joiner, T. E., Jr. (2009). Cascades of Emotion: The Emergence of Borderline Personality Disorder from Emotional and Behavioral Dysregulation. *Review of general psychology : journal of Division 1, of the American Psychological Association, 13*(3), 219. https://doi.org/10.1037/a0015687

Selby, E. A., Bender, T. W., Gordon, K. H., Nock, M. K., & Joiner, T. E., Jr (2012). Non-suicidal self-injury (NSSI) disorder: a preliminary study. *Personality disorders, 3*(2), 167–175. https://doi.org/10.1037/a0024405

Selby, E. A., Connell, L. D., & Joiner, T. E., Jr. (2010). The pernicious blend of rumination and fearlessness in non-suicidal self-injury. *Cognitive Therapy and Research, 34*(5), 421–428. https://doi.org/10.1007/s10608-009-9260-z

Selby, E. A., Franklin, J., Carson-Wong, A., & Rizvi, S. L. (2013). Emotional cascades and self-injury: investigating instability of rumination and negative emotion. *Journal of clinical psychology, 69*(12), 1213–1227. https://doi.org/10.1002/jclp.21966

Sen, R. (2016). Not All that Is Solid Melts into Air? Care-Experienced Young People, Friendship and Relationships in the 'Digital Age'. *British journal of social work, 46*(4), 1059–1075. https://doi.org/10.1093/bjsw/bcu152

Serafini, G., Canepa, G., Adavastro, G., Nebbia, J., Murri, M. B., Erbuto, D., Pocai, B., Fiorillo, A., Pompili, M., Flouri, E., & Amore, M. (2017). The Relationship between Childhood Maltreatment and Non-Suicidal Self-Injury: A Systematic Review. *Frontiers in Psychiatry, 8*. https://doi.org/10.3389/fpsyt.2017.00149

Serra, M., Presicci, A., Quaranta, L., Caputo, E., Achille, M., Margari, F., Croce, F., Marzulli, L., & Margari, L. (2022). Assessing Clinical Features of Adolescents Suffering from Depression Who Engage in Non-Suicidal Self-Injury. *Children (Basel, Switzerland), 9*(2), 201. https://doi.org/10.3390/children9020201

Seymour, K. E., Jones, R. N., Cushman, G. K., Galvan, T., Puzia, M. E., Kim, K. L., Spirito, A., & Dickstein, D. P. (2016). Emotional face recognition in adolescent suicide attempters and adolescents engaging in non-suicidal self-injury. *European child & adolescent psychiatry, 25*(3), 247–259. https://doi.org/10.1007/s00787-015-0733-1

Shaffer, D. R., & Kipp, K. (2010). *Developmental Psychology: Childhood and Adolescence, Eighth Edition*. Cengage Learning.

Shafran, R., Cooper, Z., & Fairburn, C. G. (2002). Clinical perfectionism: a cognitive-behavioural analysis. *Behaviour research and therapy, 40*(7), 773–791. https://doi.org/10.1016/s0005-7967(01)00059-6

Shahwan, S., Zhang, Y., Sambasivam, R., Ong, S. H., Chong, S. A., & Subramaniam, M. (2021). A qualitative study of motivations for non-suicidal self-injury in a sample of psychiatric outpatients in Singapore. *Singapore medical journal*. https://doi.org/10.11622/smedj.2021161

Sher, L., & Stanley, B. (2009). Biological models of nonsuicidal self-injury. In: M. K. Nock (ed.), *Understanding nonsuicidal self-injury: Origins, assessment, and treatment* (99–116). American Psychological Association. https://doi.org/10.1037/11875-006

Schacter, H. L., & Margolin, G. (2019). The Interplay of Friends and Parents in Adolescents' Daily Lives: Towards A Dynamic View of Social Support. *Social development, 28*(3), 708–724. https://doi.org/10.1111/sode.12363

Scheier, M. F., & Carver, C. S. (1985). Optimism, coping, and health: assessment and implications of generalized outcome expectancies. Health psychology : official journal of the Division of Health Psychology, *American Psychological Association, 4*(3), 219–247. https://doi.org/10.1037//0278-6133.4.3.219

Scherf, K.S., Smyth, J.M., & Delgado, M.R. (2013). The amygdala: An agent of change in adolescent neural networks. *Hormones and Behavior, 64* (2), 298-313. https://dx.doi.org/10.1016/j.yhbeh.2013.05.011

Schroeder, S. R., Rojahn, J., & Reese, R. M. (1997). Brief report: reliability and validity of instruments for assessing psychotropic medication effects on self-injurious behavior in mental retardation. *Journal of autism and developmental disorders, 27*(1), 89–102. https://doi.org/10.1023/a:1025825322955

Schuman-Olivier, Z., Trombka, M., Lovas, D. A., Brewer, J. A., Vago, D. R., Gawande, R., Dunne, J. P., Lazar, S. W., Loucks, E. B., & Fulwiler, C. (2020). Mindfulness and Behavior Change. *Harvard review of psychiatry, 28*(6), 371–394. https://doi.org/10.1097/HRP.0000000000000277

Schützmann, K., Brinkmann, L., Schacht, M., & Richter-Appelt, H. (2009). Psychological distress, self-harming behavior, and suicidal tendencies in adults with disorders of sex development. *Archives of sexual behavior, 38*(1), 16–33. https://doi.org/10.1007/s10508-007-9241-9

Siddaway, A. P., Wood, A. M., O'Carroll, R. E., & O'Connor, R. C. (2019). Characterizing self-injurious cognitions: Development and validation of the Suicide Attempt Beliefs Scale (SABS) and the Nonsuicidal Self-Injury Beliefs Scale (NSIBS). *Psychological assessment, 31*(5), 592–608. https://doi.org/10.1037/pas0000684

Singhal, A., Ross, J., Seminog, O., Hawton, K., & Goldacre, M. J. (2014). Risk of self-harm and suicide in people with specific psychiatric and physical disorders: comparisons between disorders using English national record linkage. *Journal of the Royal Society of Medicine, 107*(5), 194–204. https://doi.org/10.1177/0141076814522033

Sitnik-Warchulska, K., & Izydorczyk, B. (2018). Family Patterns and Suicidal and Violent Behavior among Adolescent Girls-Genogram Analysis. *International journal of environmental research and public health, 15*(10), 2067. https://doi.org/10.3390/ijerph15102067

Skegg K. (2005). Self-harm. *The Lancet 366*(9495), 1471–1483. https://doi.org/10.1016/S0140-6736(05)67600-3

Skinner, R., McFaull, S., Draca, J., Frechette, M., Kaur, J., Pearson, C., & Thompson, W. (2016). Suicide and self-inflicted injury hospitalizations in Canada (1979 to 2014/15). Associations longitudinales entre l'influence des parents et des pairs et l'activité physique durant l'adolescence : résultats de l'étude COMPASS. *Health promotion and chronic disease prevention in Canada : research, policy and practice, 36*(11), 243–251. https://doi.org/10.24095/hpcdp.36.11.02

Sluga, W., & Grünberger, J. (1969). Selbstverletzungen und Selbstbeschädigungen bei Strafgefangenen [Self-inflicted injury and self-mutilation in prisoners]. *Wiener medizinische Wochenschrift (1946), 119*(24), 453–459.

Smets, L., & L. Claes (2017). Non-Suicidal Self-Injury in a Flemish Population: Associations with Personality Dimensions according to DSM-5. In: E. Bell (ed.), *Understanding Self-HArm. Prevalence, Predictors and Treatment Options* (93–102). Nova Science Publishers.

Smith, C. M. (2005). Origin and uses of primum non nocere–above all, do no harm!. *Journal of clinical pharmacology, 45*(4), 371–377. https://doi.org/10.1177/0091270004273680

Smith, N. B., Steele, A. M., Weitzman, M. L., Trueba, A. F., & Meuret, A. E. (2015). Investigating the role of self-disgust in nonsuicidal self-injury. *Archives of suicide research : official journal of the International Academy for Suicide Research, 19*(1), 60–74. https://doi.org/10.1080/13811118.2013.850135

Smithuis, L., Kool-Goudzwaard, N., de Man-van Ginkel, J. M., van Os-Medendorp, H., Berends, T., Dingemans, A., ... van Meijel, B. (2018). Self-injurious behaviour in patients with anorexia nervosa: a quantitative study. *Journal of Eating Disorders*, 6(26), https://doi.org/10.1186/s40337-018-0214-2.

Sneddon, I., & Sneddon, J. (1975). Self-inflicted injury: a follow-up study of 43 patients. *British medical journal*, 3(5982), 527-530. https://doi.org/10.1136/bmj.3.5982.527

Snir, A., Rafaeli, E., Gadassi, R., Berenson, K., & Downey, G. (2015). Explicit and inferred motives for nonsuicidal self-injurious acts and urges in borderline and avoidant personality disorders. *Personality disorders*, 6(3), 267-277. https://doi.org/10.1037/per0000104

Somer, O., Bildik, T., Kabukçu-Başay, B., Güngör, D., Başay, Ö., & Farmer, R. F. (2015). Prevalence of non-suicidal self-injury and distinct groups of self-injurers in a community sample of adolescents. *Social psychiatry and psychiatric epidemiology*, 50(7), 1163-1171. https://doi.org/10.1007/s00127-015-1060-z

Somma, A., Fossati, A., Ferrara, M., Fantini, F., Galosi, S., Krueger, R. F., Markon, K. E., & Terrinoni, A. (2019). DSM-5 personality domains as correlates of non-suicidal self-injury severity in an Italian sample of adolescent inpatients with self-destructive behaviour. *Personality and mental health*, 13(4), 205-214. https://doi.org/10.1002/pmh.1462

Son, Y., Kim, S., & Lee, J. S. (2021). Self-Injurious Behavior in Community Youth. *International journal of environmental research and public health*, 18(4), 1955. https://doi.org/10.3390/ijerph18041955

Sornberger, M. J., Heath, N. L., Toste, J. R., & McLouth, R. (2012). Nonsuicidal self-injury and gender: patterns of prevalence, methods, and locations among adolescents. *Suicide & life-threatening behavior*, 42(3), 266-278. https://doi.org/10.1111/j.1943-278X.2012.0088.x

Soyyiğit Oktan, V., Saylan, E., & Toksoy, P. (2022). Could Personality and Parental Relations Be a Risk Factor for Self-Injurious Behavior? *Journal of Family Issues*, 43(6), 1669-1685. https://doi.org/10.1177/0192513X211030047

Stallard, P., Spears, M., Montgomery, A. A., Phillips, R., & Sayal, K. (2013). Self-harm in young adolescents (12-16 years): onset and short-term continuation in a community sample. *BMC psychiatry*, 13, 328. https://doi.org/10.1186/1471-244X-13-328

Stanley, B., Sher, L., Wilson, S., Ekman, R., Huang, Y. Y., & Mann, J. J. (2010). Non-suicidal self-injurious behavior, endogenous opioids and monoamine neurotransmitters. *Journal of affective disorders*, 124(1-2), 134-140. https://doi.org/10.1016/j.jad.2009.10.028

Stark, D. (2020). *The Performance Complex: Competition and Competitions in Social Life*. Oxford University Press. https://doi.org/10.1093/oso/9780198861669.003.0001

Steeg, S., Carr, M. J., Mok, P., Pedersen, C. B., Antonsen, S., Ashcroft, D. M., Kapur, N., Erlangsen, A., Nordentoft, M., & Webb, R. T. (2020). Temporal trends in incidence of hospital-treated self-harm among adolescents in Denmark: national register-based study. *Social psychiatry and psychiatric epidemiology, 55*(4), 415–421. https://doi.org/10.1007/s00127-019-01794-8

Steinbeis, N., & Crone, E. A. (2016).The link between cognitive control and decision-making across child and adolescent development. *Current Opinion in Behavioral Sciences, 10,* 28–32. https://doi.org/10.1016/j.cobeha.2016.04.009

Steinberg L. (2008). A Social Neuroscience Perspective on Adolescent Risk-Taking. *Developmental review : DR, 28*(1), 78–106. https://doi.org/10.1016/j.dr.2007.08.002

Steinhoff, A., Ribeaud, D., Kupferschmid, S., Raible-Destan, N., Quednow, B. B., Hepp, U., Eisner, M., & Shanahan, L. (2021). Self-injury from early adolescence to early adulthood: age-related course, recurrence, and services use in males and females from the community. *European child & adolescent psychiatry, 30*(6), 937–951. https://doi.org/10.1007/s00787-020-01573-w

Stoica, A. M., Stoica, O. E., Vlad, R. E., Pop, A. M., & Monea, M. (2020). The Correlation between Oral Self-Harm and Ethnicity in Institutionalized Children. *Children, 8*(1), 2. https://doi.org/10.3390/children8010002

Stone, M. H. (1987). A psychodynamic approach: Some thoughts on the dynamics and therapy of self-mutilating borderline patients. *Journal of Personality Disorders, 1*(4), 347–349. https://doi.org/10.1521/pedi.1987.1.4.347

Straiton, M., Roen, K., Dieserud, G., & Hjelmeland, H. (2013). Pushing the boundaries: understanding self-harm in a non-clinical population. *Archives of psychiatric nursing, 27*(2), 78–83. https://doi.org/10.1016/j.apnu.2012.10.008

Stumpf, H., & Parker, W. D. (2000). A hierarchical structural analysis of perfectionism and its relation to other personality characteristics. *Personality and Individual Differences, 28*(5), 837–852. https://doi.org/10.1016/S0191-8869(99)00141-5

Suchańska, A. (1998). *Przejawy i uwarunkowania psychologiczne pośredniej autodestruktywności.* [Manifestation and psychological determinants of indirect self-destructiveness] Poznan: Wydawn. Naukowe UAM.

Suchańska, A. (2001). W poszukiwaniu wyjaśnień samoniszczenia: samoniszczenie a kompetencje samoopiekuńcze. [In earch and explanations for self-destruction: self-destruction and self-care competences]. *Forum Oświatowe, 13,* 2(25), 61–73.

Sukhera, J., Wodzinski, M., Rehman, M., & Gonzalez, C. M. (2019). The Implicit Association Test in health professions education: A meta-narrative review. Perspectives on medical education, 8(5), 267–275. https://doi.org/10.1007/s40037-019-00533-8

Suyemoto K. L. (1998). The functions of self-mutilation. *Clinical psychology review, 18*(5), 531–554. https://doi.org/10.1016/s0272-7358(97)00105-0

Swannell, S. V., Martin, G. E., Page, A., Hasking, P., & St John, N. J. (2014). Prevalence of nonsuicidal self-injury in nonclinical samples: systematic review, meta-analysis and meta-regression. *Suicide & life-threatening behavior, 44*(3), 273–303. https://doi.org/10.1111/sltb.12070

Swanson, E. N., Owens, E. B., & Hinshaw, S. P. (2014). Pathways to self-harmful behaviors in young women with and without ADHD: a longitudinal examination of mediating factors. *Journal of child psychology and psychiatry, and allied disciplines, 55*(5), 505-515. https://doi.org/10.1111/jcpp.12193

Symons, F. J., Harper, V. N., McGrath, P. J., Breau, L. M., & Bodfish, J. W. (2009). Evidence of increased non-verbal behavioral signs of pain in adults with neurodevelopmental disorders and chronic self-injury. *Research in developmental disabilities, 30*(3), 521-528. https://doi.org/10.1016/j.ridd.2008.07.012

Szewczuk-Bogusławska, M., Kaczmarek-Fojtar, M., Adamska, A., Frydecka, D., & Misiak, B. (2021). Assessment of the association between non-suicidal self-injury disorder and suicidal behaviour disorder in females with conduct disorder. *BMC psychiatry, 21*(1), 172. https://doi.org/10.1186/s12888-021-03168-4

Szewczuk-Bogusławska, M., Kaczmarek-Fojtar, M., Halicka-Masłowska, J., & Misiak, B. (2021). Self-Injuries and Their Functions with Respect to Suicide Risk in Adolescents with Conduct Disorder: Findings from a Path Analysis. *Journal of clinical medicine, 10*(19), 4602. https://doi.org/10.3390/jcm10194602

Šefarová, I. (2019). Na ostrí žiletky - sebapoškodzovanie vo vzťahu k rodinnému prostrediu ako rizikovému faktoru.[On the razor blade - self-harm in relation to the family environment as a risk factor]. In: S. Démuthová, & A. Baranovská (eds.), *Kondášove dni 2019. [Kondas´ Days 2019]* (99-106). Univerzita sv. Cyrila a Metoda.

Šefarová, I. (2020). Pacienti s automutiláciou - reflexie z klinickopsychologickej praxe. [Patients with automutilation - reflections from clinical psychological practice]. In: A.Baranovská, & D. Kochanová (eds.), *Kondášove dni 2020. [Kondas´ Days 2020]* (81-87). Univerzita sv. Cyrila a Metoda.

Širilová, Z. K. (2015). Starostlivosť o seba a sebapoškodzovanie [Self-care and Self-harm]. In M. Hricová, B. Kováčová Holevová, L. Lovaš, M. Mesárošová, B. Ráczová, Z. K. Širilová, & K. Vasková (eds.) *Psychologické kontexty starostlivosti o seba [Psychological contexts of self-care]*, 145-172, Univerzita Pavla Jozefa Šafárika.

Širilová, Z. K., & Klasová, L. (2015). Rodinné prostredie a starostlivosť o seba v rámci sebapoškodzovania. [Family Environment and Self-Care in the Context of Self-Harm]. *Psychologie pro praxi, 50*(1-2), 113-123.

Širilová, Z. K., & Radoňáková, L. (2013). Emocionálna regulácia v rámci sebapoškodzujúceho správania. [Emotional regulation within the frame of self harming behavior]. *Psychológia a patopsychológia dieťaťa, 47*(4), 362-372.

Širilová, Z., & Lovaš, L. (2012). Sebapoškodzovanie – jeho výskyt a hodnotenie. [Self-injury – its occurence and assessment]. *Psychológia a patopsychológia dieťaťa, 46*(3), 261-273.

Špaňár, J., & Hrabovský, J. (1998). Latinsko/slovenský, Slovensko/latinský slovník. [Latin/Slovak, Slovak/Latin Dictionary]. 6th ed. SPN.

Tait, R. J., Brinker, J., Moller, C. I., & French, D. J. (2014). Rumination, substance use, and self-harm in a representative Australian adult sample. *Journal of clinical psychology, 70*(3), 283-293. https://doi.org/10.1002/jclp.22025

Tang, J., Ma, Y., Guo, Y., Ahmed, N. I., Yu, Y., & Wang, J. (2013). Association of aggression and non-suicidal self injury: a school-based sample of adolescents. *PloS one, 8*(10), e78149. https://doi.org/10.1371/journal.pone.0078149

Tanner, A., Hasking, P., & Martin, G. (2014). Effects of rumination and optimism on the relationship between psychological distress and non-suicidal self-injury. *Prevention Science, 15*, 860-868. https://doi.org/10.1007/s11121-013-0444-0

Tantam, D., & Whittaker, J. (1992). Personality disorder and self-wounding. *The British journal of psychiatry 161* (4), 451-464. https://doi.org/10.1192/bjp.161.4.451

Taylor, L. M., Oldershaw, A., Richards, C., Davidson, K., Schmidt, U., & Simic, M. (2011). Development and pilot evaluation of a manualized cognitive-behavioural treatment package for adolescent self-harm. *Behavioural and cognitive psychotherapy, 39*(5), 619-625. https://doi.org/10.1017/S1352465811000075

Taylor, P. J., Jomar, K., Dhingra, K., Forrester, R., Shahmalak, U., & Dickson, J. M. (2018). A meta-analysis of the prevalence of different functions of non-suicidal self-injury. *Journal of affective disorders, 227*, 759-769. https://doi.org/10.1016/j.jad.2017.11.073

Teixeira, A. M., & Luis, M. A. (1997). Suicídio, lesões e envenenamento em adolescentes: um estudo epidemiológico [Suicide, self-mutilation and poisoning in adolescents: an epidemiological study]. *Revista latino-americana de enfermagem, 5*, 31-36. https://doi.org/10.1590/S0104-11691997000500004

Terry-Short, L. A., Glynn Owens, R., Slade, P. D., & Dewey, M. E. (1995). Positive and negative perfectionism. *Personality and Individual Differences, 18*(5), 663-668. https://doi.org/10.1016/0191-8869(94)00192-U

Thomas, M. C., Kamarck, T. W., Wright, G. C., Matthews, K. A., Muldoon, M. F., & Manuck, S. B. (2020). Hostility dimensions and metabolic syndrome in a healthy, midlife sample. *International journal of behavioral medicine, 27*(4), 475. https://doi.org/10.1007/s12529-020-09855-y

Thyssen, L. S., & van Camp, I. (2014). Non-Suicidal Self-Injury in Latin America. *Salud Mental, 37*(2): 153. https://doi.org/10.17711/SM.0185-3325.2014.019

Tian, X., Yang, G., Jiang, L., Yang, R., Ran, H., Xie, F., Xu, X., Lu, J., & Xiao, Y. (2020). Resilience is inversely associated with self-harm behaviors among *Chinese adolescents with childhood maltreatment, 8*. https://doi.org/10.7717/peerj.9800

Tiggelaar, J. (1958). Automutilation and suicide. *Folia psychiatrica, neurologica et neurochirurgica Neerlandica, 61*(4), 427-444.

Tomita, T., Aoyama, H., Kitamura, T., Sekiguchi, C., Murai, T., & Matsuda, T. (2000). Factor structure of psychobiological seven-factor model of personality: A model-revision. *Personality and Individual Differences, 29*(4), 709-727. https://doi.org/10.1016/S0191-8869(99)00227-5

Tørmoen, A. J., Rossow, I., Larsson, B., & Mehlum, L. (2013). Nonsuicidal self-harm and suicide attempts in adolescents: differences in kind or in degree?. *Social psychiatry and psychiatric epidemiology, 48*(9), 1447-1455. https://doi.org/10.1007/s00127-012-0646-y

Townsend, E., Hawton, K., Altman, D. G., Arensman, E., Gunnell, D., Hazell, P., House, A., & Van Heeringen, K. (2001). The efficacy of problem-solving treatments after deliberate self-harm: meta-analysis of randomized controlled trials with respect to depression, hopelessness and improvement in problems. *Psychological medicine, 31*(6), 979–988. https://doi.org/10.1017/s0033291701004238

Tragesser, S. L., & Benfield, J. (2012). Borderline personality disorder features and mate retention tactics. *Journal of personality disorders, 26*(3), 334–344. https://doi.org/10.1521/pedi.2012.26.3.334

Trebatická, J. (2017). *Depresívna porucha v detskom a adolescentom veku.* Univerzita Komenského.

Tsang, S. K., Hui, E. K., & Law, B. C. (2012). Positive identity as a positive youth development construct: a conceptual review. *The Scientific World Journal, 2012*, 529691. https://doi.org/10.1100/2012/529691

Tschan, T., Peter-Ruf, C., Schmid, M., & In-Albon, T. (2017). Temperament and character traits in female adolescents with nonsuicidal self-injury disorder with and without comorbid borderline personality disorder. *Child and adolescent psychiatry and mental health, 11,* 4. https://doi.org/10.1186/s13034-016-0142-3

Tsirigotis K. (2016). Indirect Self-Destructiveness and Emotional Intelligence. *The Psychiatric quarterly, 87*(2), 253–263. https://doi.org/10.1007/s11126-015-9387-x

Turner, B. J., Dixon-Gordon, K. L., Austin, S. B., Rodriguez, M. A., Zachary Rosenthal, M., & Chapman, A. L. (2015). Non-suicidal self-injury with and without borderline personality disorder: differences in self-injury and diagnostic comorbidity. *Psychiatry research, 230*(1), 28–35. https://doi.org/10.1016/j.psychres.2015.07.058

Václaviková, I. (2020). Self-harm and depression: an adolescent woman with self-harming behavior and depressive symptomatology. In: *MMK 2020*, (809–817). Hradec Králove Magminitas.

Valencia, J., & Sinambela, F.C. (2021). The Relationship Between Self-Harm Behavior, Personality, and Parental Separation: A Systematic Literature Review. In: *Proceedings of the International Conference on Psychological Studies (ICPSYCHE 2020),*(10–16). Atlantis Press. https://doi.org/10.2991/assehr.k.210423.002

Valentin, A. (2006). Therapiebegrenzung oder -abbruch: Das Prinzip des "primum nihil nocere" [Limiting or withholding treatment: the principal of "primum nihil nocere"]. *Wiener klinische Wochenschrift, 118*(11-12), 309–311. https://doi.org/10.1007/s00508-006-0605-2

van den Bogaard, K., Nijman, H., Palmstierna, T., & Embregts, P. (2018). Self-Injurious Behavior in People with Intellectual Disabilities and Co-Occurring Psychopathology using the Self-Harm Scale: A Pilot Study. *Journal of developmental and physical disabilities, 30*(5), 707–722. https://doi.org/10.1007/s10882-018-9614-0

van der Kolk, B. A., Perry, J. C., & Herman, J. L. (1991). Childhood origins of self-destructive behavior. *The American journal of psychiatry, 148*(12), 1665–1671. https://doi.org/10.1176/ajp.148.12.1665

Van Liefferinge, D., Sonuga-Barke, E., Danckaerts, M., Fayn, K., Van Broeck, N., & van der Oord, S. (2018). Measuring child and adolescent emotional lability: How do questionnaire-based ratings relate to experienced and observed emotion in everyday life and experimental settings?. *International journal of methods in psychiatric research, 27*(3). https://doi.org/10.1002/mpr.1720

Vanderlinden, J., & Vandereycken, W. (1997*). Trauma, dissociation, and impulse dyscontrol in eating disorders (No. 9)*. Psychology Press.

Victor, S. E., Davis, T., & Klonsky, E. D. (2017). Descriptive Characteristics and Initial Psychometric Properties of the Non-Suicidal Self-Injury Disorder Scale. *Archives of suicide research : official journal of the International Academy for Suicide Research, 21*(2), 265–278. https://doi.org/10.1080/13811118.2016.1193078

Victor, S. E., Glenn, C. R., & Klonsky, E. D. (2012). Is non-suicidal self-injury an "addiction"? A comparison of craving in substance use and non-suicidal self-injury. *Psychiatry research, 197*(1-2), 73–77. https://doi.org/10.1016/j.psychres.2011.12.011

Vijayakumar, N., Pfeifer, J. H., Flournoy, J. C., Hernandez, L. M., & Dapretto, M. (2019). Affective reactivity during adolescence: Associations with age, puberty and testosterone. *Cortex; a journal devoted to the study of the nervous system and behavior, 117*, 336–350. https://doi.org/10.1016/j.cortex.2019.04.024

Vrouva, I., Fonagy, P., Fearon, P. R., & Roussow, T. (2010). The risk-taking and self-harm inventory for adolescents: development and psychometric evaluation. *Psychological assessment, 22*(4), 852–865. https://doi.org/10.1037/a0020583

Wang, Y. J., Li, X., Ng, C. H., Xu, D. W., Hu, S., & Yuan, T. F. (2022). Risk factors for non-suicidal self-injury (NSSI) in adolescents: A meta-analysis. *EClinicalMedicine, 46*, 101350. https://doi.org/10.1016/j.eclinm.2022.101350

Washburn, J. J., Juzwin, K. R., Styer, D. M., & Aldridge, D. (2010). Measuring the urge to self-injure: preliminary data from a clinical sample. *Psychiatry research, 178*(3), 540–544. https://doi.org/10.1016/j.psychres.2010.05.018

Washburn, J. J., Potthoff, L. M., Juzwin, K. R., & Styer, D. M. (2015). Assessing DSM-5 nonsuicidal self-injury disorder in a clinical sample. *Psychological assessment, 27*(1), 31–41. https://doi.org/10.1037/pas0000021

Watanabe, N., Nishida, A., Shimodera, S., Inoue, K., Oshima, N., Sasaki, T., Inoue, S., Akechi, T., Furukawa, T. A., & Okazaki, Y. (2012). Deliberate self-harm in adolescents aged 12-18: a cross-sectional survey of 18,104 students. *Suicide & life-threatening behavior, 42*(5), 550–560. https://doi.org/10.1111/j.1943-278X.2012.00111.x

Watkins, E., & Moulds, M. (2005). Distinct modes of ruminative self-focus: impact of abstract versus concrete rumination on problem solving in depression. *Emotion, 5*(3), 319–328. https://doi.org/10.1037/1528-3542.5.3.319

Webermann, A. R., Myrick, A. C., Taylor, C. L., Chasson, G. S., & Brand, B. L. (2016). Dissociative, depressive, and PTSD symptom severity as correlates of nonsuicidal self-injury and suicidality in dissociative disorder patients. *Journal of trauma & dissociation : the official journal of the International Society for the Study of Dissociation (ISSD), 17*(1), 67–80. https://doi.org/10.1080/15299732.2015.1067941

Weinstein, N. D. (1980). Unrealistic optimism about future life events. Journal of Personality and Social Psychology, 39(5), 806–820. https://doi.org/10.1037/0022-3514.39.5.806

Wenzel, A., & Spokas, M. (2014). Cognitiive and Information Processing Approaches to understanding suicidal behaviors. In: M. K. Nock (ed.), *The Oxford Handbook of Suicide and Self-Injury* (235–254). Oxford University Press.

Wenzel, A., Brown, G. K., & Beck, A. T. (2009). *Cognitive therapy for suicidal patients: Scientific and clinical applications.* American Psychological Association. https://doi.org/10.1037/11862-000

Wester, K. L., & Trepal, H. C. (2017). *Non-suicidal self-injury.* Routledge.

Westlund Schreiner, M., Klimes-Dougan, B., Begnel, E. D., & Cullen, K. R. (2015). Conceptualizing the neurobiology of non-suicidal self-injury from the perspective of the Research Domain Criteria Project. *Neuroscience and biobehavioral reviews, 57,* 381–391. https://doi.org/10.1016/j.neubiorev.2015.09.011

Westlund Schreiner, M., Mueller, B. A., Klimes-Dougan, B., Begnel, E. D., Fiecas, M., Hill, D., Lim, K. O., & Cullen, K. R. (2020). White Matter Microstructure in Adolescents and Young Adults With Non-Suicidal Self-Injury. *Frontiers in psychiatry, 10,* 1019. https://doi.org/10.3389/fpsyt.2019.01019

Whiteside, S. P., & Lynam, D. R. (2001). The Five Factor Model and impulsivity: Using a structural model of personality to understand impulsivity. *Personality and Individual Differences, 30*(4), 669–689. https://doi.org/10.1016/S0191-8869(00)00064-7

Whitlock, J., Exner-Cortens, D., & Purington, A. (2014). Assessment of nonsuicidal self-injury: development and initial validation of the Non-Suicidal Self-Injury-Assessment Tool (NSSI-AT). *Psychological assessment, 26*(3), 935–946. https://doi.org/10.1037/a0036611

WHO (2021). *World health organization.* https://www.who.int/about/governance/constitution

Wiederman, M. W., Sansone, R. A., & Sansone, L. A. (1999). Bodily self-harm and its relationship to childhood abuse among women in a primary care setting. *Violence Against Women, 5*(2), 155–163. https://doi.org/10.1177/107780129952004

Wolfe, K. L., Nakonezny, P. A., Owen, V. J., Rial, K. V., Moorehead, A. P., Kennard, B. D., & Emslie, G. J. (2019). Hopelessness as a Predictor of Suicide Ideation in Depressed Male and Female Adolescent Youth. *Suicide & life-threatening behavior, 49*(1), 253–263. https://doi.org/10.1111/sltb.12428

Wolff, J. C., Frazier, E. A., Esposito-Smythers, C., Becker, S. J., Burke, T. A., Cataldo, A., & Spirito, A. (2014). Negative cognitive style and perceived social support mediate the relationship between aggression and NSSI in hospitalized adolescents. *Journal of adolescence, 37*(4), 483–491. https://doi.org/10.1016/j.adolescence.2014.03.016

Wolff, J. C., Thompson, E., Thomas, S. A., Nesi, J., Bettis, A. H., Ransford, B., Scopelliti, K., Frazier, E. A., & Liu, R. T. (2019). Emotion dysregulation and non-suicidal self-injury: A systematic review and meta-analysis. *European psychiatry, 59*, 25–36. https://doi.org/10.1016/j.eurpsy.2019.03.004

Wolff, J., Frazier, E. A., Esposito-Smythers, C., Burke, T., Sloan, E., & Spirito, A. (2013). Cognitive and social factors associated with NSSI and suicide attempts in psychiatrically hospitalized adolescents. *Journal of abnormal child psychology, 41*(6), 1005–1013. https://doi.org/10.1007/s10802-013-9743-y

Wyman, P. A., Cross, W., Hendricks Brown, C., Yu, Q., Tu, X., & Eberly, S. (2010). Intervention to strengthen emotional self-regulation in children with emerging mental health problems: proximal impact on school behavior. *Journal of abnormal child psychology, 38*(5), 707–720. https://doi.org/10.1007/s10802-010-9398-x

Xie, Y., Kong, Y., Yang, J., Chen, F. (2019). Perfectionism, worry, rumination, and distress: a meta-analysis of the evidence for the perfectionism cognition theory. *Pers Individ Differ.* 139:301–312. https://doi.org/10.1016/j.paid.2018.11.028

Yakeley, J., & Burbridge-James, W. (2018). Psychodynamic approaches to suicide and self-harm. *BJPsych Advances, 24*(1), 37-45. https://doi.org/10.1192/bja.2017.6

Yang, X., & Feldman, M. W. (2017). A reversed gender pattern? A meta-analysis of gender differences in the prevalence of non-suicidal self-injurious behaviour among Chinese adolescents. *BMC public health, 18*(1), 66. https://doi.org/10.1186/s12889-017-4614-z

Yang, X., & Xin, M. (2018). "Boy Crisis" or "Girl Risk"? The Gender Difference in Nonsuicidal Self-Injurious Behavior Among Middle-School Students in China and its Relationship to Gender Role Conflict and Violent Experiences. *American journal of men's health, 12*(5), 1275–1285. https://doi.org/10.1177/1557988318763522

Ye, D., Ng, Y. K., & Lian, Y. (2015). Culture and Happiness. *Social indicators research, 123*(2), 519–547. https://doi.org/10.1007/s11205-014-0747-y

You, J., Leung, F., Lai, C. M., & Fu, K. (2012). The associations between non-suicidal self-injury and borderline personality disorder features among Chinese adolescents. *Journal of personality disorders, 26*(2), 226–237. https://doi.org/10.1521/pedi.2012.26.2.226

You, J., Ma, C., Lin, M.-P., & Leung, F. (2015). Comparing among the Experiences of Self-Cutting, Hitting, and Scratching in Chinese Adolescents Attending Secondary Schools: An Interview Study. *Behavioral Disorders, 40*(2), 122–137. https://doi.org/10.17988/BD-14-9.1

Young, M. A., Fogg, L. F., Scheftner, W., Fawcett, J., Akiskal, H., & Maser, J. (1996). Stable trait components of hopelessness: baseline and sensitivity to depression. *Journal of abnormal psychology, 105*(2), 155–165. https://doi.org/10.1037//0021-843x.105.2.155

Yu, M. and Clark, M. (2015). Investigating Mindfulness, Borderline Personality Traits, and Well-Being in a Nonclinical Population. *Psychology, 6*, 1232-1248. https://doi.org/10.4236/psych.2015.610121

Zanarini, M. C., Frankenburg, F. R., Reich, D. B., Fitzmaurice, G., Weinberg, I., & Gunderson, J. G. (2008). The 10-year course of physically self-destructive acts reported by borderline patients and axis II comparison subjects. *Acta psychiatrica Scandinavica, 117*(3), 177–184. https://doi.org/10.1111/j.1600-0447.2008.01155.x

Zerbe K. J. (1988). Walking on the razor's edge. The use of consultation in the treatment of a self-mutilating patient. *Bulletin of the Menninger Clinic, 52(6)*, 492–503.

Zhang, L., Chen, M., Yao, B., & Zhang, Y. (2021). Aggression and Non-Suicidal Self-Injury among Depressed Youths: The Mediating Effect of Resilience. *Iranian journal of public health, 50*(2), 288–296. https://doi.org/10.18502/ijph.v50i2.5342

Zubrick, S. R., Hafekost, J., Johnson, S. E., Sawyer, M. G., Patton, G., & Lawrence, D. (2017). The continuity and duration of depression and its relationship to non-suicidal self-harm and suicidal ideation and behavior in adolescents 12-17. *Journal of affective disorders, 220*, 49–56. https://doi.org/10.1016/j.jad.2017.05.050

Zuckerman, M., & Kuhlman, D. M. (2000). Personality and risk-taking: common biosocial factors. *Journal of personality, 68*(6), 999–1029. https://doi.org/10.1111/1467-6494.00124

About the Author

Slávka Démuthová was born in Martin, Slovakia in 1976. She obtained a master's degree in psychology at the Faculty of Humanities of Trnava University, Trnava. During her studies, she spent a year at the British Charity, Break (Hunstanton, UK), where, as a volunteer, she worked with children and adults with mental disabilities. In 2000, she obtained a master's degree in Psychology (Trnava University, Trnava), in 2007, she was awarded the research qualification, Ph.D. (Trnava University, Trnava) and in 2015, she qualified as an Associate Professor at the Masaryk University in Brno (the Czech Republic).

Since 2000, she has been working as an Assistant Professor at the Department of Psychology of the Faculty of Arts and Sciences of the University of Ss. Cyril and Methodius in Trnava; currently she holds the position of professor. From 2015 to 2021 she was the Head of the Department of Psychology; since 2022 she has been the Director of the Centre for Psychological Counselling and Research. She lectures in the field of developmental psychology, the history of psychology, and thanatology. Her primary areas of interest are the problems of children and youths: *Mladistvý delikvent* [The Juvenile Delinquent] (Schola Philosophica 2006), *Biologické koncepcie kriminality* [Biological Conceptions of Crime] (UCM 2012), *Keď umiera dieťa* [When the Child is Dying] (Schola Philosophica 2010), *Kapitoly z tanatológie* [Chapters from Thanatology] (UCM 2013): She is also the co-author of monographs on the perception of beauty: *Cognitive Aspects of Aesthetic Experience – Introduction* (Peter Lang Verlag 2017), *Cognitive Aspects of Aesthetic Experience – Selected Problems* (Peter Lang Verlag 2019) and *Human Facial Attractiveness in Psychological Research* (Peter Lang Verlag 2019).

In addition to her work at the University of Ss. Cyril and Methodius, she has completed several research stays and has been invited to give lectures at universities abroad: The Lund University, SE (2010); The University of Edinburgh, GB (2011); Trinity College Dublin, IRL (2013); The Hebrew University of Jerusalem, IL (2014); The University of Glasgow, GB (2015); The Cardinal Wyszyński University in Warsaw, PL (2016); Max-Planck-Institut für empirische Ästhetik (Frankfurt am Main, DE, 2017) and The University of Ljubljana, SLO (2018). Since 2010, she has regularly given lectures in Thanatology at the Masaryk University, Brno (CZ).

www.ingramcontent.com/pod-product-compliance
Ingram Content Group UK Ltd.
Pitfield, Milton Keynes, MK11 3LW, UK
UKHW041926140426
5217IPUK00014B/337